PRACTITIONERS' GUIDE TO VETERINARY DENTISTRY

Anthony D. Shipp

D.V.M., F.A.V.D.

Small Animal Practitioner,
Beverly Hills, California, USA

Peter Fahrenkrug

Dr. med. vet., Dr. med. dent., F.A.V.D.

Dentist and Veterinarian,
Hamburg, Germany

FIRST EDITION

Book Design and Layout: Dr. A. D. Shipp

Color Separations: Diversified Color Systems
3941 South Bristol Street, Suite 190
Santa Ana, California 92704

Linotronics: Southern California Printcorp
1010 East Union Street
Pasadena, CA 91106

Printed in the United States of America by

Griffin Printing, Inc.
544 West Colorado Street
Glendale, California 91204-1102

ISBN 0-9635578-0-7

FIRST EDITION

Published and Distributed by

Dr. Shipp's Laboratories
351 North Foothill Road
Beverly Hills, California 90210
Tel.: (310) 550-0107
(800) 442-0107
Fax: (310) 550-1664

CONTENTS

PREFACE

A modern veterinarian should examine the mouth of every animal that is seen, recognize the problems, know what should be done and recommend the best course of treatment. Clients should be offered all the available options so that they can decide what they want for their pet.

Many clients are very sophisticated in their knowledge of what is available to them today, and treat their pets as though they were family. Although the cost of certain procedures can be high, it should not be the responsibility of the veterinarian to determine how much the client is prepared to spend. Many clients want the very best for their pets, and the cost is secondary.

As most practicing veterinarians know, there is a great deal more to animal dentistry than just cleaning and extracting teeth. Unfortunately, advanced veterinary dentistry is still in its infancy, lagging far behind human dentistry in its breadth of knowledge and expertise among practitioners.

Even today most veterinary schools devote only a limited amount of instruction in the subject of animal dentistry. Most of what has to be learned, must come from outside lectures, conferences and textbooks. In the final analysis, it is up to veterinarians to inform and educate themselves in this ever changing and important area.

With pets living longer, eating soft sticky foods and having previously lacked good home and veterinary dental care, many of the older pets have a high incidence of dental disease. This is largely because clients were never offered modern treatment for their pets' teeth. Luckily for younger pets, this should not be the case in the future as client and veterinary awareness of animal dentistry increases. As someone said, "*the amount of pathology often found in the mouth, would never be tolerated in other parts of the body.*"

Although much has already been written about veterinary dentistry, some of this material can be overwhelming to the student or practicing veterinarian. It is the aim of the authors to present a general overview of veterinary dentistry, from basic to advanced levels, laid out under various general chapter headings. Before reading the book, however, it would be wise to read through these chapter headings and sub-headings to become familiar with the contents. The text has been carefully written and laid out to eliminate confusion for the beginner. Some material and procedures have been deliberately omitted or not elaborated on in detail because such information is available in other texts.

All key words are printed in the capital letters throughout the book, so that they are easy to locate. The index contains all these words and has been carefully cross–referenced to make it easy for the reader to find variations of the same words. The truly motivated reader should review the index, and may possibly be surprised at what he or she knows or does not know. Products and manufacturers mentioned are listed at the end of the text.

Most veterinary dental procedures and equipment have been borrowed or adapted from the human dental field. This text will explain how this is done in an easy to understand manner. For those veterinarians already practicing veterinary dentistry, there is much newly presented material. For those just beginning, this book offers an overall picture of what is current in veterinary dentistry.

We hope that this textbook will help serve the worldwide veterinary dental community in understanding this ever expanding and important field.

Anthony D. Shipp

DVM, FAVD (Fellow, Academy of Veterinary Dentistry)
Member: American Veterinary Dental Society
British Veterinary Dental Association
European Veterinary Dental Society

Beverly Hills, California, U.S.A.

Veterinary dentistry is an essential and practice building service of paramount importance for every modern veterinarian. Clinical success depends on a thorough knowledge of veterinary dentistry, the ability to perform the procedures, and use of the correct equipment and materials.

The original version of this text was published in Germany in 1984 and had the distinction of being one of the first three books on veterinary dentistry to reach a world–wide audience. The original book provided a theoretical background on diagnosis, treatment methods and dental equipment for the veterinary practitioner who had no exposure to such information during veterinary school. Practical exercises and education such as wet labs or through video programs or consulting with dentists were also recommended to the reader. The German version, now in its fifth revised edition, has been a tremendous success in Europe and has helped thousands of veterinarians discover and learn about the fascinating field of veterinary dentistry. This new knowledge has helped the pet owning population to become aware of the strides veterinarians are taking in resolving the dental problems of their pets.

During my numerous visits over the years to American conferences, congresses and clinics, I was encouraged to translate my little book into English. This turned out to be a formidable task, since the text not only had to be translated, but it had to be updated and have international application. Also, much of the equipment and materials, as well as some details in procedures, are different in Europe and the U.S.A.

I am fortunate that my friend and co-author Dr. Anthony Shipp, who practices veterinary dentistry in Beverly Hills, agreed to commit his efforts, experience and vast knowledge of veterinary dentistry into the English adaptation of this text.

Dr. Shipp, who is also my colleague in the Academy of Veterinary Dentistry, has expanded and revised the original text to more than double its original size. He has updated the text to cover the most modern treatment, techniques and materials. The chapters on Periodontics, Endodontics, Instruments and Equipment, Dental Materials and Orthodontics are of special interest.

Our joint effort provides much new material as well as simplified and concise approaches to old problems.

I would be remiss if I did not point out that before veterinary dentistry can be practiced, the theories must be understood. This involves the recognition, definition and diagnosis of dental diseases and problems. Also, it must be remembered that dental treatment is a skilled digital exercise that requires delicate craftsmanship and manual dexterity, which can only be obtained through practice under the guidance of a practitioner familiar with dental techniques.

It is our hope that this book will expand the knowledge of those already experienced in veterinary dentistry, as well as help students and practitioners who are interested in the field.

PETER FAHRENKRUG

Dr. med. vet., Dr. med. dent., FAVD (Fellow, Academy of Veterinary Dentistry)
Lecturer for Veterinary Dentistry at the Veterinary Faculty,
University of Berlin, Germany
Member: Bundesverband praktischer Tierärzte, Germany
American Veterinary Dental Society
British Veterinary Dental Association
Groupe d'Etude et de Recherche en Odonto-Stomatologie, France
Vet. Dent Science e.V., Austria
European Veterinary Dental Society

Hamburg, Germany.

ACKNOWLEDGEMENT

Special thanks to Dr. Kenneth F. Lyon of Mesa, Arizona for his time, knowledge and suggestions in helping to edit the final copy of this book. Dr. Lyon is a Diplomate of the American Veterinary Dental College and Editor–in–chief of the Journal of Veterinary Dentistry.

A.D.S.
P.F.

FURTHER ACKNOWLEDGEMENTS

Special thanks also to John Robinson, B.D.S., London, England, for his excellent suggestions while proofing the text.

We also wish to thank the following friends and colleagues in the veterinary dental and human dental professions for their advice:

Peter Emily, D.D.S., A.V.D.C.
Jean Hawkins, D.V.M., F.A.V.D., A.V.D.C.
Tom Mulligan, D.V.M., F.A.V.D., A.V.D.C.
Don Ross, D.V.M., F.A.V.D., A.V.D.C.
Stan Vogel, D.D.S.

The basic German–English translation was done by Iain Anderson, B.D.S., Hamburg, Germany.

The sketches were designed and drawn by: Peter Fahrenkrug, Angelika Schmidt, Sybille Kreynhop, Akira Fujioka (Hamburg, Germany), and Sandra Drinning and Anthony Shipp (Beverly Hills, California, U.S.A.).

Some technical sketches and photos were taken from manufacturers' manuals and other sources.

❖❖❖

CHAPTER 1

ANATOMY OF THE TOOTH AND SUPPORTING STRUCTURES

1.1 ENAMEL

Apart from variations in shape and size developed by the necessity to grasp, shear and chew different kinds of food, the mouths of household pets are very similar to those of man. The tooth is divided into the CROWN and the ROOT. The CROWN, which is the part normally visible in the mouth, is covered with enamel. The ROOT, which is the part below the gumline holding the tooth in the jawbone, is covered with cementum. ENAMEL covering the crown is about 1–2 mm thick and is the hardest substance in the body. It is highly resistant to abrasion and consists of 97% HYDROXYAPATITE crystals. The enamel is laid down in the deciduous teeth during fetal development, and in the germinal tissue of the permanent teeth in the late fetal development and shortly after birth, by special cells called AMELOBLASTS. These cells build up enamel from the inside outwards, in the form of prisms, and are themselves destroyed during eruption of the tooth. The enamel is therefore unable to regenerate when it is damaged by caries, attrition and trauma, thus must be repaired by artificial means. As a result of systemic disturbances such as physiological diseases, fever, malnutrition, poisoning, infection (especially distemper), the enamel may not be properly mineralized, resulting in ENAMEL HYPOPLASIA (partial loss of formation of enamel) or ENAMEL APLASIA (complete loss of formation of enamel).

Various drugs, especially tetracyclines, can cause discoloration of the tooth when given to pregnant bitches and to puppies under about six months of age (before tooth eruption). TETRACYCLINE STAINING is not confined to the enamel but instead predominantly involves the dentin, the matrix of which is being formed during the fetal and juvenile stages. The severity of staining depends on the time and duration of the drug administration, the type of tetracycline, and the dosage. Bleaching techniques have been used to remove such stains, but the procedure can be complex and time consuming, with variable results. Since removing stains from teeth is really cosmetic, it is not widely practiced in veterinary dentistry.

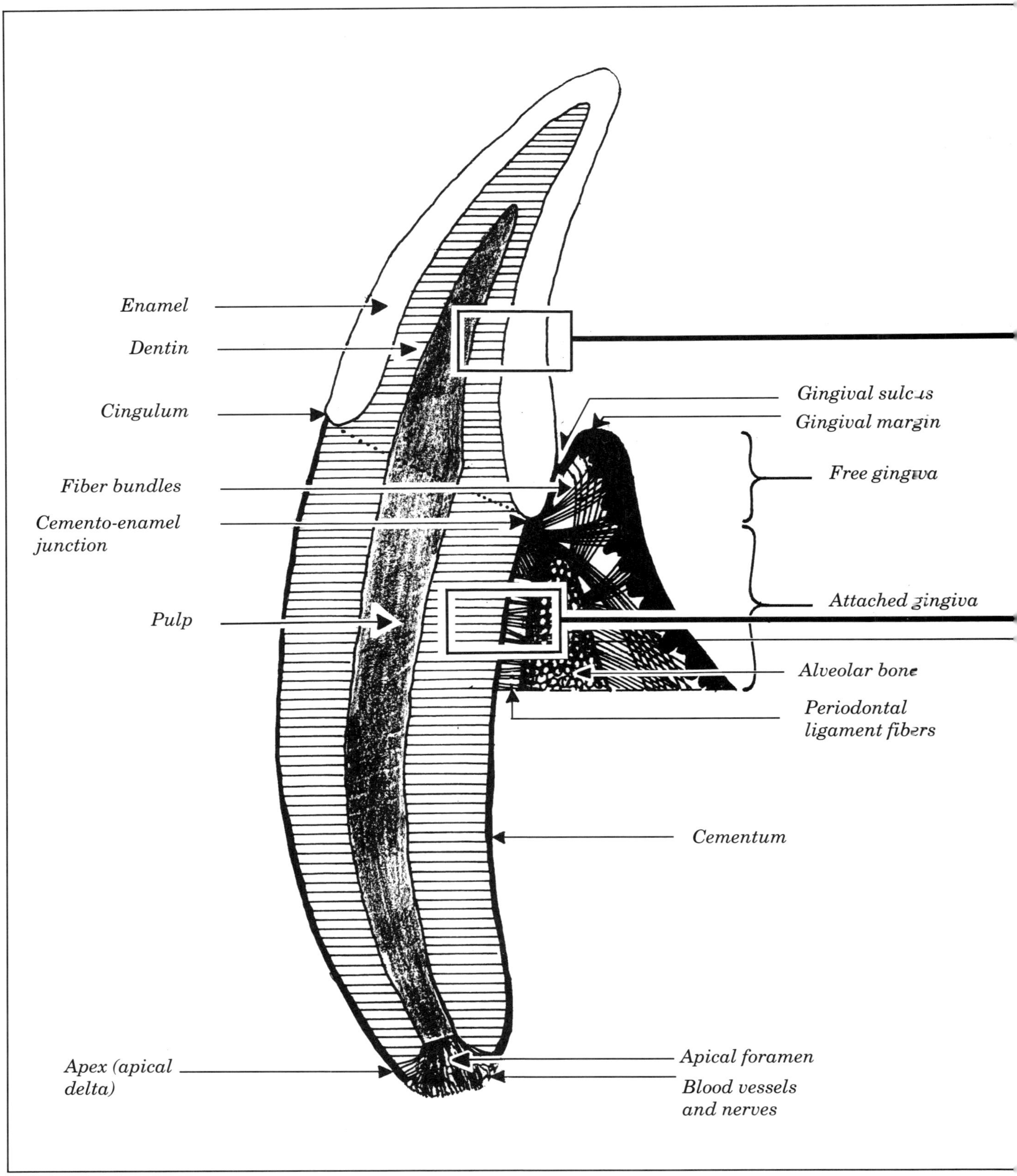

Figure 1A. Structure of tooth.

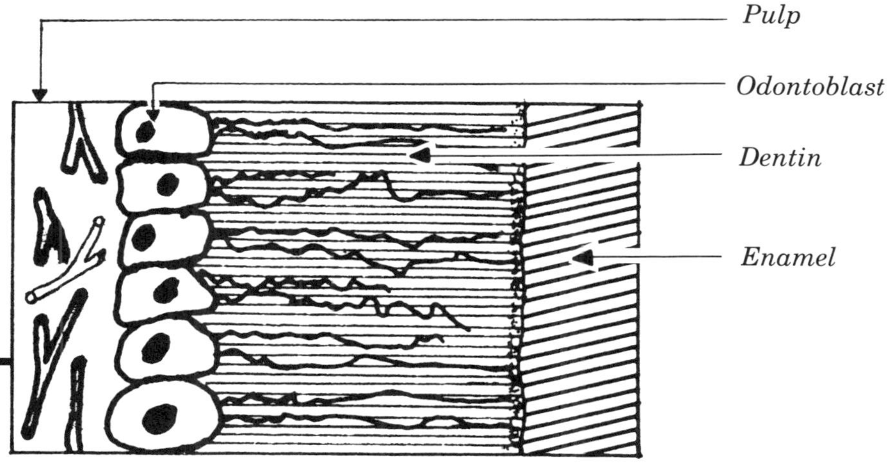

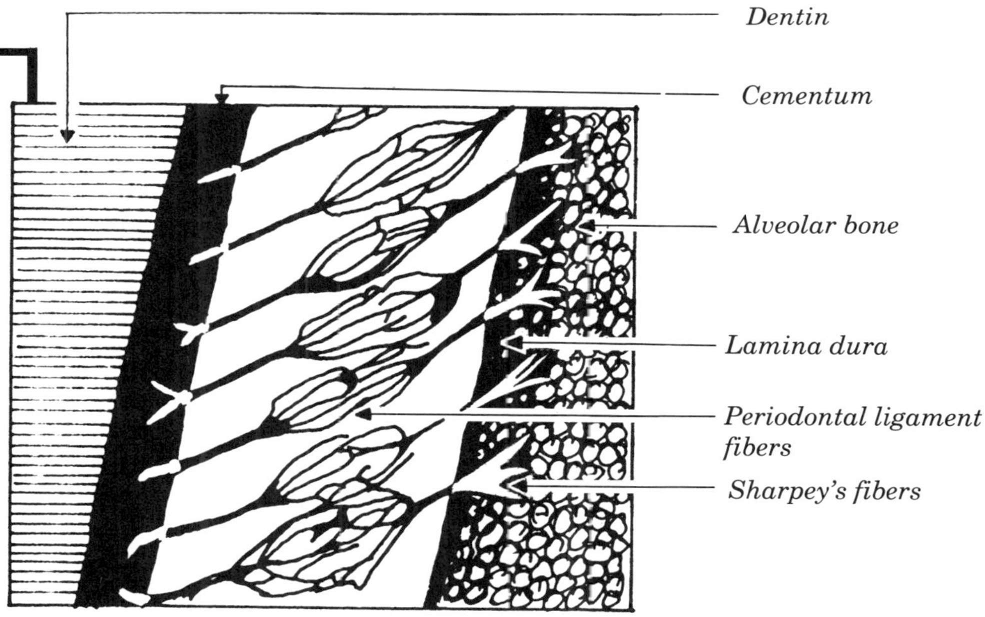

Figure 1B. Structure of tooth wall (enlarged, schematic) (top).
Figure 1C. Structure of periodontium (enlarged, schematic) (bottom).

1.2 DENTIN

Beneath the enamel of the crown and extending to the tip of the root is the DENTIN (the IVORY of ELEPHANTS' TUSKS), a substance very similar in chemical structure to bone although not morphologically similar. In that part of the root, which is supported in bone, the dentin is covered with a thin hard layer of cementum. PRIMARY DENTIN is laid down by cells called ODONTOBLASTS, starting from the inside surface of the enamel and progressing inwards towards the center of the tooth. This process, unlike that for enamel, continues throughout the life of the tooth, providing the pulp is vital.

Odontoblasts also leave extensions in the forming dentin, resulting in a radial structure of tubules. The dentin layer only becomes strong after about two years of age. Stimuli from without, such as a fracture of the enamel, a deep carious defect or even cooling (i.e., cold water), can stimulate the odontoblasts to rapidly deposit a reparative layer of dentin in order to seal and plug the tubules. This protects the pulp against chemical and thermal insults.

1.3 PULP

The PULP CAVITY is found in the center of the tooth, and its shape is similar to that of the tooth around it. For anatomical purposes the pulp cavity is differentiated into the PULP CHAMBER, found in the crown of the tooth, and the PULP CANAL (ROOT CANAL), found in the root of the tooth. The pulp cavity contains the soft tissue of the tooth, known as the PULP (or sometimes "NERVE") of the tooth. The PULP consists of an outer odontoblast layer, then a cell–free layer of supporting connective tissue, and in the middle, arteries, veins, lymph vessels and of course nerves.

Immediately after eruption, the pulp cavity is relatively wide. During the first few months after eruption, the thickness of the dentin rapidly increases inwards, by deposition of SECONDARY DENTIN, so as to strengthen the tooth. By one to one and a half years of age, the diameter of the pulp cavity becomes greatly reduced. With advancing age, the pulp cavity becomes so reduced that only a thin thread–like space remains, or it may even be completely obliterated (see tooth changes with age, 2.3).

A multi–rooted tooth may have one or more accessory pulp canals in each root. These small canals branch off the main pulp canal out through the dentin, to the surface of the root. The majority of the vessels and nerves leave the tooth through the APICAL FORAMEN, the opening at the tip (or APEX) of the root of adult teeth. Recent confirmation by *HENNET* has indicated that the apical foramen in some adult dogs is in fact a large APICAL DELTA (multiple exit holes rather than one large one) and that the pulp branches into many smaller canals at the apex (Fig. 2). The NERVOUS INNERVATION in the TOOTH is through the maxillary and mandibular branches of the trigeminal nerve.

1.4 PERIODONTIUM

The PERIODONTIUM consists of the *cementum*, the *periodontal ligament*, the *alveolar bone*, the *gingivae*, and the *epithelial attachment* (Figs. 1, 1A, 1B). CEMENTUM, which covers the root, is similar in structure, although not morphology, to bone. It contains no blood and lymph vessels, has no innervation, and does not undergo physiological resorption or remodeling. Cementum is continuously deposited throughout life. It contributes to the process of repair after the root surface has been damaged. The cementum helps to anchor the tooth to the bone, and is therefore a part of the supporting tissues of the tooth called the periodontium. The PERIODONTAL LIGAMENT (PERIODONTAL MEMBRANE) fibers are anchored in the cementum of the root. These fibers are oriented outwards, and slightly upwards and towards the alveolar crest, ending in the bone that supports the teeth, the ALVEOLAR BONE. The ALVEOLUS (SOCKET) has a lining of denser bone, the LAMINA DURA, to which the periodontal ligament fibers attach. Underneath the lamina dura is the supporting CANCELLOUS ALVEOLAR BONE. The lamina dura is visible on dental radiographs as a dense white line, called the LINEA ALBA. The ends of the periodontal ligament fibers, which are embedded in the root cementum and in the alveolar bone periosteum, are called SHARPEY'S FIBERS. The periodontal ligament fibers are elastic, which allows for a small amount of tooth movement, and protects the tooth against sharp forces like a shock absorber. The PERIODONTAL (ligament) SPACE is the space between the external surface of the root (cementum), and the lining of the ALVEOLAR PROCESS (alveolar bone socket into which the tooth fits). The periodontal space, which is about 0.25 mm wide, is normally taken up with the periodontal ligament fibers, connective tissue, blood vessels and nerves.

The gingivae and the epithelial attachment (see gingiva and mucosa, 1.5) form a seal around the teeth and although not the main supporting tissues of the teeth, do give some support to the teeth.

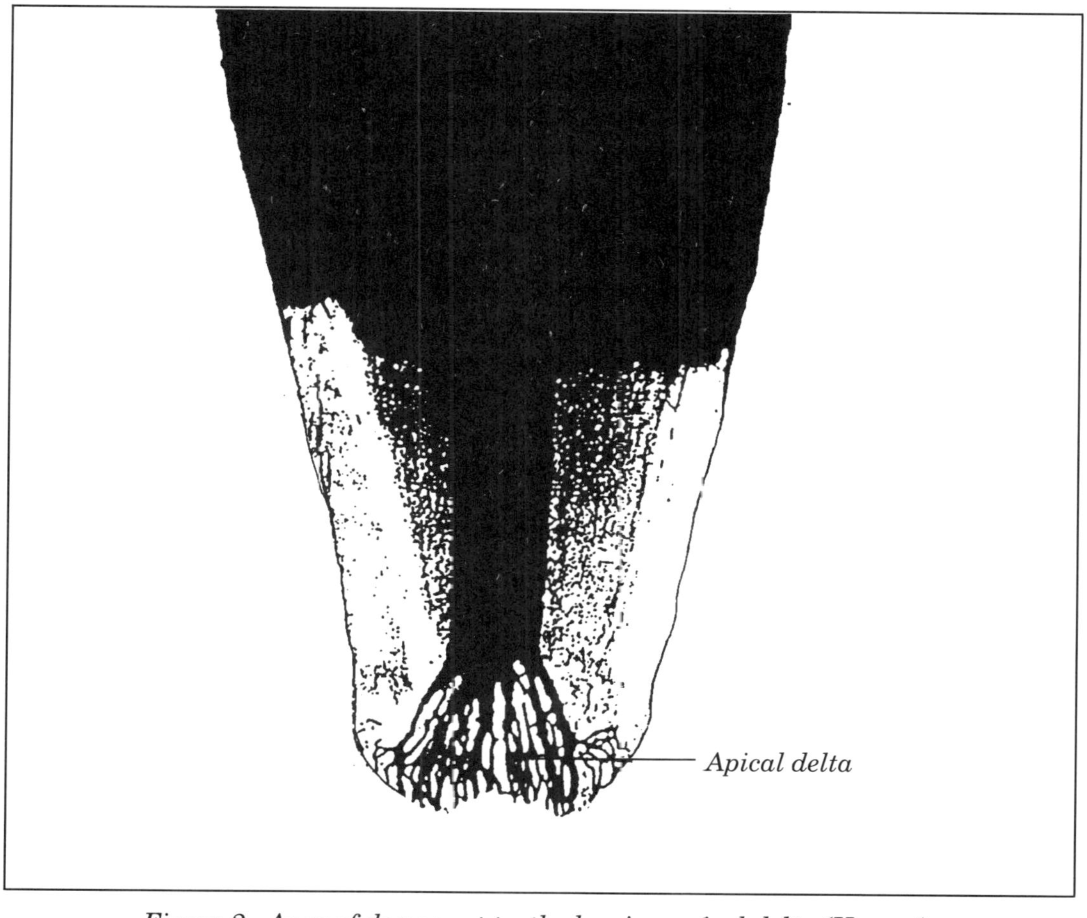

Figure 2. Apex of dog or cat tooth showing apical delta (Hennet).

1.5 GINGIVA AND MUCOSA

Gingival tissue is anatomically divided into *non–attached* (marginal or free), *attached* and *interdental gingiva*, based on location and whether or not it is bound to underlying tooth structures or to periosteum.

The CORONAL (towards the crown) part of the gingiva is known as the NON–ATTACHED (FREE or MARGINAL) GINGIVA, since it has no attachment to the tooth or to the bone. The edge of the free gingiva is called the GINGIVAL MARGIN. The space between this free edge of gingiva and the tooth is called the GINGIVAL SULCUS (also called GINGIVAL POCKET or GINGIVAL CREVICE). It is only a potential space, since the free gingiva under normal conditions fits tightly to the surface of the tooth. The V–shaped sulcus can be probed with a periodontal probe and normally should be no more than 1–3 mm in depth, depending on the age, size, breed and species of animal. The fibers in the region of the CEMENTO–ENAMEL JUNCTION (CEJ, CERVICAL LINE), which is where the cementum approximates the enamel, are embedded in the coronal part of the GINGIVA or GUMS.

The ATTACHED GINGIVA, which is attached by similar fibers called DESMOSOMAL FIBERS (DESMOSOMES), is held tightly to the outer surface of the alveolar bone and is heavily keratinized. Desmosomes (and HEMIDESMOSOMES) are also found in the "RESTS OF MALLASSEZ," which are epithelial cells, found in the periodontal ligament. The point at the bottom of the gingival sulcus, where the free gingiva starts and the attached gingiva ends, is called the DENTINOGINGIVAL JUNCTION or EPITHELIAL ATTACHMENT. It is normally at, or slightly above, the cemento–enamel junction and is where the JUNCTIONAL EPITHELIUM attaches. This is an important landmark since it is where periodontal disease starts to attack the periodontium. The gingiva between the teeth is called the INTERDENTAL GINGIVA or INTERDENTAL PAPILLA.

In an APICAL DIRECTION (APICALLY) (towards the tip of the root), the attached gingiva is continuous with the loose, less keratinized, darker red ALVEOLAR MUCOSA (mucosa lying over the alveolar bone). The line of demarcation between the attached gingiva and the alveolar mucosa is called the MUCOGINGIVAL JUNCTION or MUCOGINGIVAL LINE and is clearly visible.

The remainder of the mucosa of the mouth, which is not lying over alveolar bone, is known as the ORAL MUCOSA. The oral mucosa can be subdivided into the BUCCAL MUCOSA (inside the cheeks), the LABIAL MUCOSA (inside the lips), the VESTIBULAR MUCOSA (lining the vestibule of the mandible), the SUBLINGUAL MUCOSA (under the tongue), the PALATINE MUCOSA (covering the hard and soft palate) and the PHARYNGEAL MUCOSA (covering the pharynx).

A fold of mucosa and connective tissue, called the FRENULUM MAXILLARIS, is located in midline above the central maxillary incisors. This fold passes from the ROSTRAL (towards the nose or anterior) alveolar mucosa to the rostral labial mucosa. It helps to stabilize the upper lip in the midline. Two other folds of mucosa and connective tissue, each called the FRENULUM MANDIBULARIS, are located BUCCAL (towards the cheeks) to the mandibular canine teeth. These folds pass from the alveolar mucosa to the labial mucosa just caudal to the mandibular canine teeth. The frenulae help stabilize the lower lips. Another fold of mucosa, called FRENULUM LINGUAE, runs in midline from the rostral floor of the mouth to the anterior body of the tongue. This helps to stabilize the tongue in midline.

ABNORMAL PROLIFERATIVE SUBLINGUAL MUCOSA is sometimes found in the dog under the tongue, running parallel to its surface. These folds of mucosa and connective tissue protrude laterally from the base of the tongue, and run from the area of the frenulum linguae attachment to the CAUDAL (towards the tail, or posterior) part of the base of the tongue. ABNORMAL PROLIFERATIVE BUCCAL MUCOSA is sometimes found lateral to the cheek teeth. These mucosal and connective tissue lesions protrude medially from the buccal mucosa just caudal to the commissures of the lips. Both types of lesions develop from self–inflicted trauma and are abnormal. They require surgical removal (see sublingual and buccal mucosa resection, 10.16), (Photos 95, 96).

CHAPTER 2

Eruption and Dentition

2.1 ERUPTION OF THE TEETH

The eruption of the DECIDUOUS (TEMPORARY) TEETH, and their replacement by the permanent teeth, is a complicated process whose physiology is still poorly understood. The deciduous teeth have a complete root system similar to permanent teeth. During the development of the PERMANENT TOOTH the TOOTH FOLLICLE (GERMINAL TISSUE, TOOTH GERM), which is located near or between the roots of the deciduous tooth it will replace, increases in size, pressing on the roots of the deciduous tooth. This results in resorption of the deciduous tooth root and eventual loss of the tooth. This pressure results in cells differentiating into ODONTOCLASTS (or DENTINOCLASTS), which then resorb the deciduous tooth root.

2.2 ERUPTION DEFECTS

Abnormal eruption is often seen, especially in dogs. The result of deciduous tooth roots either not being resorbed at all, or sometimes only minimally resorbed, allows the deciduous tooth to remain firmly anchored or retained in the mouth. These problems arise from dislocation of the tooth germ following trauma, abnormal position or orientation of the tooth germ, or growth disturbances in the jawbone.

Attempts to remove a RETAINED DECIDUOUS TOOTH may result in a fracture of the tooth, with a part of the root remaining in the bone. It was once thought that this root fragment would eventually be resorbed, but is now considered not the case. The remaining root tip becomes covered with epithelium, and remains clinically inactive in the bone until such time as bone resorption brings it to the surface. Sometimes the retained root tip becomes infected and may cause a fistula to develop. Since the periodontium becomes obliterated and the root sclerosed, the fragmented root tip is often difficult to visualize on a radiograph. To what extent the tooth is actually resorbed requires more research. However, at this time, it is suggested that complete removal of the retained deciduous tooth *root* should be performed, which often requires a gingival flap to access the root (see gingival flap and ostectomy, 10.11). Care must be taken not to damage the permanent tooth, which lies extremely close to the deciduous root.

In cats and dogs, the deciduous dentition should have been completely shed by the seventh month, or slightly later in the smaller breeds of dogs. The most common eruption problem, especially in dogs, is the retention of the deciduous canine teeth. These teeth are often firmly anchored in the jaw and in direct contact with the completely erupted permanent canine teeth (Photo 1). The deciduous canine teeth possess long and delicate roots, making complete extraction difficult. To prevent serious complications (e.g., cyst, fistula, abscess, misalignment of a permanent tooth) removal of the tooth by ostectomy of the surrounding bone should be considered. When a root tip remains, it is still occupying space adjacent to the permanent tooth, and therefore can affect the path of eruption of the permanent tooth.

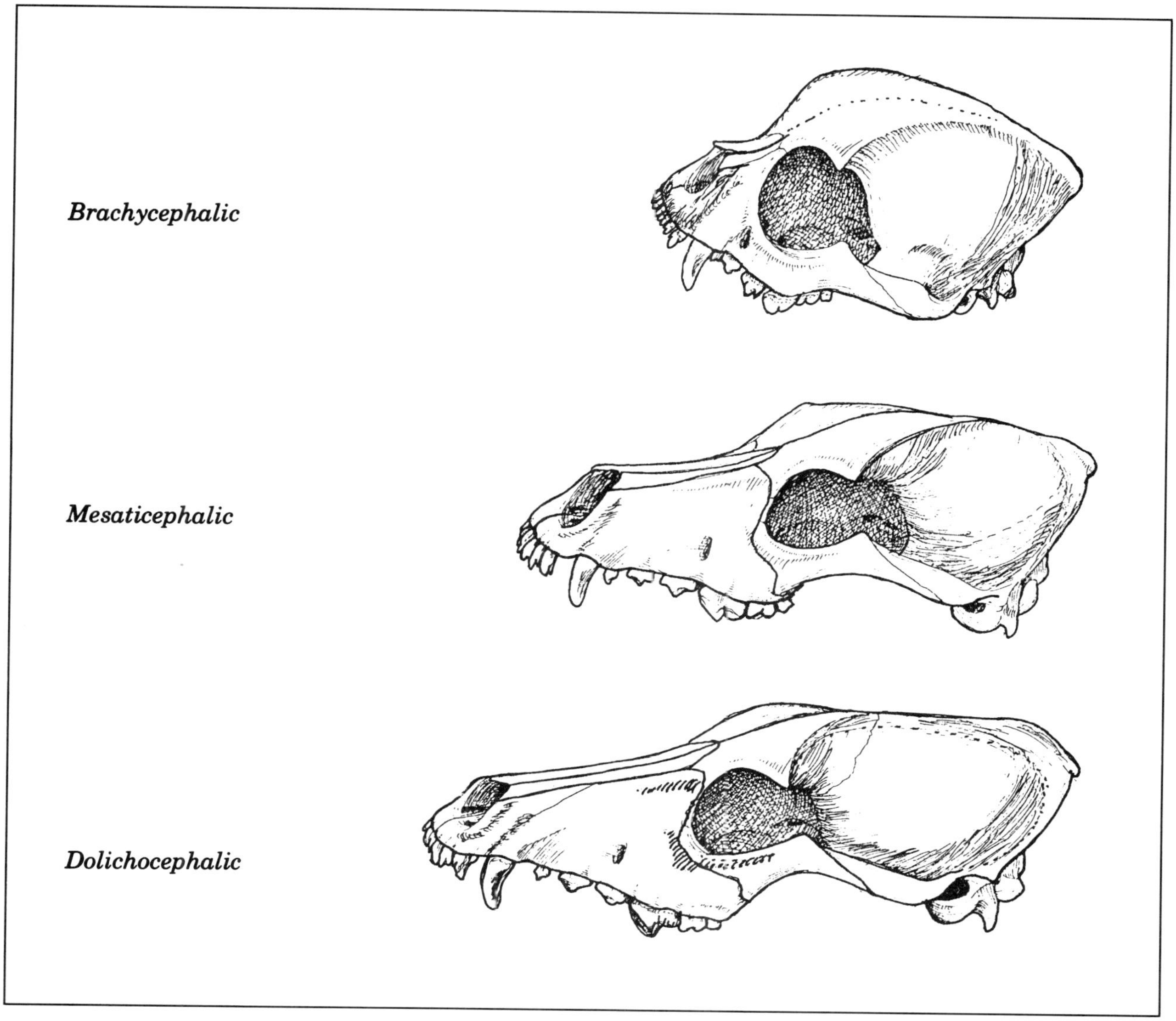

Figure 3. Breed variations in skull type (modified after Miller).

When deciduous teeth erupt in the wrong position, the improper interlocking of the maxillary and mandibular teeth can change the growth pattern of the jaws, which would otherwise be genetically sound. If malocclusion is noticed, early extraction of some or all of these deciduous teeth, as early as six to eight weeks of age, may prevent a future problem (see retained deciduous teeth, 9.5). If the deciduous teeth are extracted early (see interceptive orthodontics, 9.24) and there is still an abnormal jaw length after JAW GROWTH has been completed, then the problem must be considered genetic. Completion of jaw growth varies tremendously depending on the breed and skull type (Figure 3). For the average size skull, growth is considered to stop at about 12 to 15 months of age and for very large skulls, growth may continue for as long as 30 months. In some small breeds growth continues longer than the average. Generally the lower jaw (mandible) continues to grow later than the upper jaw (maxilla). Retained deciduous teeth should probably be considered a genetic problem, although at present this has not been confirmed.

The absence of teeth or the impaction of permanent teeth is seen less often than retained teeth. If however a permanent tooth is absent, the deciduous tooth will often be retained. The absence of the permanent tooth must be confirmed by dental radiographs (Photo 5).

Occasionally a retained deciduous tooth will conceal a NON–ERUPTED PERMANENT TOOTH. Providing this is found soon after eruption of the permanent teeth, extraction of the retained deciduous tooth will often allow the non–erupted permanent tooth to erupt. If after about four weeks no change is seen, the crown of the permanent tooth should be exposed surgically (see impacted or retained teeth exposure, 10.13).

In the horse, the first maxillary premolars known as the WOLF TEETH, and in the human, the third maxillary and mandibular molars known as the WISDOM TEETH, do not always erupt. While in some cases the tooth germinal tissue is never laid down, in most cases the crowns of the teeth are fully developed, but are impacted and often malpositioned.

2.3 TOOTH CHANGES WITH AGE

While the *outer shape* of the tooth does not change with age, except through abrasion and trauma, new dentin is laid down in the pulp cavity throughout the life of the animal. Before performing crown restoration or root canal procedures, it is important to know the size and shape of the pulp cavity. The surest method to evaluate this is to radiograph the tooth, but size estimates based on the age of the dog can be highly reliable.

The LUMEN (the internal pulp space) of the pulp cavity of permanent teeth rapidly decreases in size until about two years of age. The lumen gradually becomes smaller in cats and dogs after two years of age, and a thin thread–like or completely obliterated pulp can be expected in older pets. Thus the shape and size of the crowns of adult teeth can be safely reduced (e.g., for crown preparation) without fear of exposing the pulp tissue.

In younger animals, especially under one year of age, the lumen is much larger, and considerable care must be taken during surgical crown reduction to avoid exposing the pulp tissue. Root canal treatment at a young age also provides further difficulties, which will be discussed in more detail in the appropriate sections (see vital pulpotomy, 7.12 and root canal preparation, 7.13). The following illustration demonstrates these changes by means of cross–sections of the canine tooth of the Beagle dog.

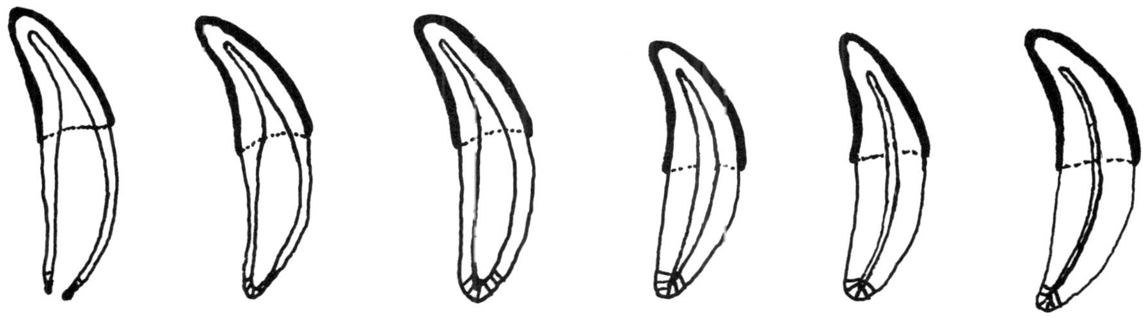

Figure 4. Schematic representation of the root canal system at varying ages (canine tooth).

2.4 DENTITION OF THE DOG

The dog (Canis familiaris) is a carnivore and possesses a dentition less adapted for chewing, than for gripping, killing its prey, tearing off and shearing manageable chunks of meat to swallow. The perpendicular arrangement of the mandibular condyles allows only minimal lateral grinding movement unlike herbivores and rodents. The temporomandibular joint provides a stable hinge, contributing to a powerful grip with the jaws. By stabilizing the prey with the front legs, the dog uses the powerful action of the teeth and jaws to tear the prey into pieces. Smaller bones can be broken by the powerful shearing action of the carnassial teeth.

The FANGS and CARNASSIALS (of the dog) are often confused:

Fang = canine tooth = eye tooth = cuspid.
Carnassial = SECTORIAL (CUTTING) = maxillary fourth premolar and mandibular first molar.

DENTAL FORMULA (DOG):

Deciduous dentition	2	x	$\frac{\textbf{3dI 1dC 3dP}}{\textbf{3dI 1dC 3dP}}$	=	**28 teeth**
Permanent dentition	2	x	$\frac{\textbf{3I 1C 4P 2M}}{\textbf{3I 1C 4P 3M}}$	=	**42 teeth**

The six single–rooted INCISORS in each jaw are arranged in an arch. The roots converge towards the midline. The crown of the maxillary incisors is comprised of a central CUSP (POINT of the tooth) and two smaller MESIAL (surface nearest the midline) and DISTAL (surface furthest from midline) LOBES, while the crown of the mandibular incisors is comprised of a central cusp and a small distal lobe.

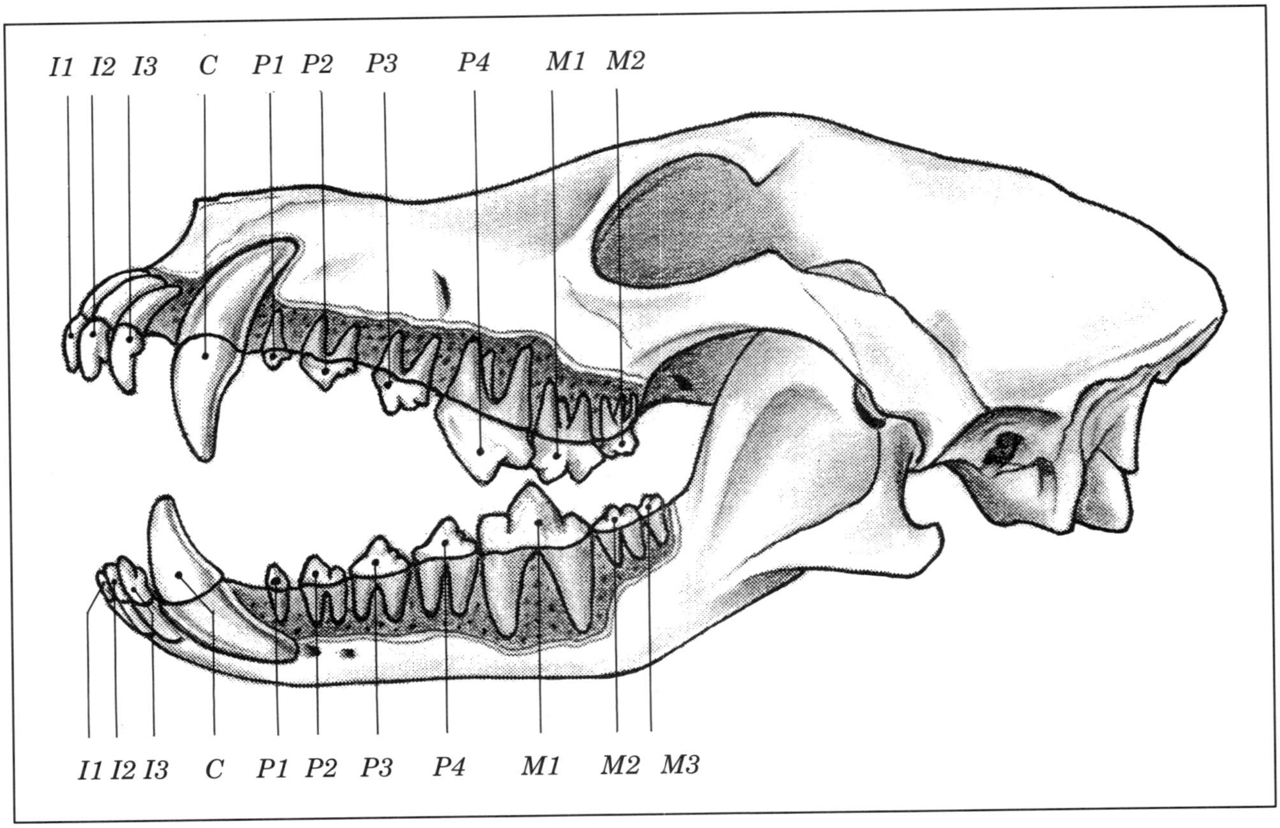

Figure 5. Permanent dentition of the dog.

The four CANINE TEETH have a convex curvature, and are oval with slightly flattened sides. The root extends distally to the level of the MESIAL (ROSTRAL) ROOT of the second premolar.

The first PREMOLARS are single–cusped and single–rooted. Their small size and occasional absence indicates an evolutionary change. The second, third and fourth premolars all have one small and one large cusp. In the *maxilla* the second and third premolars have two roots, and the fourth has three roots (one palatal and two buccal). In the *mandible,* the second, third and fourth premolars all have two roots.

The two maxillary MOLARS each have three roots, while the mandibular first two molars only have two roots. The vestigial, and often absent, third mandibular molar has only one root.

All teeth have a horizontal ridge of enamel around their circumference, just above the free gingiva, called the CINGULUM (Figure 1). This ridge aids in deflecting food and debris off the gingiva, and helps to prevent accumulation of debris in the gingival sulcus thus damaging the delicate epithelial attachment.

The space between teeth is known as the INTERDENTAL SPACE. When this space is wider than normal, it is called a DIASTEMA. Such a space is found between the canine teeth and the first premolars. The space between the maxillary third incisors and the canine teeth is known as an OCCLUSAL SPACE. This space permits the normal dental interlock of the mandibular canine teeth.

The deciduous teeth differ from their permanent successors in their coloration and smaller size. The opacity of the enamel gives deciduous teeth a whiter appearance. In some dental records they are represented by "d" for deciduous.

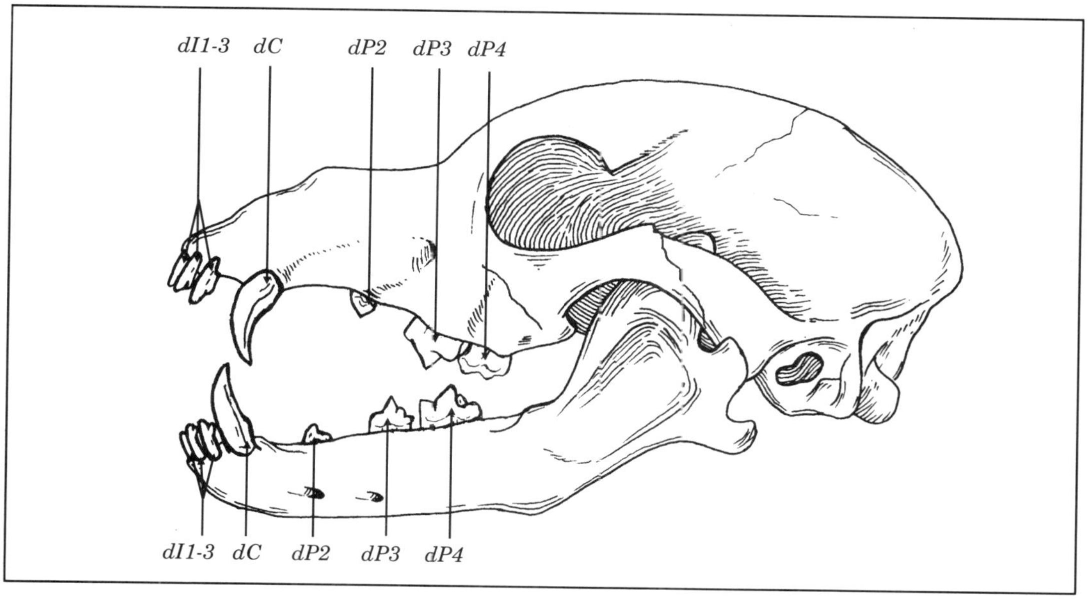

Figure 6. Deciduous dentition of the dog.

The carnassial teeth of the puppy are dP3 in the maxilla and dP4 in the mandible. Although there are only three deciduous premolars in each quadrant, they are numbered dP2, dP3 and dP4 (see cat premolar numbering sequence, 2.6). Maxillary dP4 resembles anatomically a permanent molar, and is not the carnassial. The first of the deciduous teeth are normally lost around the third month, and the last around the seventh month. This exfoliation varies from breed to breed, with the smaller breeds usually taking the longest.

The position of the teeth and their OCCLUSION (how the teeth come together) should be the same in all breeds. However, due to the skull shapes of certain breeds, malocclusions develop. Long skulled (dolichocephalic) breeds, such as the Collie, have widely spaced teeth with INTERDENTAL (INTERPROXIMAL) CONTACT (contact between neighboring teeth) between the maxillary fourth premolars and molars, between the mandibular molars, and sometimes between the incisors. In normal occlusion, the mandibular canine tooth occludes equidistantly between maxillary lateral incisor and canine tooth. When the mouth is closed the canine teeth usually do not make contact, except in short–skulled (brachycephalic) breeds.

One of the breed characteristics of Boxers and Pekingese is a PROGNATHISM (UNDERSHOT JAW) (OVERBITE) where the mandibular incisors, canine teeth and premolars occlude *in front* of their maxillary counterparts (see prognathism, 9.20). The opposite is a BRACHYGNATHISM (OVERSHOT JAW) (UNDERBITE) where the mandibular incisors, canine teeth and premolars occlude *behind* their maxillary counterparts. This is often seen in Collies and Shelties (see brachygnathism, 9.19). These are both genetic functional deficiencies of varying degrees caused by breeding (and fashion) and do not occur naturally.

When the permanent teeth become FULLY ERUPTED (five to seven months of age), the root apices begin to close. Root development continues for two to three years, with a reduction in size of the pulp chamber. Enamel on the crown is not replaced if it is damaged, worn down or malformed. If any wear (attrition) encroaches on the pulp chamber, TERTIARY or REPARATIVE DENTIN is formed and the pulp regresses away from (apically) the crown surface (see caries, 6.3).

2.5 DENTITION OF THE CAT

The carnivorous dentition of the cat is similar to that of the dog, although with fewer teeth.

DENTAL FORMULA (CAT):

Deciduous dentition 2 x $\frac{\text{3dI 1dC 3dP}}{\text{3dI 1dC 2dP}}$ = **26 teeth**

Permanent dentition 2 x $\frac{\text{3I 1C 3P 1M}}{\text{3I 1C 2P 1M}}$ = **30 teeth**

The permanent dentition erupts between the third and sixth months of life. The incisors become larger from midline to lateral, and do not have central and lateral lobes, as in the dog. Incisors appear small and rudimentary, but are important for grooming.

In the permanent dentition of the *maxilla,* the two canine teeth are larger than those in the mandible. In the maxilla, there are three premolars, P2, P3 and P4 (see cat premolar numbering sequence, 2.6). Sometimes P2 may be absent. The largest and most powerful is P4, the carnassial tooth, and is the only tooth with three roots. The only maxillary molar, appears rudimentary and has two roots, one buccal and one palatal. In the *mandible* there are only three posterior teeth on each side, and all are double–rooted. These are P3, P4 and M1, the carnassial, which is the largest mandibular tooth. The molars have no deciduous counterparts.

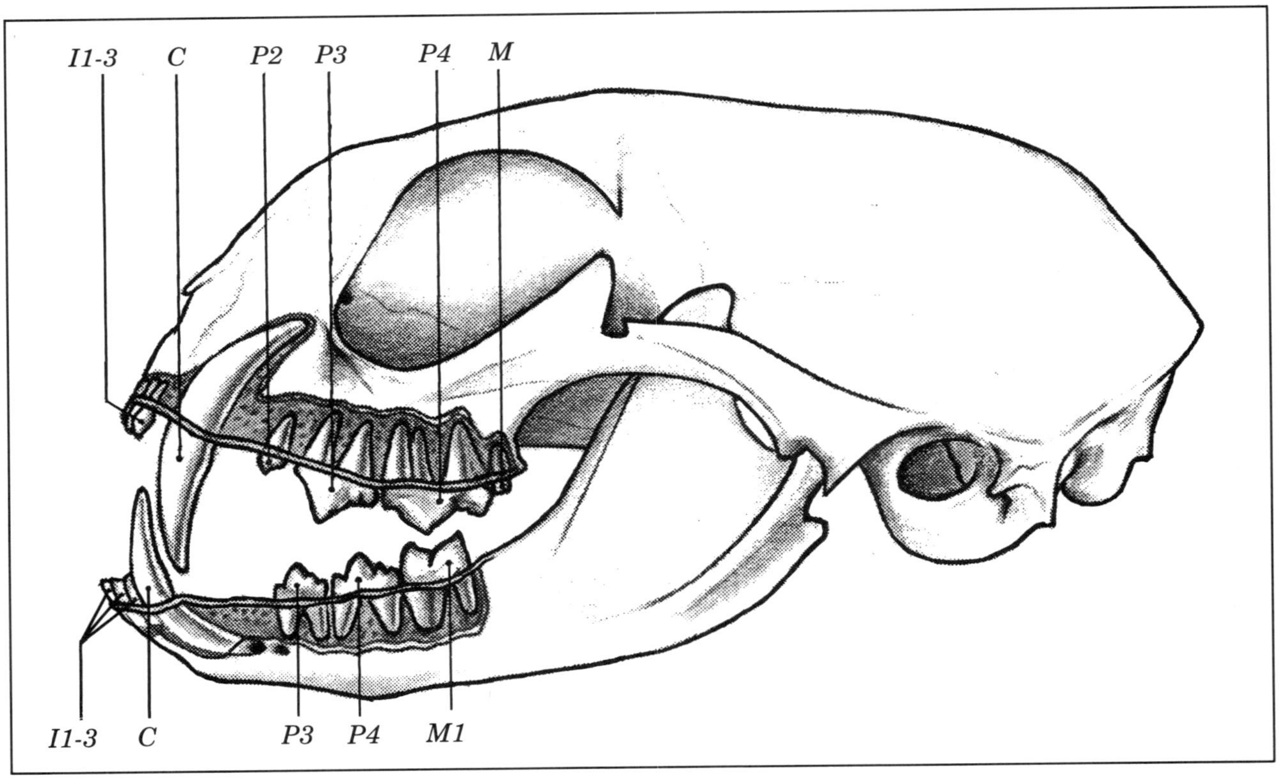

Figure 7. Permanent dentition of the cat.

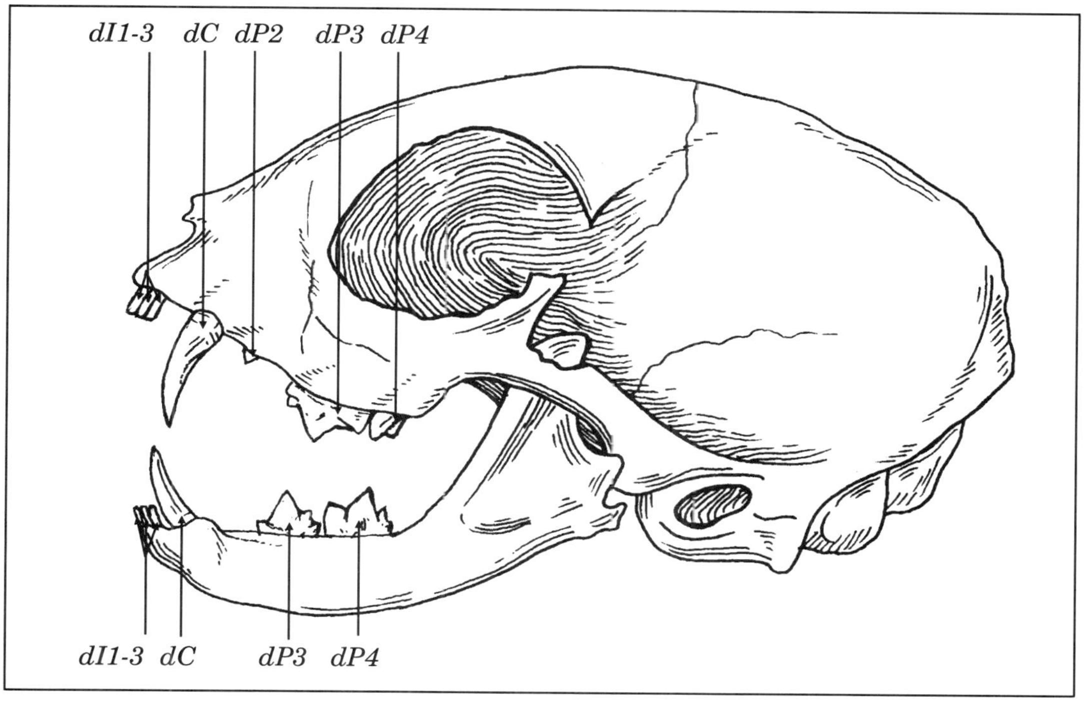

Figure 8. Deciduous dentition of the cat.

2.6 CAT PREMOLAR NUMBERING SEQUENCE

There is still confusion concerning the correct numbering sequence of the premolars of cats.

Most European and now most American veterinary dentists call the *last* (most distal) maxillary and mandibular premolars, the *fourth* premolar. Based on evidence from paleontological studies of the teeth of old skulls, it is believed that all species of carnivores originally had four premolars. The basic rules of comparative odontology for all mammals state that:

1. Permanent molars have no deciduous predecessors.
2. First premolars are not replaced and as such are permanent teeth when present.
3. Deciduous incisors, canine teeth and premolars (with the exception of the first maxillary premolars and first and second mandibular premolars in cats) are replaced with permanent counterparts.
4. Maxillary and mandibular carnassial teeth are designated as such by their SECODONT (cutting) shape and shearing interaction.

The last or most caudal premolar in the cat should thus be called a fourth premolar. This is based also on the anatomic shape and function of the tooth, and the recommendations of the Nomina Anatomica Veterinaria (NAV). Therefore, the preceding premolars should be numbered three and two (maxilla), and three (mandible), which means that in the cat there are no *maxillary* first premolars and no *mandibular* first and second premolars. Since these same principles also apply to the cat (and dog) *deciduous* dentition, it is suggested that the same numbering sequence be used for these teeth.

There has been confusion and controversy surrounding the appropriate numbering sequence for cat teeth. It is hoped that in the near future the premolar numeration will be standardized throughout the world. The use of the Triadan system (see charting the dentition, 2.15) should lead to standardization.

It should be noted that numbering of the feline premolars in this book is based on the European classification, the maxillary premolars being the *second, third* and *fourth*, and the mandibular premolars being the *third* and *fourth*.

2.7 DENTITION OF LAGOMORPHS AND RODENTS

For a long time lagomorphs (rabbits, hares and pikas) were classified as rodents. The resemblance between lagomorphs and rodents is only superficial, having been based more on their feeding habits. Pikas are rabbit–like animals with short bodies, no tail, round ears and hind legs only slightly longer than the fore legs. The most commonly known rodents include guinea pigs, hamsters, mice, rats, gerbils, chinchillas, ferrets, beavers, squirrels and porcupines. Both lagomorphs and rodents possess incisor teeth that are continuously erupting gnawing teeth, and there is a space (DIASTEMA) between the incisors and premolars.

The great difference between rodent and lagomorph dentition is based on the number of maxillary incisors. Lagomorphs have two additional small rudimentary maxillary incisors, often referred to as "PEG TEETH," caudal to the large incisors (Photo 59). This double dentition places lagomorphs into a group called DUPLICIDENTATA or double dentition. Rodents do not have these second maxillary incisors, and thus are classified as SIMPLICIDENTATA or simple dentition.

When lagomorphs chew, the jaw moves laterally, a reflection of the development of their jaw musculature. According to the composition of the blood, lagomorphs are actually more closely related to ungulates (hoofed animals) than rodents. The front feet of lagomorphs are not used for seizing objects as in rodents, being used more for defense and attack. Most importantly there are no evolutionary links between lagomorphs and rodents. Lagomorphs and rodents only illustrate convergent evolution based on gnawing teeth. There are many mammals that possess gnawing teeth, which are unrelated to each other. The duplicidentata consist of the rabbit–like leporides (the genus is called Lepus) or LAGOMORPHS, with 13 species, most having a DIPHYODONT DENTITION (deciduous and permanent teeth). The simplicidentata consist of the TRUE RODENTS, the Rodentia, with 344 species, most having a MONOPHYODONT DENTITION (no deciduous teeth).

The incisors of all lagomorphs and rodents are open-rooted and erupt continuously. The cheek teeth of most rodents, except some such as the hamster, gerbil, mouse and rat, are also open–rooted. This CONTINUOUS ERUPTION throughout their life is counterbalanced by constant wear from the opposing teeth in normal occlusion. The rate of eruption is identical to the rate of attrition. The incisors develop a sharp CHISEL EDGE since only the labial, mesial and distal surfaces are covered with enamel, the rest being dentin (see crown reduction of rodents, 7.18). This enamel on these surfaces covers the crown and root within the alveolus. During gnawing, the softer dentin on the non–enamel side is eroded faster than the enamel side, leaving a sharp chisel edge. The rate of growth of the incisor teeth varies considerably in rodents and lagomorphs. The American Pocket Gopher (thomomys bottae) shows an incisor growth of about 4.4 mm per week in the maxilla, and 6.9 mm per week in the mandible (nearly 1 mm per day!).

It is extremely important for continually erupting teeth to occlude with each other. Lack of contact permits these teeth to rapidly overgrow, leading to an inability to eat, starvation and death (see crown reduction, rodents, 7.18). The name *rodent* comes from the Latin "rodere," meaning "to gnaw."

The premolars and molars have flattened occlusal surfaces that make occlusal contact similar to the human. However the buccal cusps of the maxillary premolars and molars are slightly angled and longer than the lingual cusps. Conversely the lingual cusps of the mandibular premolars and molars are slightly angled and longer than buccal cusps. Since lateral jaw movement is possible, these teeth are very effective for grinding food. Excessive wear of the posterior teeth is prevented through vertical RIDGES OF ENAMEL.

Although rabbits and hares have very similar dentitions, they do differ in the eruption times, which *KEIL* (1966) attributed to the differing lifestyles. The eruption of the permanent dentition of hares (which flee the nest) is earlier than that of rabbits (which remain longer with the family). In both animals the deciduous dentition is not functional and is lost in the third to fifth week of life during the lactation period. In spite of this, the deciduous teeth show considerable wear due to a type of "grinding" movement. There appears to be some controversy about whether lagomorphs have a deciduous dentition. This may be explained by the fact that at birth the deciduous dentition may have already been lost in some breeds. The changing of teeth and the development of the dentition may not have always been investigated thoroughly in some species and breeds.

2.8 DENTITION OF THE RABBIT (LAGOMORPH)

HABERMEHL (1975) showed that the deciduous dentition is complete at birth.

Often the tip of the first permanent incisor (I1) is also present at birth so that three incisors are visible per side in the maxilla. In the third to fifth weeks, M1 and M2 appear in the maxilla, followed by P2, P3, P4, and then M3.

In the lower jaw, P3 and P4 are replaced first, followed by M1, M2, and M3.

DENTAL FORMULA (RABBIT):

Deciduous dentition	**2**	**x**	$\frac{\textbf{2dI 3dP}}{\textbf{1dI 2dP}}$	=	**16 teeth**
Permanent dentition	**2**	**x**	$\frac{\textbf{2I 3P 3M}}{\textbf{1I 2P 3M}}$	=	**28 teeth**

All of the teeth have OPEN–ROOT APICES, thus allowing for CONTINUOUS ERUPTION of all the teeth. The rabbit incisor grows about 2.0 mm per week in the maxilla, and about 2.4 mm per week in the mandible.

The premolars tilt caudally and the molars tilt rostrally. The crowns of the mandibular arcade are longer rostrally than they are caudally, giving a gentle backward slope to the line of occlusion.

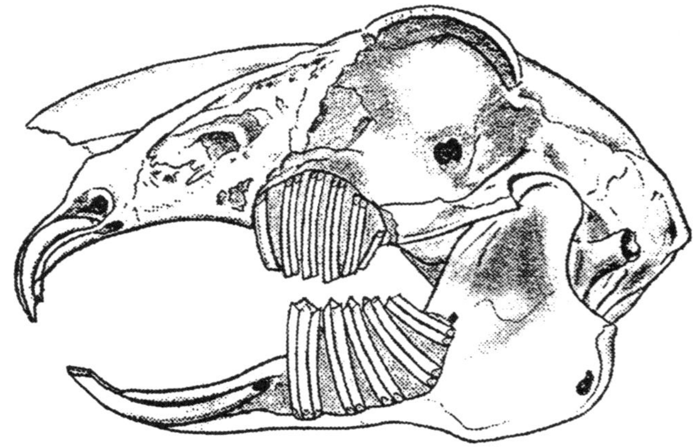

Figure 9A. Rabbit dentition (lateral view).

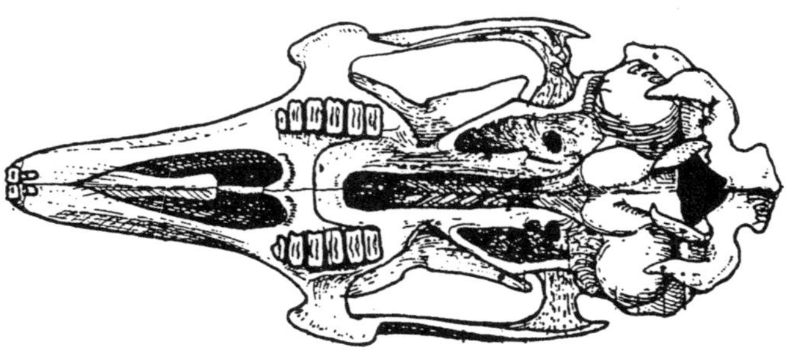

Figure 9B. Rabbit dentition (ventro–dorsal view).

2.9 DENTITION OF THE HARE (LAGOMORPH)

Although the hare has the same permanent dentition as the rabbit, the deciduous dentition consists of only 12 teeth.

As with the rabbit, none of the teeth have a closed apex, thus allowing for continuous eruption of all the teeth. This continuous eruption is made possible by the unusual form of the supporting tissue, as *EMMEL* (1938) was able to demonstrate in the squirrel. The connective tissue does not make a direct connection between the tooth and bone, but provides a tightly woven sheath between tooth and bone, holding it in place without rigid fixation. Since the tooth is resilient, this sheath allows the tooth to absorb pressure during mastication without being luxated.

DENTAL FORMULA (HARE):

Deciduous dentition	2	x	$\frac{\text{1dI 3dP}}{\text{2dP}}$	=	12 teeth
Permanent dentition	2	x	$\frac{\text{2I 3P 3M}}{\text{1I 2P 3M}}$	=	28 teeth

2.10 DENTITION OF THE GUINEA PIG (RODENT)

According to *HABERMEHL* (1975) the guinea pig has no deciduous dentition, and the deciduous incisors demonstrated by *KEIL* (1966) are considered to be fetal.

DENTAL FORMULA (GUINEA PIG):

Deciduous dentition			None		
Permanent dentition	2	x	$\frac{\text{1I 1P 3M}}{\text{1I 1P 3M}}$	=	20 teeth

The posterior teeth of the guinea pig consist of ridged enamel. Each tooth has three layers that lie close together in zig–zag folds.

The occlusal surfaces of the posterior teeth segments rise and fall, thus increasing the surface area.

All the teeth have open–root apices, allowing for continuous eruption.

2.11 DENTITION OF THE HAMSTER (RODENT)

The Golden Hamster (mesocricetus auratus) is a Murid, relating to the family muridae, which is comprised of mice and rats. It is a common patient in veterinary practice. The hamster only has a permanent dentition, consisting of incisors and molars. The tips of the maxillary incisors appear at the age of three days, and within 21 days the full dentition has erupted. The number of molars varies between two and three in each posterior segment.

DENTAL FORMULA (HAMSTER):

Deciduous dentition			None		
Permanent dentition	2	x	$\frac{\text{1I 3(2)M}}{\text{1I 3(2)M}}$	=	16 (12) teeth

The posterior teeth have roots with closed apices, and therefore do not continuously erupt. According to *KITTEL* (1972) they have two longitudinal rows of cusps. These cusps become rounded through normal occlusal erosion, and eventually disappear completely.

2.12 DENTITION OF THE RAT (RODENT)

The white laboratory rat is an albino breed of the gray wild rat (rattus norvegicus), and is a Murid. It is widely used as an animal study model for the evaluation of drugs and other medical research. In human dental research, rats are the most frequently used animals to study naturally or artificially induced caries. The primary similarity between the teeth of the rat and the human is the shape of the molar teeth. However rat molars have thinner enamel on the occlusal surfaces than human molars. The rat has no deciduous dentition and a very reduced permanent dentition.

DENTAL FORMULA (RAT):

Deciduous dentition **None**

Permanent dentition $\mathbf{2 \times \frac{1I \quad 3M}{1I \quad 3M} = 16\ teeth}$

At the age of 8 to 10 days, the incisor teeth begin to erupt, and within 18 days the first molars appear. The second molars are visible within about 21 days followed by the third molars at about the 35th day.

The incisor teeth have open–root apices resulting in continuous eruption. The molars have closed root–apices, therefore do not show further growth after complete eruption. They are slowly worn down by attrition as the animal ages. The height of the molar crowns is relatively short. The occlusal pattern shows cusps with enamel and uncovered ridges and fissures.

2.13 DENTITION OF THE HUMAN

Original permanent dental pattern of *placental mammals*: $2 \times \frac{3I\ IC\ 4P\ 3M}{3I\ IC\ 4P\ 3M}$

During the phylogenetic development of species, the dentition has changed significantly in shape and number of teeth according to the needs of the species. While cats and dogs have retained, almost unchanged, the dentition of predatory animals of three million years ago, the PRIMATES, including the human, have developed a set of teeth and jaws of a more omnivorous nature. Early placental mammals originally had 44 teeth. Evolution has reduced this number to 32 teeth in the human.

DENTAL FORMULA (HUMAN):

Deciduous dentition $\mathbf{2 \times \frac{2dI \quad 1dC \quad 2dM(dP)}{2dI \quad 1dC \quad 2dM(dP)} = 20\ teeth}$

Permanent dentition $\mathbf{2 \times \frac{2I \quad 1C \quad 2P\ 3M}{2I \quad 1C \quad 2P\ 3M} = 32\ teeth}$

The deciduous teeth in the human are commonly known as "BABY TEETH," "MILK TEETH" or "PRIMARY TEETH." They start to erupt at about six months of age, and are fully developed by two and a half years of age. The milk teeth consist of two incisors, one canine tooth and two "milk molars." This latter terminology appears confusing since the permanent molars have no deciduous predecessors. "Milk molars" are in reality premolars, although morphologically and functionally they resemble molars.

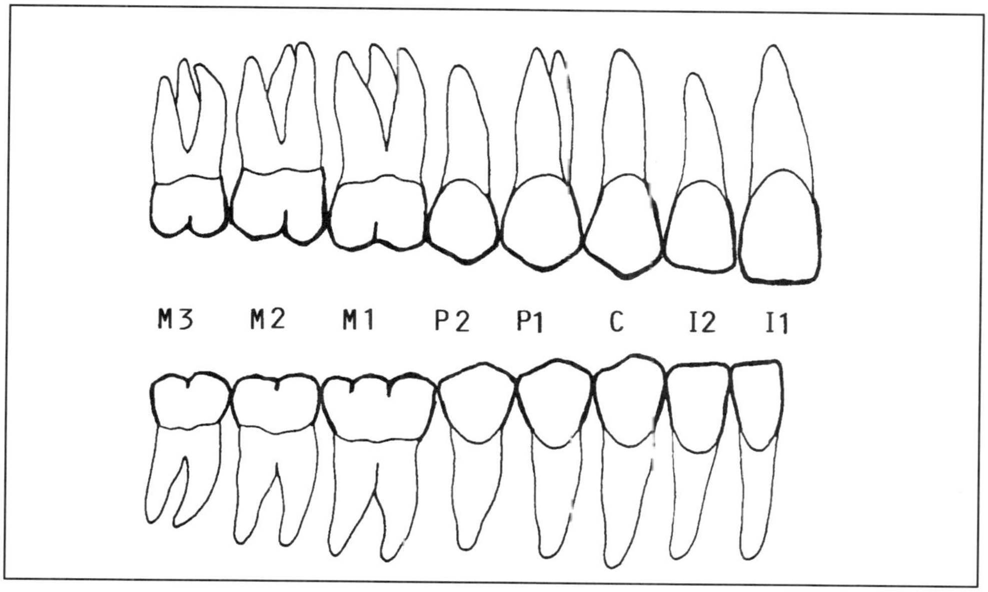

Figure 10. Human dentition.

The permanent teeth begin to erupt at about six years of age. The first permanent teeth to appear are the first molars, followed by the mandibular central incisors, maxillary central incisors, mandibular lateral incisors, maxillary lateral incisors, mandibular canine teeth, first premolars, second premolars, maxillary canine teeth, second molars and third molars. The incisors and canine teeth *develop* lingual to the deciduous teeth but normally *erupt* into the exact same position as the deciduous teeth. The premolars develop between the roots of the deciduous "milk molars," i.e., directly underneath.

By the age of twelve years, all teeth except the "wisdom teeth" (maxillary and mandibular third molars) should be erupted and in use. The "wisdom teeth" normally erupt between the eighteenth and twenty–second year, although occasionally decades of delay may occur.

The incisor teeth have chisel–shaped cusps, and their functions include cutting food and assisting in producing distinct speech. They are single rooted.

The canine teeth, which in most animal species are long and pointed, are reduced in the human and resemble more closely the height and shape of the incisors. This evolutionary change to meet the needs of human eating habits is called INCISIVATION of the canine teeth. The mandibular canine teeth in ruminants have changed in a similar evolutionary manner. The canine teeth, CUSPIDS, show a slight tendency to pointed cusps in most humans. These teeth are single–rooted.

The premolar teeth are adapted for grinding and crushing of food. The evolutionary change of the cusps to a shape similar to the molar teeth is called MOLARIZATION. The premolars usually have one root, except the maxillary first premolar, which usually has two roots (palatal and buccal). The maxillary second premolar occasionally has two roots. Although the premolars are known as BICUSPIDS, the maxillary premolars have two cusps and the mandibular premolars generally have two cusps, but the lingual cusp is commonly diminished in size.

The molar teeth are grinding teeth, having large crowns and broad chewing surfaces. They are known as MULTICUSPIDS, having from three to five cusps. The maxillary molars have three roots, one palatal and two buccal (mesial and distal), and the mandibular molars have two roots, mesial and distal. The maxillary and mandibular third molars are known as the "WISDOM TEETH," and do not always erupt due to impaction or to pathology. In 25 percent of humans, one or more wisdom teeth never develop.

The shape and function of the temporomandibular joint allows a chewing action, which is a combination of the up and down action of dogs and cats, and the extreme sideways movement of ruminants, herbivores and rodents. In order to allow for proper digestion, humans can bite, chew and masticate most different sorts of diets, which indicates their omnivore characteristics.

Since veterinary dentists will invariably be reading human dental textbooks to further their knowledge, it is important to have a basic understanding of the human dentition.

2.14 NOMENCLATURE OF TEETH

Incisors — dentes incisivi — symbol: I.

Apart from ruminants, which have no maxillary incisors, most animals have three incisors in each jaw quadrant, called (from the midline, distally) central, middle, and lateral incisors. They are also called one, two and three respectively.

Canine teeth — dentes canini — symbol: C — also known as "EYE TEETH," "FANGS" or "CUSPIDS."

Canine teeth are present in pigs, and all carnivores. Among the equine species, canine teeth are normally only present in stallions. Mares have only rudimentary, non–erupting canine teeth. The maxillary canine teeth of ruminants are absent, while those in the mandible resemble incisors in both form and function, having evolved from canine teeth.

Premolars — dentes premolares — symbol: P — also known as "BICUSPIDS."

Premolars have deciduous predecessors, except the first premolar in dogs and some species such as guinea pigs. However, it is thought that in dogs the deciduous first premolar *does* start to differentiate from the dental lamina, but disappears without ever calcifying. Cats have no maxillary first and mandibular first and second deciduous or permanent premolars (see cat premolar numbering sequence, 2.6).

Molars — dentes molares — symbol: M — also known as "MULTICUSPIDS."

Molars have no deciduous predecessors.

In general, most vertebrate animals have from four to seven posterior teeth (premolars and molars) on each quadrant. Each quadrant consists of two to four premolars and one to three molars, depending on the species.

2.15 CHARTING THE DENTITION

In order to represent various dentitions, and to uniquely identify different teeth for archival purposes or in publications, various methods have been developed. They are all based upon the principle of the QUADRANT with a vertical line separating the left and right sides of the skull, and a horizontal line separating the maxilla and mandible. The division into left and right sides is from the frontal viewpoint of the operator, for example, the patient's right side appears on the left side of the chart.

Examples:	$\underline{9\,\rvert}$	=	1st upper right molar.
	$\overline{\lvert\,1}$	=	1st lower left incisor.

The ANATOMICAL CHARTING pattern names the teeth as I1–I3, C, P1–P4, M1–M3 in each quadrant. Whether the tooth is upper (maxillary) or lower (mandibular), left or right, is determined by the position of the number.

Examples:	P^4	=	Upper right 4th premolar.
	$_3I$	=	Lower left 3rd incisor.

To denote deciduous teeth, the letter "d" precedes the number of the tooth. (In some classifications "d" follows the number of the tooth.)

Example:	d^3I	=	Upper left deciduous 3rd incisor.

TRIADAN introduced an extension to the world–wide FDI (Federation Dentaire Internationale) system in 1972. In the FDI system each tooth in the human is uniquely identified by two digits. The first digit in the *permanent dentition* represents the QUADRANT (1, 2, 3 or 4) from the front on viewpoint of the operator, numbered in a clockwise direction, starting in the upper right quadrant of the patient.

Upper right quadrant	=	1
Upper left quadrant	=	2
Lower left quadrant	=	3
Lower right quadrant	=	4

Upper Right	Upper Left	
1	2	(MAXILLA)
Lower Right	**Lower Left**	
4	3	(MANDIBLE)

In the *deciduous dentition* the quadrants are numbered five to eight, so that a unique identification for each deciduous tooth is possible. The *individual teeth* are numbered from the midline distally. To indicate a particular tooth, the number of the quadrant followed by the number of the tooth is given. The human upper right first incisor is therefore number 11, pronounced one–one (not eleven), the lower left wisdom tooth (3rd molar) 38, pronounced three–eight.

Since the animal dentition often has more than nine teeth in each quadrant, the VETERINARY TRIADAN CHARTING SYSTEM (Figure 11) uses a two–digit number for each tooth, with the single digit numbered teeth being preceded with a zero. For a dog then, the upper right first incisor is 101, pronounced one–zero–one and the lower left third molar is 311, pronounced three–eleven. The Triadan system has been proven in practice, since with a little experience, rapid orientation is possible, and since no special characters are required as in other systems, it can be easily written on typewriters and word processors.

A DENTAL CHART recording the conditions that you diagnose and treat is very important, not only for your own reference, but also for medico–legal purposes. Many such charts are available (e.g., from Dr. Shipp's Laboratories). Cat and dog *diagnostic dental charts* should indicate the occlusion problems, the degree of periodontal disease, and the exact oral or dental problem. *Treatment dental charts* should indicate exactly what was done and include information on anesthesia/sedation, endodontics, exodontics, oral surgery, orthodontics, periodontal surgery, prophylaxis, radiographs and restorations.

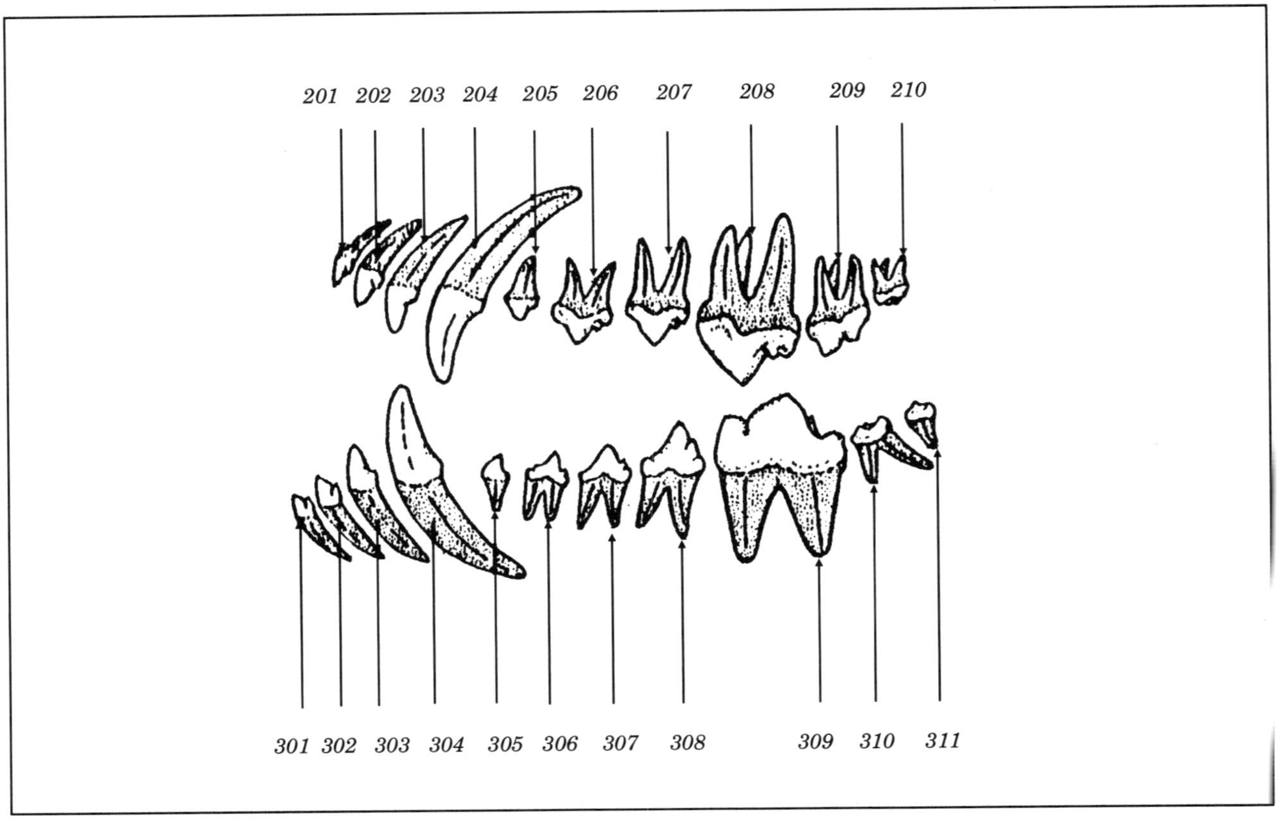

Figure 11A. Triadan numbering system – dog.

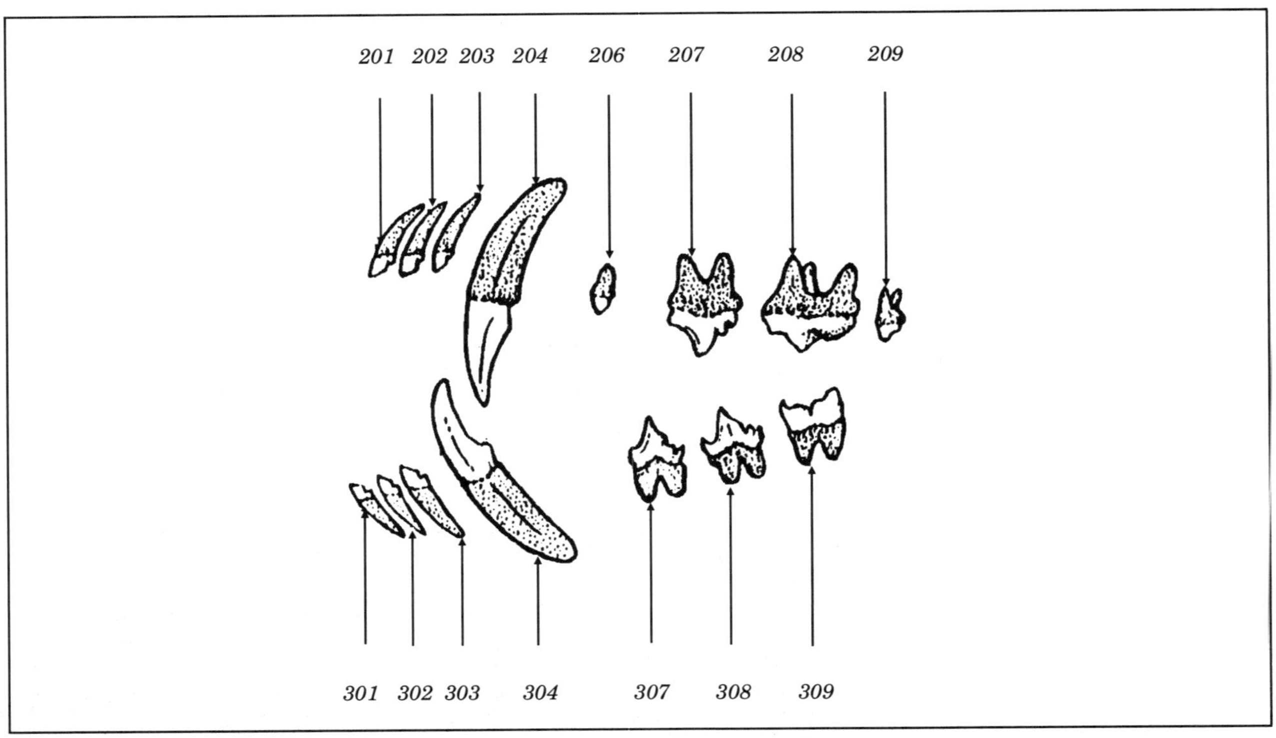

Figure 11B. Triadan numbering system – cat.

All charts should have a schematic drawing of the teeth. These should be accurately marked so that a referring veterinarian (or even the client) can understand what was diagnosed and treated. Copies should be given to the client and the referring veterinarian, and are excellent practice builders.

2.16 TOPOGRAPHY OF THE TOOTH

In order to uniquely identify each SURFACE OF THE TOOTH for documentation and record keeping, the following descriptions are used:

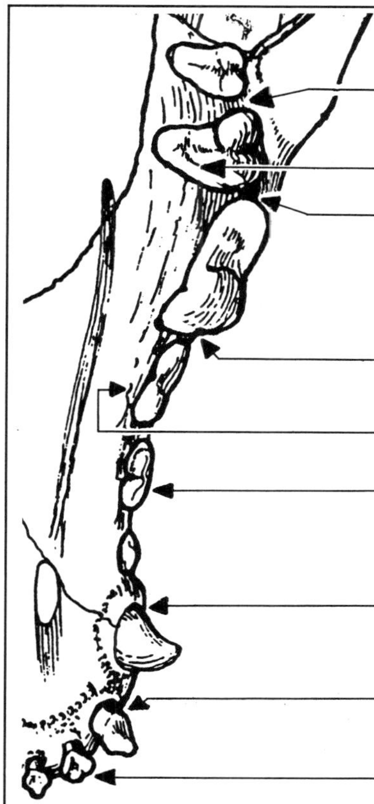

SURFACE	DEFINITION
PROXIMAL (INTERPROXIMAL)	— between the teeth
OCCLUSAL	— occluding or masticating surface
DISTAL	— posterior or caudal (interproximal surface farthest from the central incisor)
MESIAL	— anterior or rostral (interproximal surface nearest the central incisor)
PALATAL; (LINGUAL-mandible)	— towards the palate (towards the tongue)
BUCCAL (LABIAL-mandible)	— towards the cheeks (towards the lips)
MARGINAL	— border or edge near the gingival margin
CERVICAL	— neck of tooth
INCISAL	— cutting edge

Figure 12. Topography of the tooth (ventral aspect of the maxilla).

CHAPTER 3

DENTAL INSTRUMENTS AND EQUIPMENT

3.1 BASIC EQUIPMENT

Although there is an enormous amount of equipment that one can buy, most of it is not expensive. A reasonable investment can set you up initially. There are many sources of used equipment, such as used medical equipment suppliers and dentists who are upgrading or selling their current equipment.

3.2 DENTAL BASE UNIT

There are several complete dental base units on the market, or you can make up your own fixed unit from component parts. Complete MOBILE DENTAL UNITS (e.g., Schein's Vet Base) have a built–in water reservoir and air compressor, a high–speed handpiece, a low–speed handpiece, an air–water syringe, an on/off switch, a water volume knob, a pressure gauge and a foot switch. Mobile units require the water reservoir to be filled periodically, the noise of the compressor is constantly in the room and the unit takes up space. Some mobile units (e.g., VRx Products iM3) contain additional features such as a sonic scaler, a light–cure unit and a suction hose. Although the compressor is very quiet, it may be removed from the base and placed outside the room.

FIXED DENTAL UNITS similar to those found in dental offices, are better for the serious veterinary dentist since they are more sophisticated and allow you more options. Usually there is an extra four–hole connector for additional instruments (e.g., sonic scaler, air driven endo–file or just a second high–speed handpiece). Each hose can have its own adjustments for air and water, and on/off switches. FIBER OPTICS, which allow illumination of the operating site by providing a light source at the head of the handpiece, is an optional extra. The units can be mounted on a swivel arm that reaches over to the operating area. These units take up less space and are more convenient. The compressor can be placed outside the operating room, thus eliminating the noise, and an air hose can be led into the room to connect to the unit. Water is "hard wired" into the unit, so no filling of a reservoir with water is required.

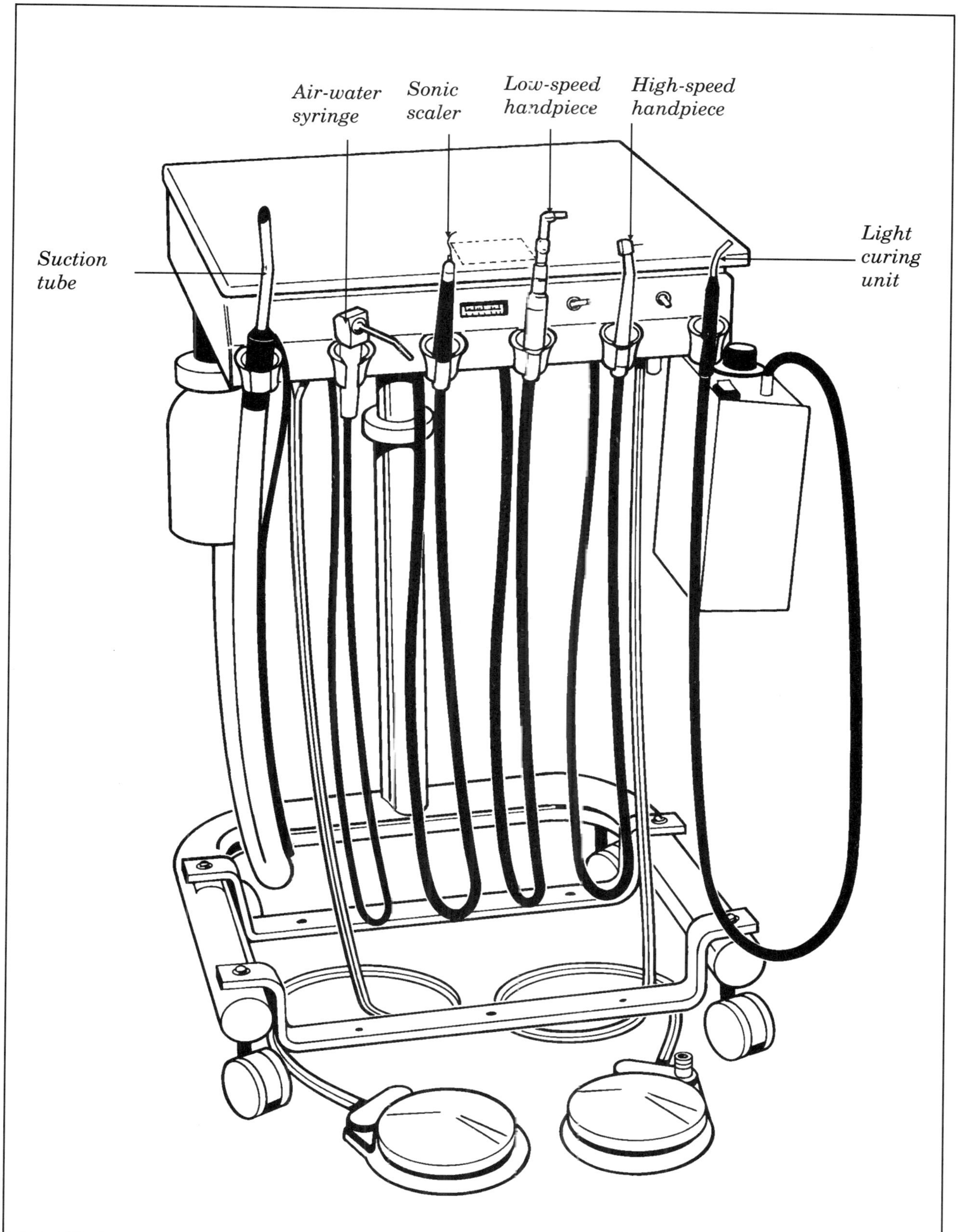

Figure 13. Mobile air–driven dental unit (VRx Products iM3).

3.3 HANDPIECES

An AIR–DRIVEN DENTAL HANDPIECE is a useful addition to any well–equipped small animal practice, since it can be used for simple or for complex dental procedures, and can be used for several non–dental functions. It can be used in general surgery (e.g., drilling holes for fixation of fractured bone segments), for the cleaning, sharpening and polishing of surgical instruments, or in avian medicine for the removal of leg rings and for beak trimming. The three basic instruments that are needed, are a high–speed handpiece, a low–speed handpiece and an air–water syringe. Remember to lubricate the handpieces routinely on a daily or weekly basis depending on the amount of use. It is a good idea to have backup handpieces in case of breakage or servicing. The TURBINE of a high–speed handpiece has very limited tolerances and is delicate, therefore do not allow it to drop on the floor. A new turbine is expensive. The latest turbines have ceramic rotors and are lubrication free.

3.4 HIGH–SPEED HANDPIECE (CONTRA ANGLE)

This handpiece uses various shapes of high–speed burs (*friction grip* or FG) and is used for most dental drilling. The end of the handpiece has a contra angle making it possible to get into confined or awkward places. Other features that are useful are a built-in FIBER OPTIC LIGHT SOURCE, an AUTOCHUCK (for quick changing of burs), and a handpiece SWIVEL (e.g., Star Dental's 430 SWL).

High–speed handpieces can be dangerous, with speeds between 300,000 and 400,000 rpm. The turbine in the head of the instrument is driven directly by air. They should be used with care, and practice is recommended. The handpiece must be held firmly to prevent the bur from slipping into adjacent soft tissue. Handpieces should be held like a pen, with the thumb and first two fingers holding the instrument, and the third and fourth fingers being the "FINGER REST," supporting the hand on the adjacent teeth in the arch. Without this support good workmanship is impossible.

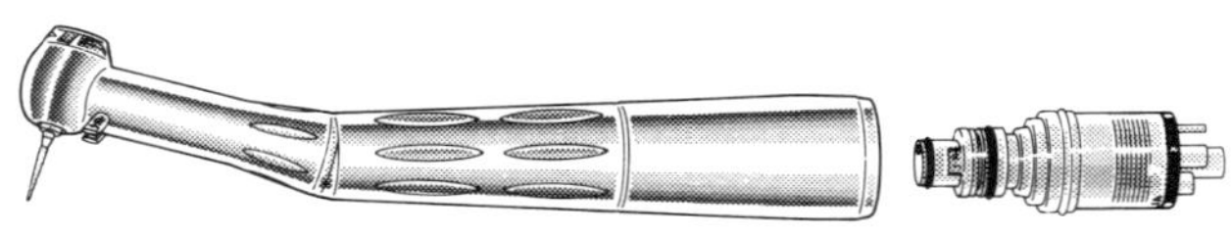

Figure 14. Contra angle high–speed turbine handpiece.

3.5 LOW–SPEED HANDPIECE (CONTRA ANGLE ATTACHMENT AND STRAIGHT ATTACHMENT)

This handpiece uses various shapes of low–speed burs (RA, *right angled,* latch type burs used with a contra angle attachment, and HP, *hand piece*, long shank friction grip burs used with a straight handpiece attachment), cutting discs, polishing wheels, contra angles and prophy angles. The low–speed handpiece is useful in reducing bone (OSTEOTOMY), sectioning and reducing crowns with a diamond disc, shaping and remodeling acrylic splints and orthodontic devices, drilling dentin (i.e., cavities) and polishing teeth.

Low–speed handpieces often have variable speeds that can be adjusted by turning a knob on the handpiece, or by reduction gear attachments that fit on the end. The lower speed is between 5,000–6,000 rpm, and should be used for drilling dentin, polishing teeth and for implant drilling. The faster speed is between 20,000–30,000 rpm, and should be used for some osteotomies, shaping acrylic orthodontic devices, and sectioning and reducing crowns. The actual speed can be variably controlled with the foot switch. The *slower* the speed the *less* chance there is of thermal necrosis of the tooth or the bone structure. Since most low–speed handpieces do not have a built–in water spray, water should be sprayed on tooth and bone structures that are being drilled.

The rotating source in a low–speed handpiece is in the base of the instrument. This can be either air driven or electrical. A mechanical drive or shaft passes from this source through different attachments to the bur.

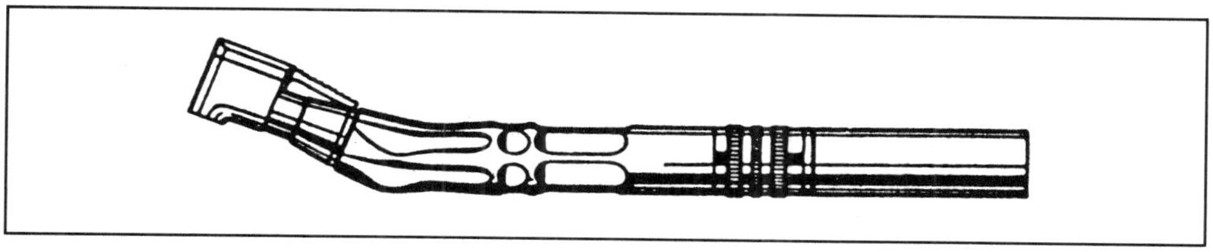

Figure 15. Contra angle low–speed handpiece attachment.

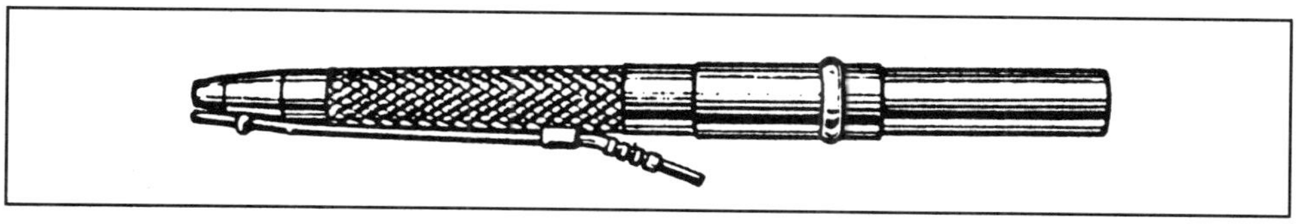

Figure 16. Straight low–speed handpiece attachment.

For those just beginning or those with limited funds, an ELECTRIC MINI–DRILL can be used to accomplish most dental procedures. These drills do not turn as fast as air–driven high–speed handpieces (electric drills turn from approximately 30,000 rpm up to 100,000 rpm with a special handpiece) and usually have no water cooling and fiber optic capability. Different types of contra angles can be attached to the handpiece, enabling reasonably satisfactory results (Fig. 17).

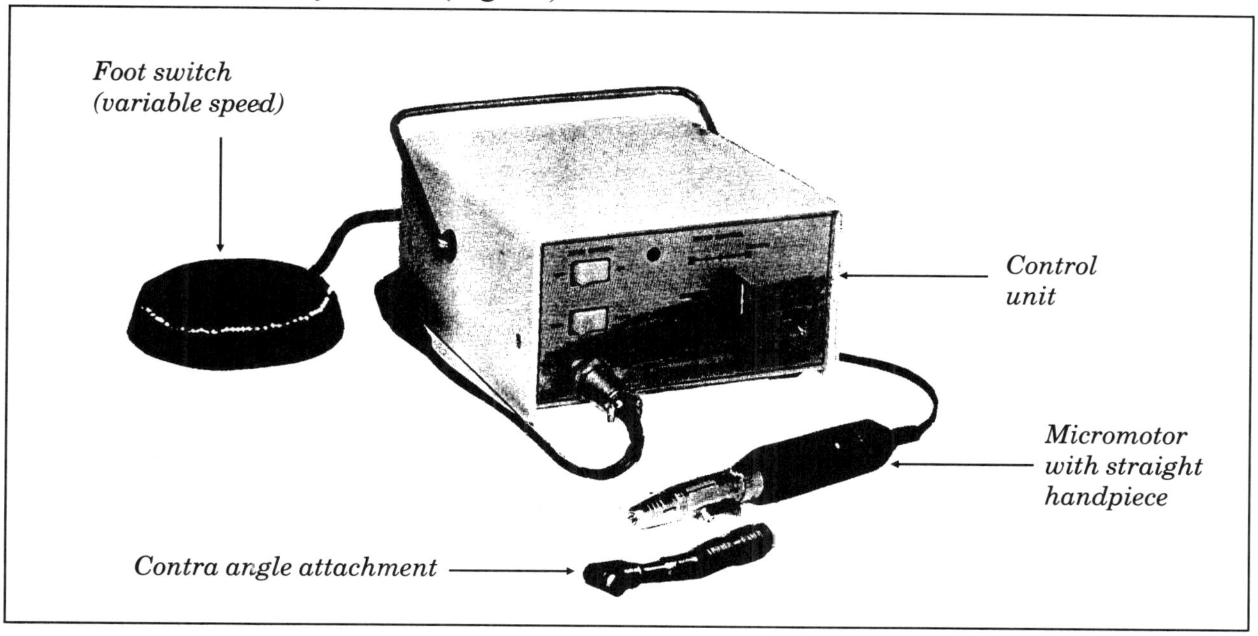

Figure 17. Electric mini–drill unit with micromotor (Schein).

3.6 PROPHY ANGLE

The prophy angle is an attachment used on the low–speed handpiece for polishing teeth. Most prophy cups rotate and sometimes inadvertently catch facial hair in the shaft of the cup. A prophy angle with a cup that oscillates (back and forth about 90 degrees) is more beneficial (e.g., Medidenta's Prophy–Matic). There are many different PROPHY CUPS available and soft ones are recommended. PROPHYPASTES are made in different ABRASIVE grades (GRITS) and flavors. Although flavor is not important for the anesthetized pet, a very palatable malt–flavored prophypaste is available for animals (e.g., CET malt flavored ANIMAL PROPHYPASTE). This can also be used periodically as part of home dental care. The abrasive grade best suited for general use has a medium grit.

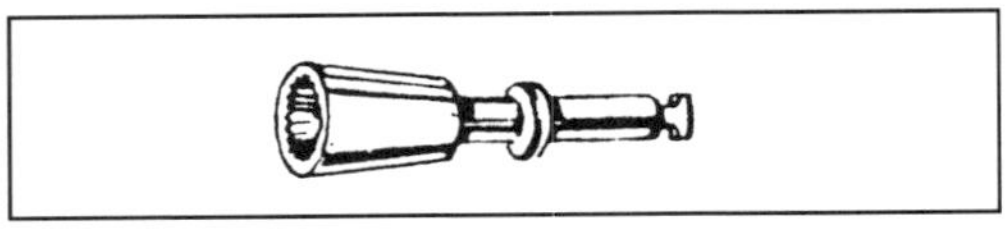

Figure 18. Polishing (prophy) cup.

3.7 AIR/WATER SYRINGE (THREE–WAY SYRINGE)

The air/water syringe is used to clean and dry the teeth and mouth before, during and after dental procedures. The two control buttons allow the operator to use air and water separately, or as a spray by combining both air and water (see Fig. 13).

3.8 SCALERS (MECHANICAL AND HAND)

Scalers are used to clean the teeth. There are four basic types, the ULTRASONIC SCALER (e.g., Cavitron), the SONIC SCALER (air driven, e.g., Titan), the ROTO–SONIC SCALER (which is a six–sided bur used in an air–driven high–speed handpiece) and the HAND SCALER. There are several different tips for the ultrasonic and sonic scalers. Generally a pointed and a chisel tip will suffice. Roto–Pro burs are manufactured in four shapes, *perio*, *flame*, *regular* and *round* (Fig. 19). It is best to have all shapes, but those most commonly used are the *perio* and *flame*.

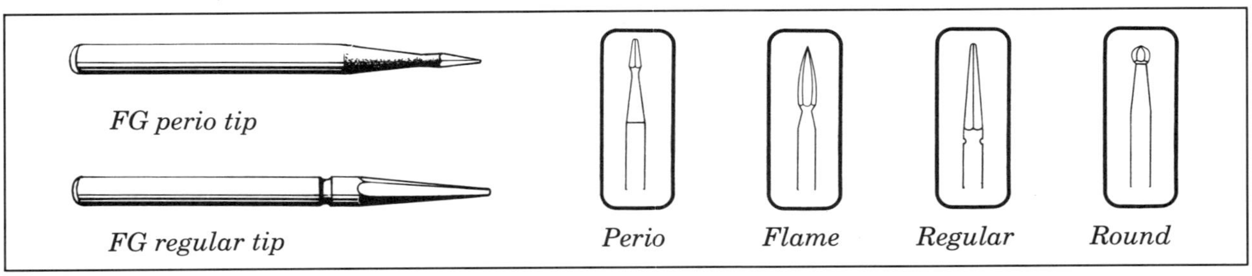

Figure 19. Roto–Pro cleaning burs (Ellman).

All mechanical scaling instruments can *potentially* cause damage to the tooth surface, therefore care should always be used. Mechanical scaling instruments are extremely tactile sensitive, and with practice they can be used very safely and effectively. The secret is to keep the tip moving and use gentle pressure.

It is important to remember that ultrasonic scalers should not be used subgingivally because of possible thermal damage. The sonic scalers and Roto–Pro burs can be used subgingivally. There are many advantages of the Roto–Pro bur. It performs scaling the most rapidly, the air jet lifts the gingival tissue and gives visibility to what you are doing, the water spray flushes out the debris, and the rotation of the bur gives some smoothing effect to the tooth surface. The *perio* bur is best used subgingivally and on the crowns of small teeth, the *flame* and *regular* bur on the crowns of large teeth, and the *round* bur on the occlusal surfaces of the posterior teeth. Roto–Pro burs are also useful to reduce the "FLASH" (jagged or rough edges) of composite and glass ionomer restorations, as well as reduce the tooth and bone around gingivectomy and gingival flap sites. The Roto–Pro bur should always be used at maximum high–speed, since the cleaning action is only achieved at this speed. This six–sided bur, when rotating at 300,000 – 400,000 rpm, sets up a vibrating effect of approximately 25,000 cycles per second, similar to the ultrasonic scaler. Remember, this instrument is very tactile sensitive, so keep the tip moving while applying gentle pressure and use plenty of water. The bur will wear down with use but is generally good for four to six prophies.

Studies by *MARTIN and LIE* indicate that the Roto–Pro bur produces more roughness on the tooth than hand instruments, but less than the ultrasonic instruments.

HAND SCALERS are made in many configurations for human use. They are used to scale the crown of the tooth and should only be used a short distance subgingivally. Large and small "sickle–shaped" scalers are necessary for most veterinary work, as well as a variety of odd–angled scalers for use in those hard to reach areas on small teeth. A dental catalog can help you choose what you need. Scalers generally have two cutting edges, a flat cutting surface, sharp pointed tips and a triangular cross section.

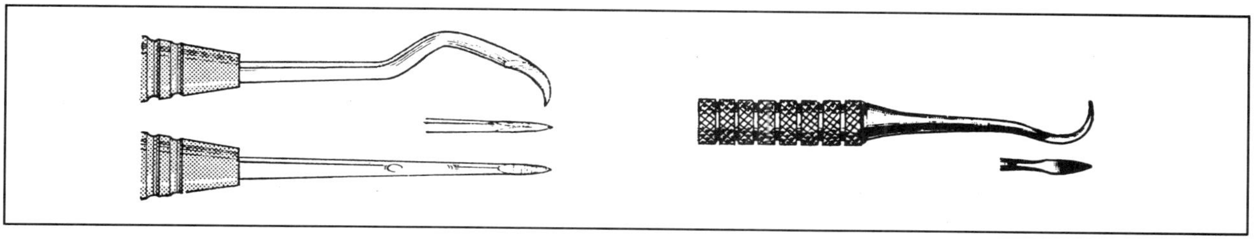

Figure 20. Scalers.

3.9 CURETTES (CURETS)

Curettes are basically similar to scalers, but differ slightly in their shape. Although the UNIVERSAL CURETTE has two cutting edges at 90–degree angles (similar to scalers), the most commonly used curette is the GRACEY CURETTE (11/12 and 13/14). This curette has only one cutting edge at a 60– to 70–degree angle to the cutting surface, a curved cutting surface (to hug the curved surface of the root), a rounded tip (to prevent damage to the subgingival tissues) and a "half–round" shaped cross–section. This is the instrument of choice for removing deep subgingival calculus (concretion), root planing the cementum, and for removing the soft tissue of the periodontal pocket. Since there are many useful curette sizes and shapes, use a catalog to help you decide.

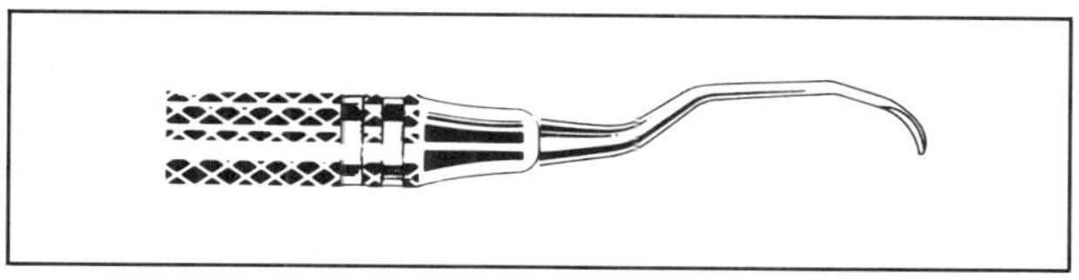

Figure 21. Curette.

Scalers and curettes must be kept sharp. This can either be done professionally (ask your local dental distributor or dental hygienist for advice) or they can be sharpened yourself. Several types of ARKANSAS SHARPENING STONES (flat, conical and rotary) are available, or sharpening kits are available (e.g., Dental instrument sharpening kit, VRx Products).

3.10 EXPLORER

This instrument's sharp explorer point is used to discover early carious defects, subgingival deposits, broken enamel edges, surface defects and the smoothness of the root surfaces after root planing. In endodontics it is used to locate the pulp canal orifice.

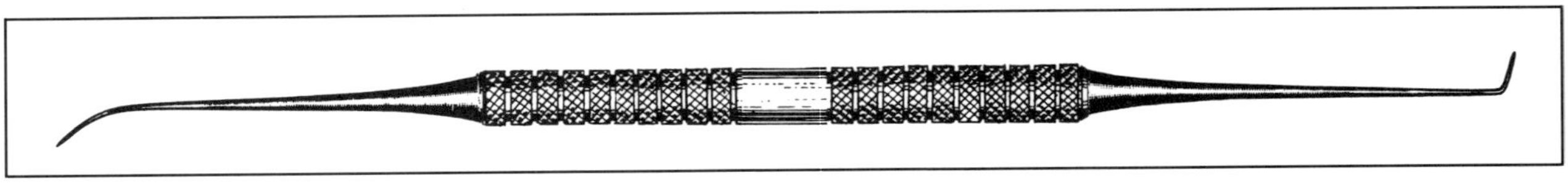

Figure 22. Explorer.

3.11 PERIODONTAL PROBE

This instrument is used to measure the gingival sulcus depth and to determine the depth of periodontal pockets. Color–coded probes, with varying millimeter increments, make probing measurements easier.

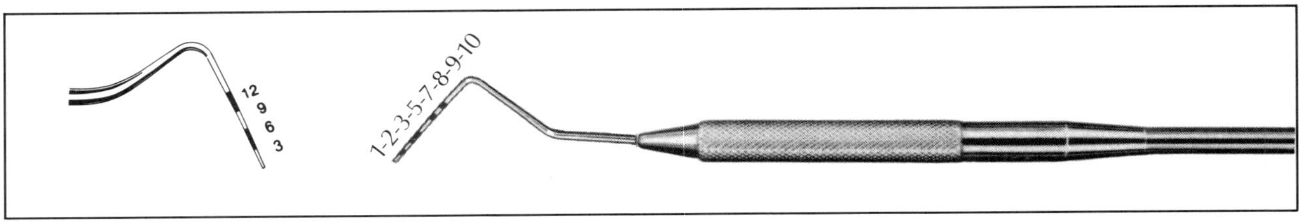

Figure 23. Periodontal probe.

3.12 DENTAL COTTON PLIERS (COLLEGE PLIERS)

These are used for placing objects into the mouth or for removing objects from the mouth. Holding cotton pledgets for the application of medicaments, and cleaning and drying of tooth surfaces with cotton pledgets are also accomplished with dental cotton pliers. Cotton pliers with a quick release lock are useful for holding gutta–percha and paper points.

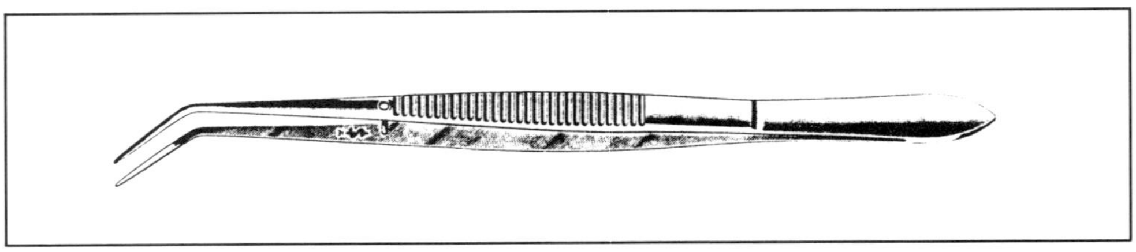

Figure 24. Dental cotton pliers.

3.13 MIRROR

The dental mirror is used to examine poorly visible areas of teeth and oral tissues. Different sizes are available, e.g., #3 and #5. The Fahrenkrug double-ended mirror has the advantage of two sizes in one instrument.

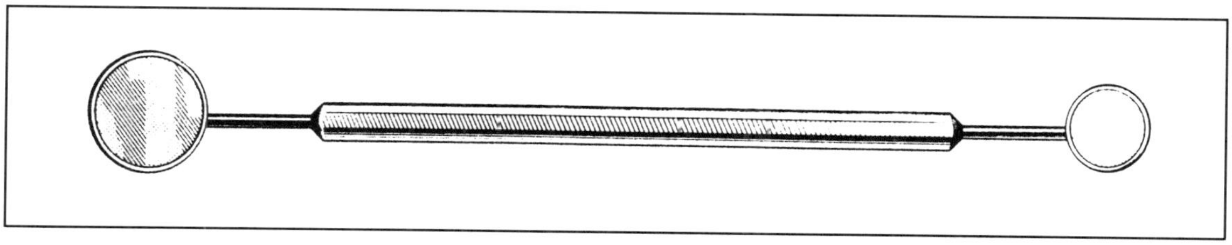

Figure 25. Double-ended mirror (Fahrenkrug).

3.14 EXTRACTION INSTRUMENTS

For successful extraction of teeth several types of *dental elevators, periosteal elevators, extraction forceps, chisels* and *burs* will be needed.

3.15 ELEVATORS (ROOT)

Straight–root and curved–root elevators

Straight–root elevators are the most commonly used and are available in several sizes, measuring 2–4 mm in width at the tip. Most of these have large handles, which are necessary to exert the inward pressure required to properly elevate the root, and some have small serrated ridges on the cutting edge, in order to sever the periodontal ligament.

A special curved–root elevator is available (Fahrenkrug elevator) for removing curved rooted teeth, such as the canine teeth (Fig. 26 B).

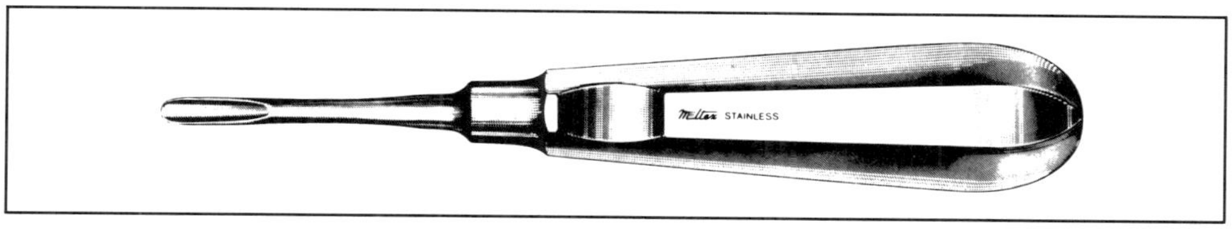

Figure 26 A. Straight–root elevator.

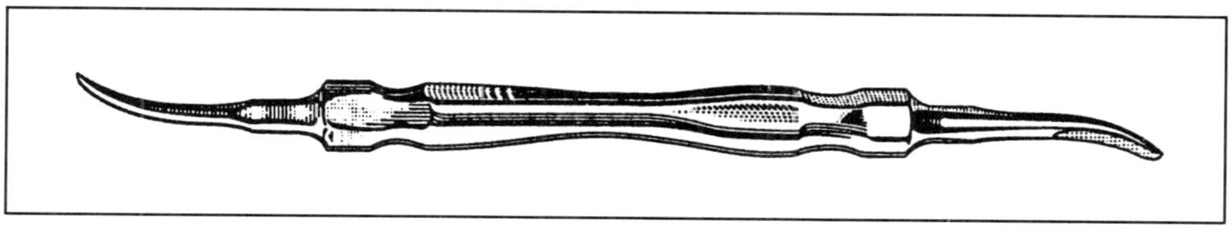

Figure 26 B. Curved–root elevator (Fahrenkrug elevator).

Root–tip elevators

Root–tip elevators are necessary to remove the root tips of small teeth and broken roots. These have small pointed, straight or slightly curved tips and usually a moderately large handle.

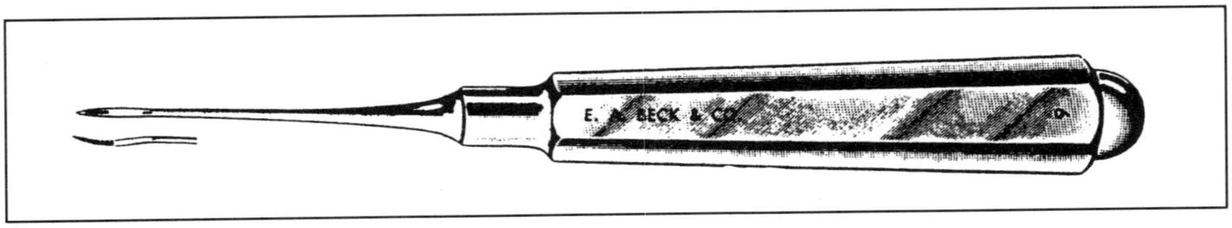

Figure 27. Root–tip elevator.

Root–tip picks

Root–tip picks have very fine pointed tips and often a small diameter handle. They are used to remove small pieces of broken root tips. Although some root–tip elevators and picks have a curve in the shaft, just before the tip, these are not so useful since the necessary pressure cannot be directed effectively.

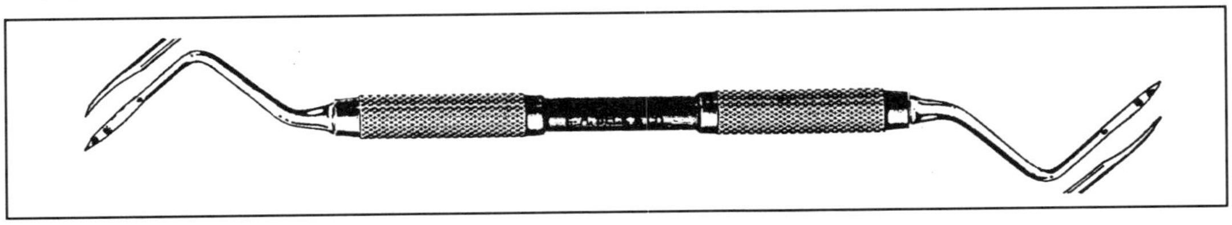

Figure 28. Root–tip pick.

3.16 ELEVATORS (PERIOSTEAL)

In order to extract some teeth, such as deciduous and permanent canine teeth, a gingival flap may have to be raised to access the root. A periosteal elevator is used to elevate the intact gingiva and periosteum. Periosteal elevators are made in different shapes and sizes and a variety should be available to cover all possibilities.

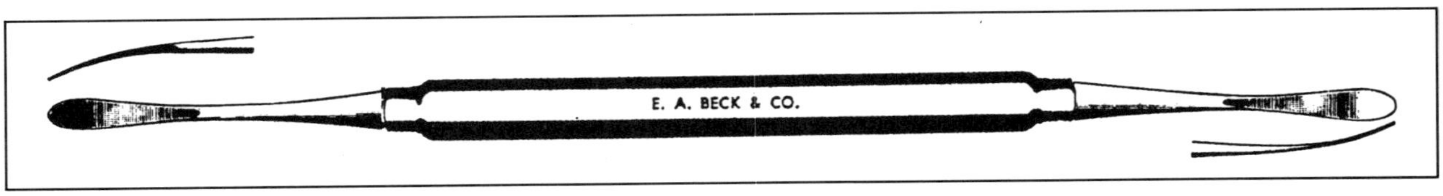

Figure 29. Periosteal elevator.

3.17 EXTRACTION FORCEPS (TOOTH AND ROOT)

These can be divided into and TOOTH EXTRACTION FORCEPS. The beaks of *tooth extraction forceps* do not meet, so that even when the forceps are fully closed a space remains between them. The beaks of *root extraction forceps* are generally longer and thinner than tooth forceps, and come together at the tips when closed. For human dentistry a wide variety of extraction forceps has evolved resulting in several different forceps for each tooth. A sensible selection for a small animal practice is depicted (Fig. 30–36).

Forceps should be chosen with respect to the size and position of the tooth to be extracted. Especially *unsuitable* for animals are the human molar forceps (Fig. 35). These are designed with a ridge which grips under the FURCATION of the human roots (area where the roots branch). This ridge applies an uneven pressure to the small and brittle animal teeth resulting in splintering or fracture.

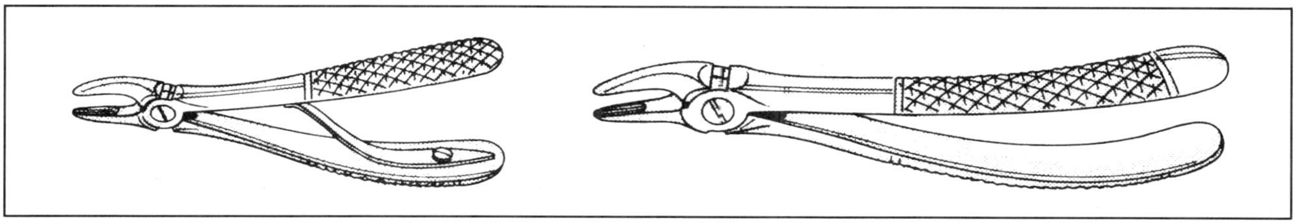

Figure 30. General extraction forceps (small and large).

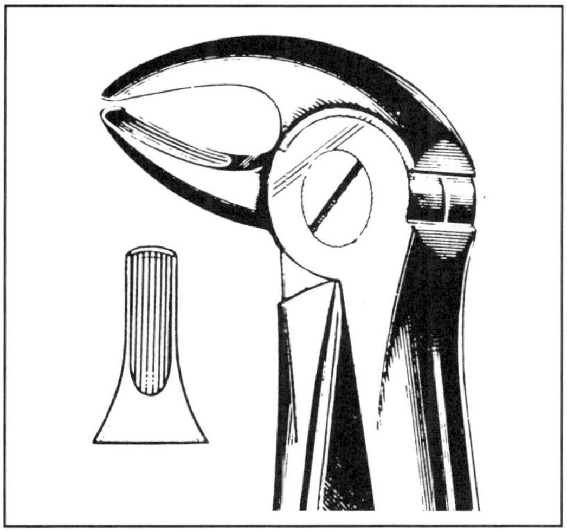

Figure 31. Extraction forceps (right angled).

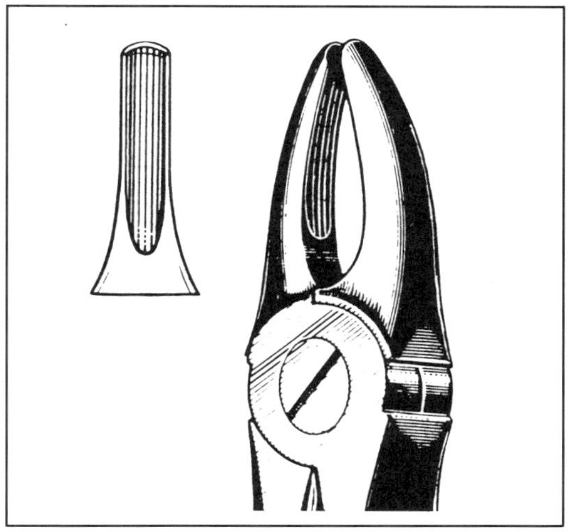

Figure 32. Extraction forceps (straight).

Especially useful for extracting the small delicate teeth and broken roots of animals, are the STIEGLITZ fragment and root extraction forceps (Fig. 34), (Photo 10).

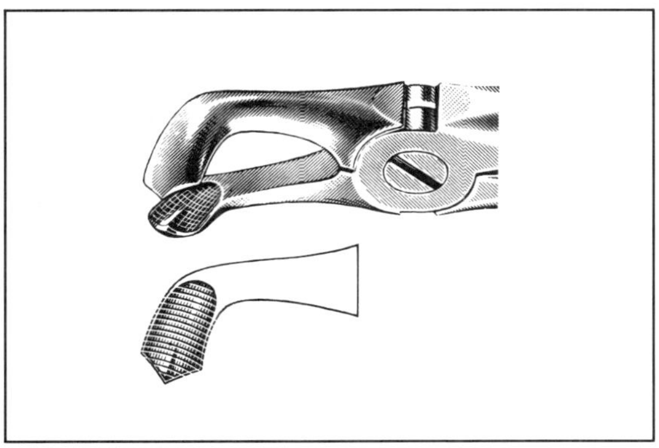

Figure 33. Extraction forceps with groove (Beware – not suitable for animals – teeth may fracture).

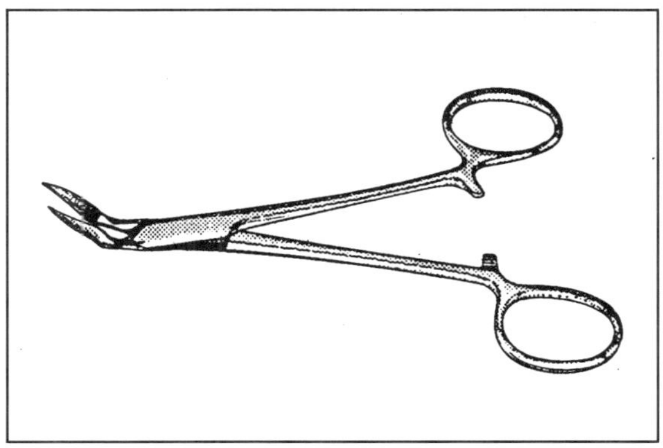

Figure 34. STIEGLITZ fragment and root extraction forceps (45° angle).

Dietrich tartar removal forceps resemble extraction forceps, but are designed to remove large deposits of calculus from the teeth, prior to scaling.

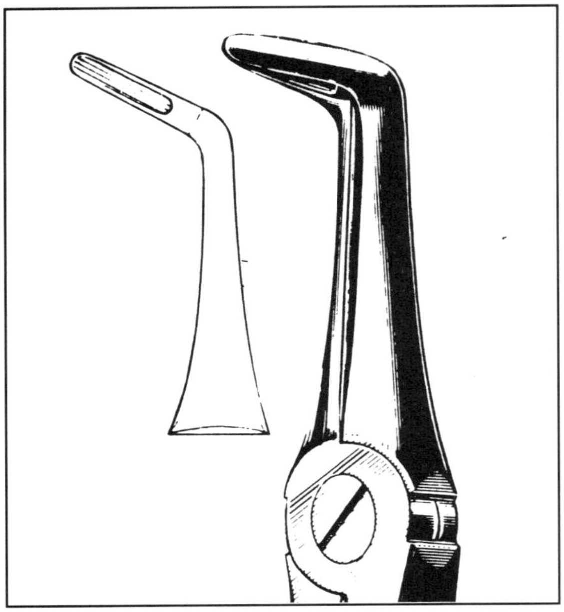

Figure 35. Extraction forceps (angled).

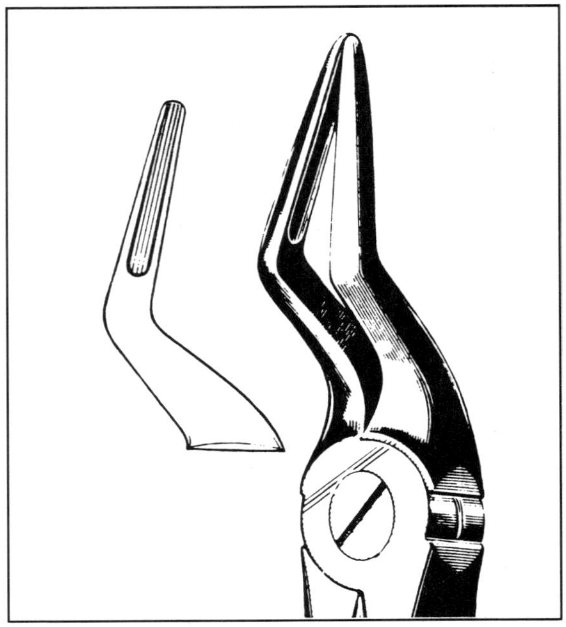

Figure 36. Extraction forceps (semi–angled, bayonet–type).

3.18 CHISELS (BONE) AND BURS (BONE)

It is often necessary to remove alveolar bone around the root of a tooth, such as a large canine tooth. A high–speed or a low–speed handpiece should be used with either bone cutting drills or carbide burs (round or fissure). Adequate amounts of sterile saline or water must be used to prevent thermal bone damage. Round BONE CUTTING BURS usually have five cutting blades.

Hand chisels and a mallet can be used if rotary equipment is not available, but there is a great risk of fracturing the bone.

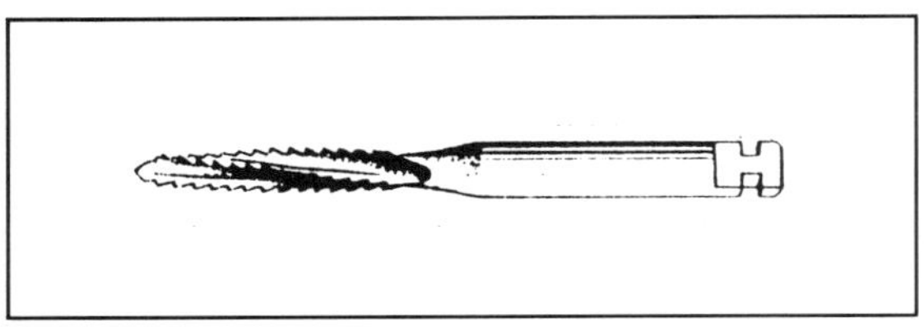

Figure 37. Bone cutting drill.

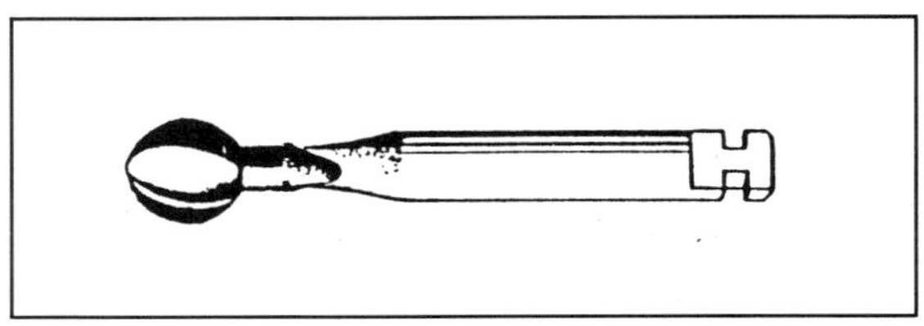

Figure 38. Bone cutting bur (round).

3.19 EQUIPMENT FOR CAVITY PREPARATION AND FILLING

Burs

A cavity is prepared using a high–speed (and sometimes a low–speed) handpiece, and a selection of burs. Initial preparation of the cavity, and also the removal of enamel margins of fractured teeth, is achieved with either a DIAMOND TIPPED or a TUNGSTEN CARBIDE BUR.

Basic carbide burs should include:

ROUND	No's ¼, ½, 1, 2, 4, 6, 8.
INVERTED CONE	No's 33½, 34, 35, 37.
PLAIN TAPER FISSURE	No's 169–172.
CROSSCUT TAPER FISSURE	No's 699–703.
PLAIN (straight) FISSURE	No's 1156–1158.
CROSSCUT (straight) FISSURE	No's 556–558.

There are other less commonly used burs that may prove useful, such as:

END CUTTING	No's 957 and 958.
PEAR SHAPE	No 1930.
CHAMFER TIPS	No 288 E.

Figure 39. Round bur (tungsten carbide).

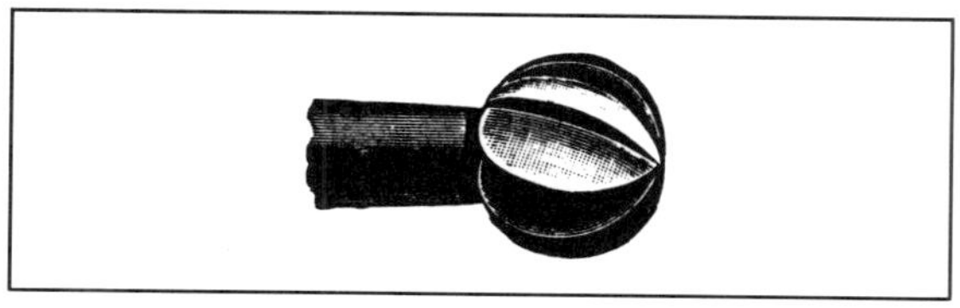

Figure 40. Straight fissure bur (tungsten carbide).

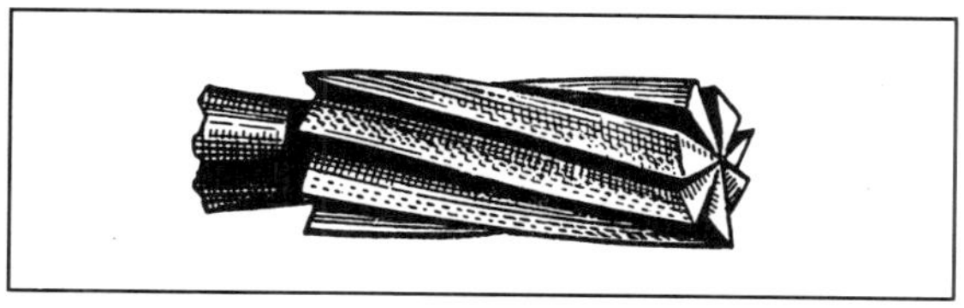

Figure 41. Inverted cone bur (tungsten carbide).

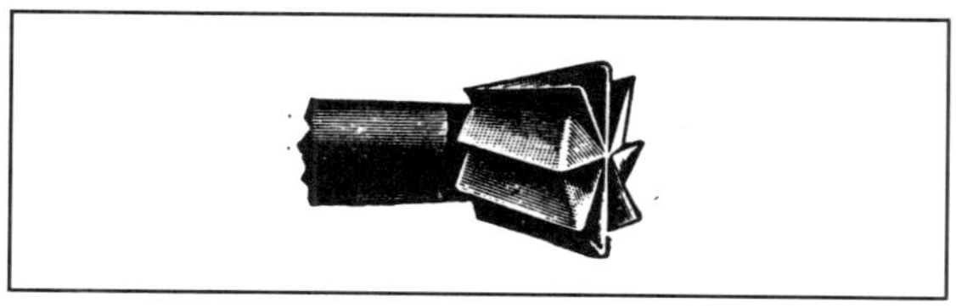

Figure 42. Diamond bur (round).

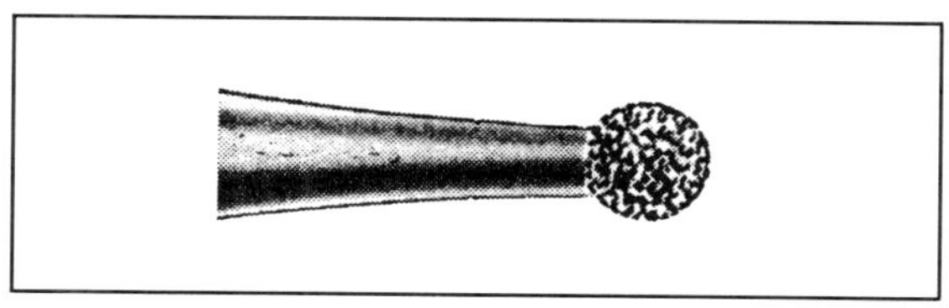

Figure 43. Diamond bur (tapered).

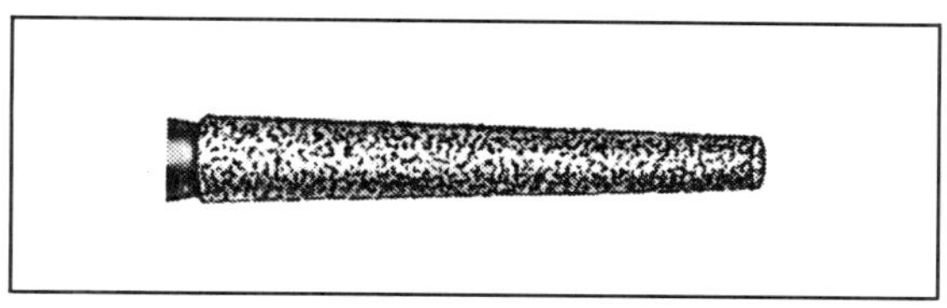

It is best to look in human dental catalogs, contact a dental distributor or go to a human dental exhibition to help decide what you need. Crosscut fissure burs cut quickly and minimize clogging of the bur. Some fissure burs have an "L" following the number. This indicates a longer than normal cutting end, which can be very useful at times. There are also long shaft burs, which are often denoted "surgical." These burs are also very useful when additional shaft length is needed due to tooth or to bone morphology. Diamond burs are manufactured in all different shapes, sizes and textures. Round and tapered diamonds are the most useful in coarse, medium, fine and extra fine textures. Diamond burs are especially useful for cutting enamel and will make fast work of dentin in cases of gross reduction. They are also good for bulk reduction of composites and for sectioning teeth.

There are several different abbreviations of the types of burs:

HP	=	Handpiece (very long shafted burs that fit in the low–speed handpiece).
RA	=	Ratchet (RATCHET END that clips into a low–speed LATCH–TYPE contra angle).
RA Surgical	=	Same as RA but with a long shank.
FG	=	FRICTION GRIP (friction grip end that fits into a high–speed handpiece).
FG Surgical	=	Same as FG but with a LONG SHANK.
FG SS	=	Same as FG but with a SHORT SHANK.
Mini burs	=	Designed for mini high–speed handpieces often used in pedodontic work. These burs are not available in all sizes and shapes.

Dentin is softer than enamel and should be removed using a tungsten–carbide bur. A *round* bur is the best for caries removal. A *straight* or a *tapered fissure* bur is recommended for preparation and smoothing of cavity walls and for tooth sectioning. An *inverted cone* bur is used for preparation of the cavity floor, smoothing the cavity lining and the production of undercuts that improve retention of restoration materials. FINISHING BURS are less sharp than regular cutting burs and have more FLUTES or CUTTING BLADES (12 – 40) than a REGULAR CUTTING BUR (6–8 flutes). Finishing burs are used to reduce excess amalgam, composite and glass ionomer and give the surface an initial polish. A 40 fluted long–tapered or a flame finishing bur is useful for some of the delicate finishing procedures required in veterinary dentistry.

Cavity filling instruments

Cavity liners, bases and cements are applied using a variety of plastic and stainless steel FILLING and PLUGGING INSTRUMENTS. A human dental catalog is useful to decide which instruments suit your needs.

Mixing instruments

A GLASS SLAB and a CEMENT SPATULA are required for mixing some cements, while other materials such as liners, bases, composites, glass ionomers and core build–up materials are best mixed with a spatula on disposable and hygienic WAX PAPER pads. Because more force is required when mixing cements, the wax paper could be damaged, causing some paper and wax particles to be incorporated into the material. Glass slabs can also be chilled to help slow down the curing rate of some materials.

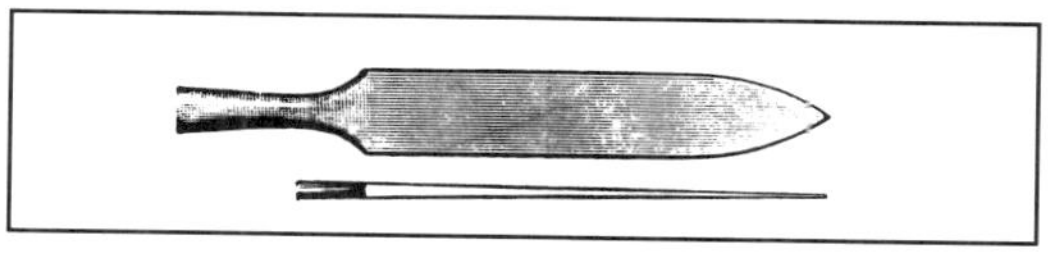

Figure 44. Cement spatula.

Amalgam instruments

An AMALGAM CARRIER and various AMALGAM PLUGGERS, CARVERS and BURNISHERS are used to transport the amalgam to the cavity and pack, shape and smooth the amalgam. The old method of mixing amalgam was with a MORTAR and PESTLE. A more accurate and safer (no toxic fumes) method of mixing amalgam is to use an AMALGAMATOR. This is an electric amalgam mixing (triturating) machine designed to use measured amounts of amalgam (metals and mercury) in a capsule.

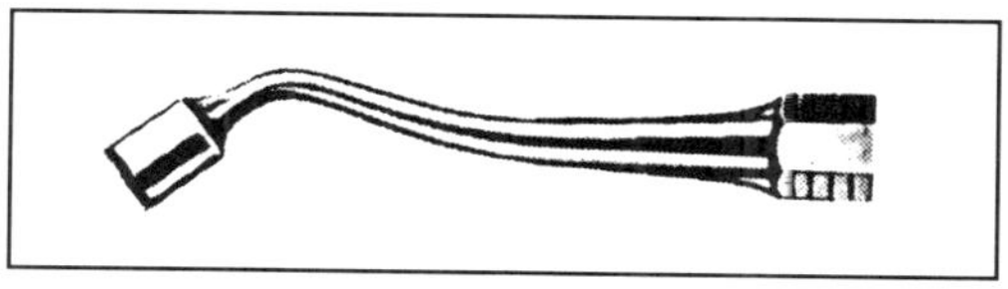

Figure 45. Amalgam plugger.

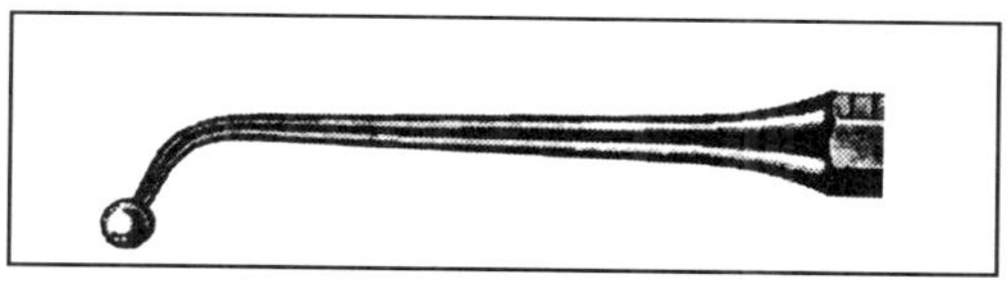

Figure 46. Amalgam burnisher.

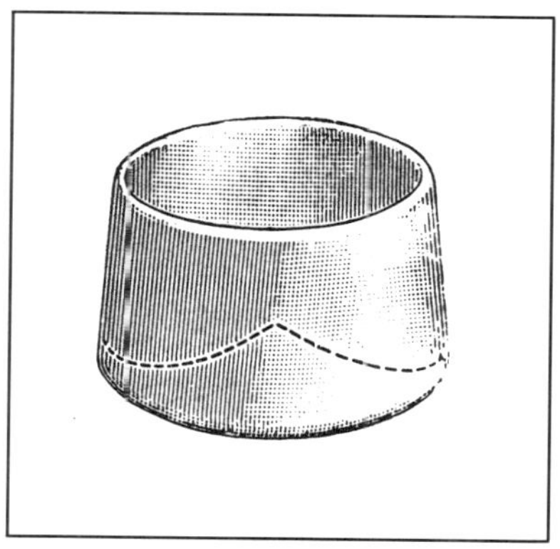

Figure 47. Amalgam mortar.

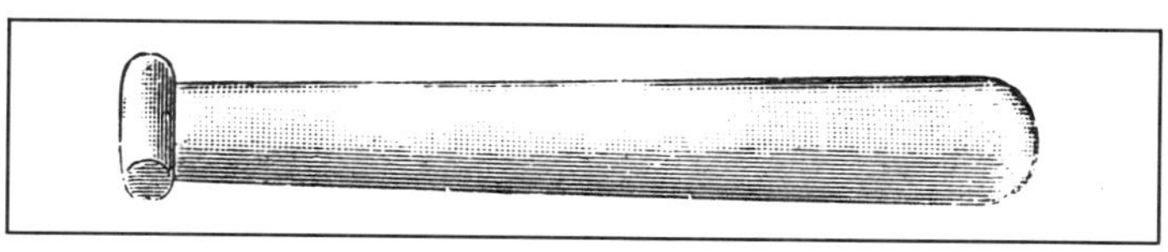

Figure 48. Amalgam pestle.

3.20 ROOT CANAL (ENDODONTIC) INSTRUMENTS

There are several special instruments required for root canal treatment and these can be listed by their function.

Exploring (e.g., explorers) – Used to locate the canal orifice and to determine or assist in obtaining patency of the pulp chamber (see explorer, 3.10). (Small endodontic reamers such as a #08 or #10 can also be used to explore.)

Debridement (e.g., barbed broaches) – Used to remove the pulp, debris and other foreign material from the root canal.

Shaping (e.g., reamers and files) – Used to shape and clean the canal laterally and apically. Gates–Glidden drills and Peeso reamers (drills) can also be used to enlarge the canal orifice and improve straight line access.

Obturating (e.g., lentulo spiral paste fillers, spreaders and pluggers) – Used to fill and pack the canal.

DIMENSIONS OF REAMERS AND FILES

All of these instruments are used for human dentistry and are completely adequate for cats and *most* breeds of dogs. However, the canine teeth of medium to large breeds of dogs may have root canal lengths of 40 mm or more and require longer instruments. Special H–files, broaches and lentulo spiral paste fillers are currently available to veterinary dentists in lengths up to 60 mm. Human reamers, K–files and H–files are made in lengths of 21 mm, 25 mm (28 mm) and 31 mm. A set of human reamers and files (31 mm length and with ISO diameter sizes 10–80), broaches and lentulo spiral fillers are adequate for most veterinary cases, in addition to the 60 mm instruments mentioned above.

These *lengths* refer to the total length of the instrument, from tip to hub, although the actual cutting–edge length is only on the first 16 mm from the tip.

Reamers and files are numbered and color coded according to the *size* of their diameter in millimeters at the tip, or actually 0.5 mm from the tip, where the first spiral begins. These size numbers are internationally known as ISO sizes (International Standards Organization). The tip diameter was originally known as D1 but is now known as D0. The tip diameter (D0) of *K–files* starts at size 06, *reamers* at 08 and *H–files* at 10, and go up to size 140. These tip diameters progress in 0.05 mm increments up to size 60 (0.60 mm at the tip) and then increase in 0.10 mm increments up to size 140 (1.40 mm at the tip).

The point where the spiral cutting edge ends (16 mm from the tip) is known as D16 (formerly D2). Since these instruments are tapered and the diameter always increases at a rate of 0.02 mm per running millimeter of file length, the diameter at D16 is always 0.32 mm larger than that of the tip. This means that a size 10 file has a 0.10 mm diameter at the tip and a 0.42 mm diameter 16 mm from the tip.

The 60 mm H–type files (Schein) have a cutting length of 30 mm, but H-files 55 mm and smaller all have the standard 16 mm cutting length.

The COLOR CODING for the handles of the FILES and REAMERS was developed for easy selection. Nine colors are used starting with pink (06), gray (08) and purple (10). Six colors then follow which repeat every six sizes. They begin with *white* for size 15, *yellow* (20), *red* (25), *blue* (30), *green* (35), *black* (40), and then repeat with white for size 45, and so on (see Table 1). A helpful rhyme (mnemonic) to remember the repeating order of these six colors is "When You Reach Black Go Back." Many files and reamers have the number stamped on the top of the handle.

Size	Handle Color Code	DO mm	D16 mm
06	Pink	0.06	0.38
08	Gray	0.08	0.40
10	Purple	0.10	0.42
15	White	0.15	0.47
20	Yellow	0.20	0.52
25	Red	0.25	0.57
30	Blue	0.30	0.62
35	Green	0.35	0.67
40	Black	0.40	0.72
45	White	0.45	0.77
50	Yellow	0.50	0.82
55	Red	0.55	0.87
60	Blue	0.60	0.92
70	Green	0.70	1.02
80	Black	0.80	1.12
90	White	0.90	1.22
100	Yellow	1.00	1.32
110	Red	1.10	1.42
120	Blue	1.20	1.52
130	Green	1.30	1.62
140	Black	1.40	1.72

TABLE 1. Size, color and diameter of endodontic instruments. (All dimensions are in millimeters, with a diameter tolerance of ± 0.02 mm.)

Broaches (Barbed)

Endodontic barbed broaches are thin, flexible, usually tapered and pointed, metal hand instruments, made from drawn wire and have tiny barbs projecting from the shaft. They are used for engaging and removing the soft tissue from the root canal and pulp chamber. They are very susceptible to breakage in the root canal and must be used with care. Because of the barbs they are very difficult to remove if they lock into the dentin and/or break.

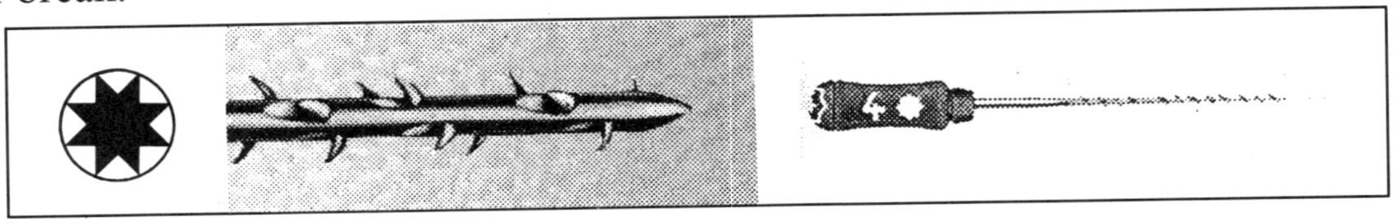

Figure 49. Barbed broach.

Reamers

K–type reamers (or just *reamers*) are made from stainless steel wire onto which is machined either a three– or four–sided, tapered, pyramidal blank. The blank portion of the wire can be a square, a rhombus or an equilateral triangle in cross section. When twisted into a series of spirals to produce less than a quarter to less than a tenth of a spiral per millimeter of length, depending on the size, a reamer is produced. There are from 0.28 to 0.80 cutting FLUTES per millimeter of operating head. They are used to enlarge root canals by a rotary cutting action.

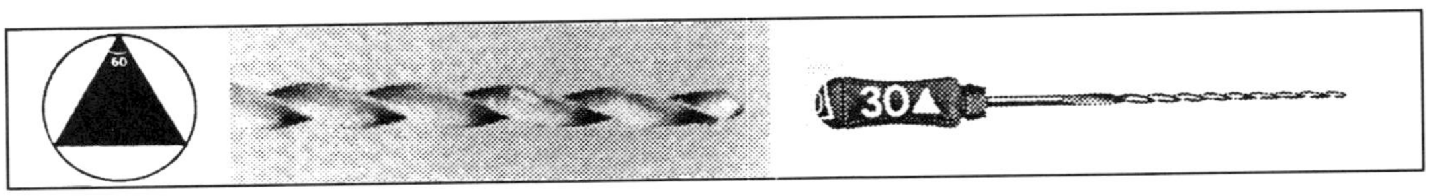

Figure 50. K–type reamer.

K–type files (K–files)

K–type files (K–files) are manufactured from similar blanks to K–type reamers, but are twisted to produce from a quarter to more than a half of a spiral per millimeter length, depending on size. There are from 0.88 to 1.97 cutting FLUTES per millimeter of operating head. They are used to enlarge the root canal by a quarter to a half turn rotary push and pull stroke.

The main difference between K–type files and reamers is the number of spirals or cutting flutes per millimeter. For example, a size 30 *reamer* may have 15 flutes per 16–mm blade, and a size 30 *file* may have 22 flutes per 16–mm blade. The tendency today is for *files* to be twisted from *square* cross–section blanks, and *reamers* to be twisted from *triangular* cross–section blanks (except those less than 0.30 mm in diameter, which are usually twisted from square blanks).

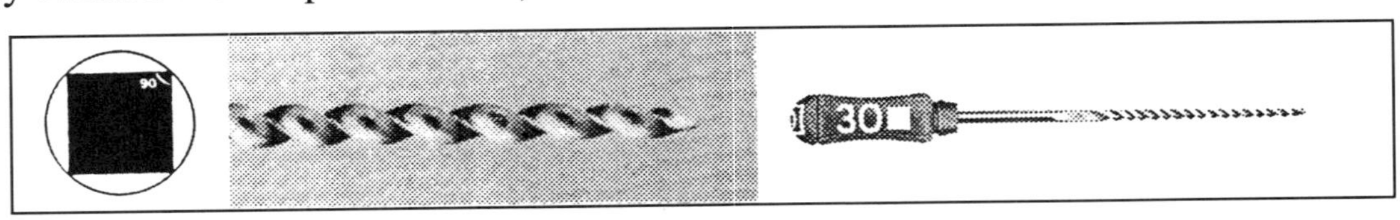

Figure 51. K–type file.

H–type files (H–files) (Hedstrom files)

H–type files (H–files or Hedstrom files) are made by machine–grinding the FLUTES of the file into the metal stock of the operating head, so as to form a series of intersecting cones successively larger from the tip towards the handle. The helical angle of the cutting edge of the usual H–type file is close to 90 degrees, or nearly perpendicular to the instrument's central axis. These tapered and pointed metal files have spiral cutting edges arranged so that cutting occurs principally on the pulling stroke. They are used to enlarge and smooth the canal walls by either a cutting or an abrasive action.

Theoretically H–files should never be rotated and then pulled, as they are likely to bind and break. However the experienced endodontist can use both reamers and files with a push turn (reaming) and a pull stroke (filing) in one continuous motion. Frequent irrigation of the canal with sodium hypochlorite, hydrogen peroxide and CHELATING AGENTS such as EDTA, greatly assists the procedure. RC Prep is a lubricating gel–like preparation of EDTA (dentin softener) and urea peroxide (antibacterial agent).

Certain precautions should always prevail throughout instrumentation. Never turn the instruments more than a quarter to a half turn, do not force an instrument that binds, debride and inspect the blade frequently, irrigate and lubricate frequently, recapitulate frequently and use rubber or plastic stops on the shaft of the instrument to maintain the working length and thus prevent penetrating the apex (see root canal preparation, 7.13).

"H–type" and "K–type" are generic classifications based on a manufacturing process and do not imply a manufacturer's brand or line of instruments. There are also modifications and variations of these instruments including tip design, cross–sectional design, and depth or angle of the cutting edges. Power–driven filing instruments are also available including sonic, ultrasonic and mechanical.

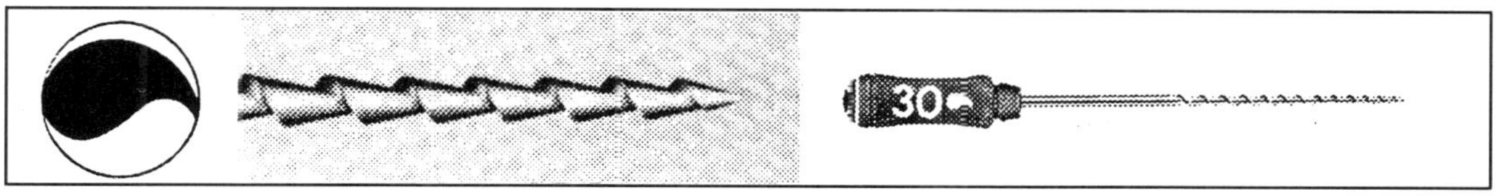

Figure 52. Hedstrom file.

Gates–Glidden drill (G–type reamer)

This is a drill that has a long, thin shaft that ends in an elliptical, flame–shaped cutting head with a safe tip to guard against perforations. It is always used with a latch–type contra angle attachment in a low–speed handpiece and runs in a clockwise direction. There are six sizes, with size 1 equivalent to a size #50 file or reamer. The instruments increase in 0.20 mm increments (size 2 = #70, size 3 = #90, size 4 = #110, size 5 = #130 and size 6 = #150). The number of rings on the shank, indicates the size of the drill (i.e., one ring = size 1, 2 rings = size 2, etc.).

The long shaft is designed to break at the neck, near the handpiece, so that the protruding end can be easily grasped for removal. (Sizes 1 and 2 however are more susceptible to breaking just behind the cutting head, because of the thin shaft, so be very careful when using these sizes.)

The Gates–Glidden drill is used primarily in the coronal third of the canal for enlarging the orifice, and cleaning and shaping the cervical third of the root canal in step–back procedures.

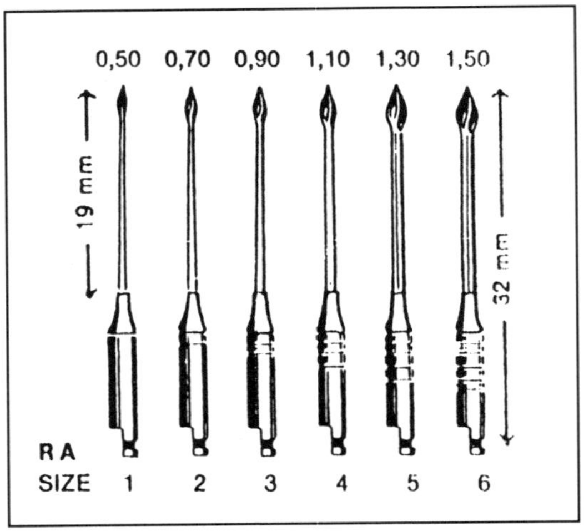

Figure 53. Gates–Glidden drills.

Peeso reamer drill (P–type reamer)

This drill is similar to a Gates–Glidden drill, except the cutting end has long parallel sides rather than an elliptical shape. There are also six sizes with size 1 starting at file or reamer size #70, then increasing at 0.20 mm increments. As with Gates–Glidden drills the number of rings on the shank indicates its size.

Although the Peeso reamer drill is designed primarily for parallel post preparation and undercuts that need reduction, it is also useful in improving the straight–line access to the root canal.

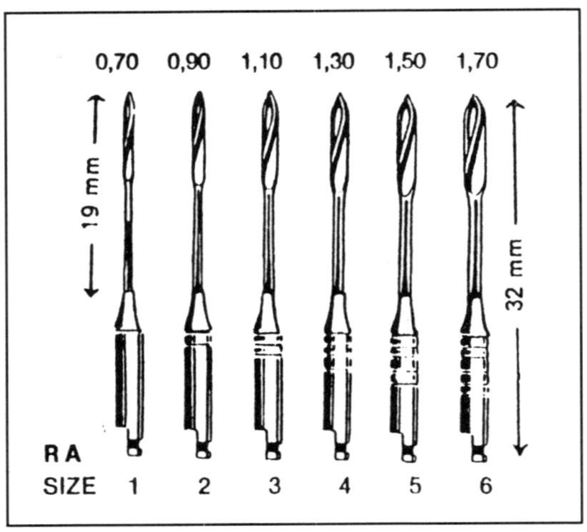

Figure 54. Peeso reamer drills.

Lentulo spiral paste filler (Lentulo spiral) (Lentulo) (Spiral filler) (Paste carrier)

This is a twisted–wire instrument that is used in a low–speed contra angle handpiece to spin sealer, filler cement or calcium hydroxide paste, down the canal (Photo 43). To introduce the material with this instrument, the lentulo is either dipped in the material and spun down the canal, or picked up off a spatula held close to it as it spins the material down the canal. When using a lentulo, caution must be exercised to confirm clockwise rotation to introduce the material (counterclockwise when removing the spiral). Also, the speed should be slow and care should be used to avoid locking the lentulo tip in the apical area of the root canal. It is wise to hand fit the lentulo into the canal, and then mark the depth before putting it in the handpiece. The length of the lentulo should be sufficient to introduce the material close to the apex, with the diameter as large as possible which will fit near the apex.

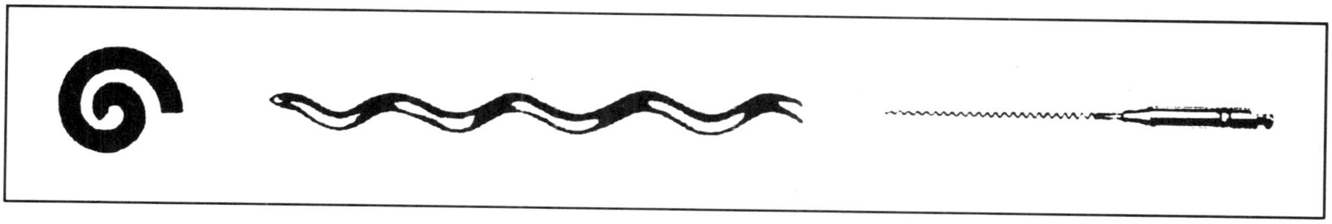

Figure 55. Lentulo spiral filler.

Spreaders and pluggers (condensers)

These instruments are used to spread, adapt and condense the gutta–percha in order to create space for the accessory gutta–percha points. *Spreaders* create LATERAL CONDENSATION (compaction) and *pluggers* create VERTICAL CONDENSATION (compaction). The instruments can be "*handled,*" having a shank that attaches to a metal handle, or "*finger–type,*" which have a plastic hub. "Finger type" instruments are non–annealed stainless steel, and are therefore more flexible for curved root canals. Spreaders are pointed at the tip, whereas pluggers have flat ends. All of these instruments taper at a greater rate than standardized endodontic reamers and files.

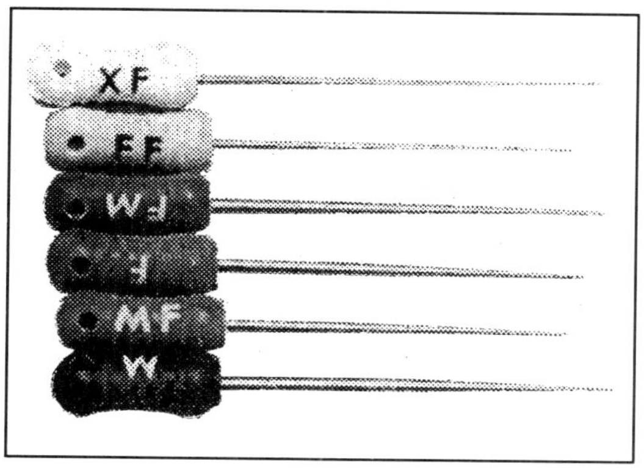

Figure 56. Spreaders.

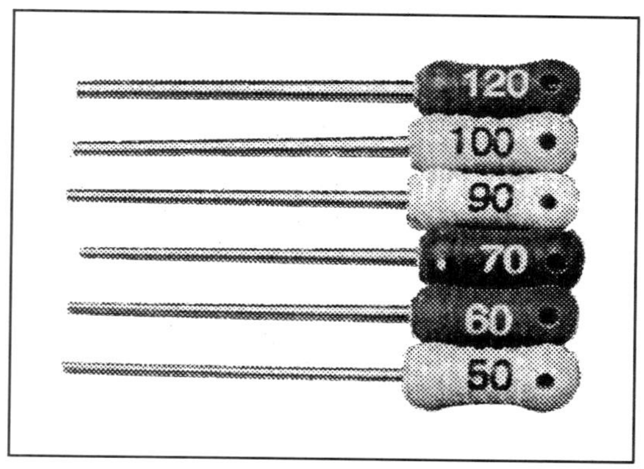

Figure 57. Pluggers.

3.21 OPERATORY EQUIPMENT

The surgery table is usually adequate for dental procedures, although some veterinarians use modified units with good drainage or a sink, or even have custom made tables. The important thing is to have a comfortable working surface with adequate drainage.

Although the majority of dental equipment is small, there is much available. Shelves, drawers and cupboards should all be close by and neatly arranged.

The delicate nature of dental work necessitates a comfortable working position. The operator and assistant should be in a sitting position, opposite each other, with the animal at elbow height. A human dentist's chair on wheels, with a back and arm support, is a worthwhile investment for the serious veterinary dentist.

Since the areas being worked on are small, it is extremely important to have good lighting. An overhead surgery light, as well as a high intensity, low–heat light, is recommended. Although you may have excellent sight, it is still important to see the teeth close up. Magnifying glasses make all the difference and there are many available on the market. It is best to purchase a pair that is light and comfortable, and has a flip–up frame to save having to remove them when not needed. A magnifying power of one and a half to two times is adequate with a focal distance of 12–14 inches. An extra pair of more powerful (three times magnification) glasses is a good idea for the examination of very small teeth. Expensive binocular–type glasses are not really necessary and become heavy when used for prolonged periods.

3.22 ANESTHESIA

Apart from simple operations such as checking or removing some orthodontic appliances, general inhalent anesthesia, with a cuffed endotracheal tube, will be required for most dental procedures. The inflatable cuff of the endotracheal tube prevents water, debris and bacteria from entering the lungs. Atropine may be used as premedication in cases of excess salivation.

With the advent of inhalent anesthetics such as ISOFLURANE ("Aerrane"), dental procedures are feasible on all ages and conditions of pets with extreme safety. Older animals or those at high risk should have mask induction only with isoflurane. Most cats and dogs can be anesthetized using mask induction. Large dogs may require two or three people to hold them down, but induction only takes a few minutes. The safety factor is increased and recovery is very rapid, with the pet usually fully recovered in 10–20 minutes from cessation of the anesthesia. The client is always reassured and impressed when their pet goes home fully awake.

Large animals and those that are difficult to handle, usually require preanesthetic sedation. Intravenous Valium and Ketamine HCl (50/50) works well (use just enough to be able to intubate). The pet may take a few hours to become fully recovered, but the drug combination is very safe.

If you are not currently using Isoflurane, but are using Halothane, Metafane or other inhalent anesthetics, consider changing to Isoflurane. Although it is ideal to purchase an Isoflurane vaporizer, the Halothane vaporizer can be easily cleaned out with chloroform and used for Isoflurane (contact Anaquest for instructions). The anesthetic dose and oxygen flow is similar to Halothane. Unfortunately, the extra cost of Isoflurane is often a limiting factor in the choice of drug used. (This should be dramatically reduced when the patent expires.)

Preanesthetic work–ups should be performed as deemed necessary, which include a thorough examination, blood tests, X–rays, EKG and urinalysis.

Close monitoring of the heart rate, respiratory rate, blood pressure and blood oxygen levels also add to the safety of the anesthetic procedure. There is a large selection of monitoring equipment available, and can often be obtained inexpensively as used equipment from human hospitals or medical suppliers. Some procedures, such as a triple root canal and restoration, can take one to two hours, thus this equipment enables you to do your work safely while it constantly monitors the patient.

CHAPTER 4

PERIODONTICS

PERIODONTICS or PERIODONTOLOGY is the study and treatment of diseases of the tooth supporting structures (Periodontium). The PERIODONTIUM includes:

1. The cementum on the root of the tooth.
2. The periodontal ligament.
3. The alveolar bone.
4. The epithelial attachment.
5. The gingivae.

Periodontal disease, from early to advanced stages (Photos 20, 21), is a very common finding in small animal practice, often affecting 80 percent or more of cats and dogs over two years of age. Clients are usually aware of bad breath (HALITOSIS) in their pets, but often do not notice gingivitis, calculus, caries, odontoclastic resorptive lesions or broken teeth. It is important to thoroughly examine the mouth of *every pet* that you see, and inform the owner of your findings. Your thoroughness will boost your image as a veterinarian, not to mention your income.

4.1 PERIODONTAL DISEASE (DEFINITION AND ETIOLOGY)

PERIODONTAL DISEASE can be classified as simple *gingivitis*, chronic *periodontitis*, and other diseases of the periodontium. GINGIVITIS is limited to GINGIVAL INFLAMMATION with *no* loss of gingival attachment or *no* bone resorption. It can be the initial stage of periodontal disease and is reversible. Many, but not necessarily all, cases of gingivitis progress to periodontitis. PERIODONTITIS is a chronic disease characterized by gingival inflammation, PERIODONTAL POCKET FORMATION, bleeding and suppuration from the gingiva, tooth mobility, alveolar bone resorption and finally, tooth loss (Photo 22). Periodontitis is the result of progression of the inflammatory process from the gingiva to deeper structures of the periodontium. Characteristics of the disease are loss of GINGIVAL and PERIODONTAL ATTACHMENT and DESTRUCTION or LOSS of ALVEOLAR BONE (Photo 23). The direction of bone loss or bone destruction is determined using the cemento-enamel junction (CEJ) as a plane of reference.

When the bone loss occurs on a plane *parallel* to the CEJ, it is called HORIZONTAL BONE LOSS. When the bone loss occurs *apical* to the crest of the surrounding bone, either in an *angular* or a *right angle* direction to the CEJ, it is called VERTICAL BONE LOSS. *Horizontal bone loss* is usually seen as a SUPRA–BONY POCKET, whereas *vertical bone loss* is usually seen as a SUB–BONY (INFRA-BONY) POCKET around the proximal aspect of one tooth. The result in both cases is the formation of a TRUE PERIODONTAL POCKET, which is an abnormal SUBGINGIVAL POCKET apical to the epithelial attachment of the gingiva. Bone loss in animals is most commonly horizontal. Some cases of periodontitis may progress to acute periodontal abscesses. Most forms of gingivitis and periodontitis are initiated primarily by BACTERIA and their TOXINS that colonize the gingival sulcus and attach to tooth surfaces.

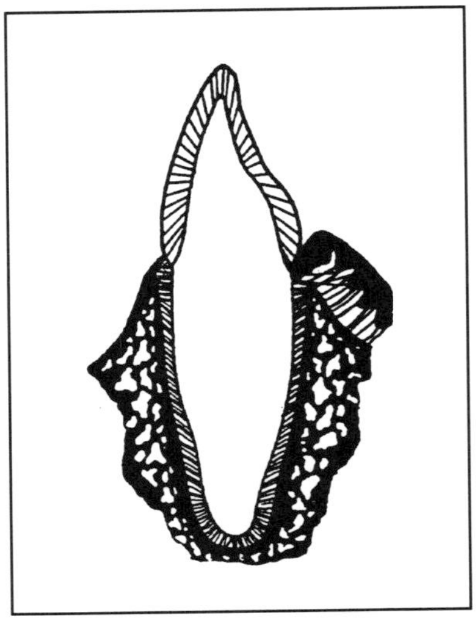

Figure 58.

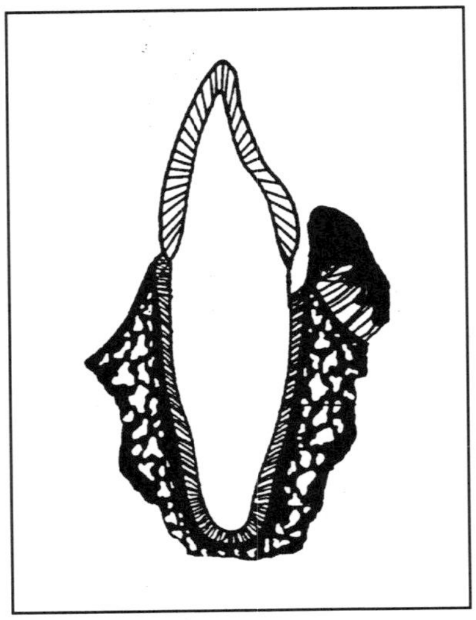

Figure 59.

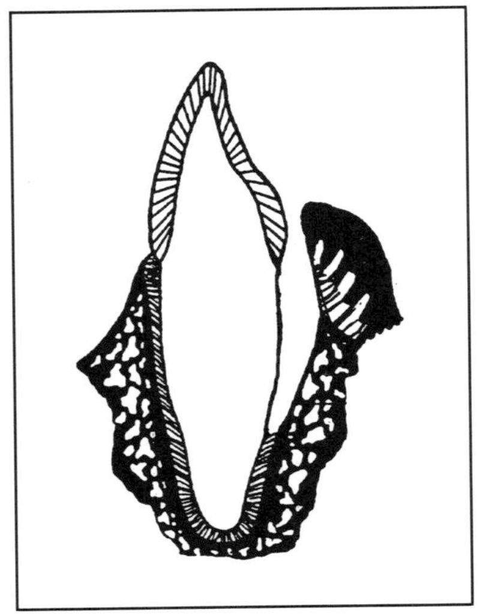

Figure 60.

Figure 58. Healthy periodontium. Sulcus depth normally 1–3 mm.

Figure 59. Moderate periodontal disease. Periodontal pocket, gingival inflammation and moderate horizontal bone loss. Pocket is above the bone. (Supra–bony pocket.)

Figure 60. Severe periodontal disease. Deep periodontal pocket, gingival inflammation and severe vertical bone loss. (Sub–bony (infra–bony) pocket.)

PERIODONTAL DISEASE is caused by a number of factors. The most common factors are lack of oral hygiene and nutritional problems. Domestic animals are generally fed prepared food and have no chance to clean their teeth and gums through catching and tearing apart their prey. Thus, plaque and calculus tend to form rapidly, unless home dental care is performed. Calculus accumulates more easily on teeth that are badly positioned or are retained (Photo 1), have enamel defects, or are positioned so as to allow food and hair to become trapped. Plaque and calculus contain massive numbers of bacteria and their toxins, and contribute to gingivitis and periodontitis. It should be noted that the amount of calculus on the teeth is not related to the degree of periodontal disease. There can often be large amounts of calculus found on the teeth with minimal gingivitis. Conversely, there can be severe gingivitis and periodontitis with little or no calculus accumulation.

Periodontal disease is further influenced by:

1. Hormone imbalance (e.g., pregnancy).
2. Medication (e.g., phenytoin for epilepsy).
3. Vitamin deficiency (e.g., scurvy, malabsorption syndrome).
4. Metabolic and infectious diseases of the blood system.
5. Diabetes mellitus.
6. Feline viral diseases (e.g., FeLV, FIP, FIV).
7. Heavy metal poisoning (e.g., lead).

Long standing periodontal disease is commonly seen in geriatric patients. It should be stressed that the chronic reservoir of infection in the periodontium may eventually spread systemically by passing through the gingival tissues into the bloodstream. Chronic bacterial ENDOCARDITIS, NEPHRITIS, HEPATITIS and PNEUMONIA can result. The sooner these patients are treated the better. There is usually more risk of a geriatric patient dying from these diseases than from the anesthetic necessary to perform the procedure, providing the safest anesthesia protocols are followed (see anesthesia, 3.22).

4.2 PLAQUE

Plaque is a soft, sticky, white material that adheres to the PELLICLE, an acellular membrane of mucoproteins, which accumulates on the tooth surface both supragingivally and subgingivally. The plaque is comprised mostly of bacteria, salivary glycoproteins, extracellular polysaccharide–like glucans and fructans and exfoliated epithelial cells. The metabolic by–products of plaque production diffuse into the gingival epithelium, leading to inflammation of the gingiva (gingivitis) and stimulation of leukocyte movement into the epithelium.

4.3 CALCULUS (TARTAR)

Calculus is a hard, creamy white to brown substance formed *supragingivally* on the tooth surface, and is caused by the mineralization of plaque and the calcification of necrotic micro–organisms (Photo 22). Continuous growth of calculus occurs through more plaque deposition and mineralization. MINERALIZATION occurs by the precipitation of calcium phosphate and calcium carbonate. Calculus is found most commonly near the salivary duct openings. The PAROTID and ZYGOMATIC DUCT OPENINGS are located on the alveolar/buccal mucosa junction above the maxillary fourth premolars and the first molars. The MANDIBULAR and SUBLINGUAL DUCT OPENINGS are located at the ventral end of the frenulum linguae.

4.4 CONCRETION (CONCREMENT) (SUBGINGIVAL CALCULUS)

Concretion is the name given to the *subgingival* calculus (Photo 21). It is harder and develops more slowly than calculus, and adheres more tightly to the cementum than calculus does to the enamel. Concretion is usually dark brown to green, the coloration being caused by blood cell pigments and bacteria, and is formed by mineralization from the *sulcular fluid*. Calculus is formed by mineralization incorporating the *saliva*. Concretion is composed of 80 percent inorganic material, calcium phosphate, calcium carbonate and magnesium phosphate integrated into a mesh. The remaining 20 percent of organic material includes keratin, mucopolysaccharides, amino acids and mucin.

4.5 GINGIVITIS

Gingivitis is an inflammation of the gingival margin, which does not directly affect the more apical parts of the periodontium. Symptoms include swelling, bleeding, lymph node involvement, fever and malaise. Surveys indicate that about 80 percent of cats and dogs have some degree of gingivitis, stressing the need for veterinary dental care and home dental care.

4.6 CHRONIC HYPERPLASTIC GINGIVITIS

Chronic hyperplastic gingivitis is a proliferation of the epithelium, connective tissue and blood vessels of the gingival tissues. The gingival margin is red and swollen (Photo 22).

4.7 NECROTIZING GINGIVITIS

Necrotizing gingivitis is a destructive inflammatory gingival condition, characterized by necrotic lesions along the gingival margin. The ulcers produced are usually covered by yellow–white or gray debris, are painful to touch and bleed easily. The condition can be either acute or chronic and is caused by a combination of bacteria, spirochetes, pre–existing gingivitis, stress and other factors.

4.8 GINGIVAL RECESSION

Gingival recession is the regression of the gingival margin and attached gingiva away from (apically) its normal position (Photo 1). It is usually the result of chronic gingivitis, periodontal disease or trauma. The attached gingiva is important for the health of the periodontium, and therefore as much as possible must be preserved. In some cases the attached gingiva may be difficult to differentiate from the oral mucosa. A simple IODINE TEST can resolve this problem. By painting iodine on to the area with a swab, the mucosa will stain brown, because it contains glycogen. The attached gingiva does not contain glycogen, and will not stain brown. The decision as to whether to treat gingival recession is dependent largely on the amount of remaining attached gingiva, the degree of periodontal involvement and its location. Surgical corrections vary depending on these and other factors, although often in small animals more frequent professional prophylaxis and good home care give better long term results.

4.9 FIBROMATOSIS

Fibromatosis is a massive proliferation of the gingival collagen fibers, which can completely cover the tooth. This condition is typically seen in epilepsy patients being treated with phenytoin.

4.10 PERIODONTAL ABSCESS

A periodontal abscess is a localized accumulation of purulent exudate within the wall of a periodontal pocket. Periodontal abscesses may be either acute or chronic, and are a result of inflammatory and infectious processes in the periodontal pocket. Abscesses also result from trauma and subsequent introduction of infection into the gingival sulcus. In animals this is often the result of damage occurring during prophylaxis, dislodged calculus being left in the pocket after prophylaxis, or hair impaction from self–grooming which is pushed further into the sulcus by mastication. If left untreated, periodontal abscesses can progress to severe periodontal disease and osteomyelitis.

4.11 PERIODONTOSIS

Periodontosis is the non–infectious form of periodontal disease; i.e., a primary non–inflammatory degenerative periodontal disease. There is recession of the gingiva with bone loss and mobility of the tooth. This condition is usually a normal part of the aging process, and is only pathological when it occurs at an early age. This form of periodontal disease seldom occurs in animals. Cats occasionally show this condition.

4.12 LYMPHOPLASMACYTIC GINGIVITIS–STOMATITIS COMPLEX (LPGS)

LPGS in cats (sometimes called LYMPHOCYTIC PLASMACYTIC GINGIVITIS or FELINE GINGIVITIS–STOMATITIS COMPLEX) is a chronic inflammation of the gingiva, generally around all of the teeth, but particularly in the premolar and molar region. Sometimes the gingiva is cherry red and bleeds easily on probing. There is often severe inflammation of the oral mucosa (STOMATITIS), especially towards the pharynx. Although the predominant cells found on biopsy are lymphocytes, plasma cells and neutrophils, these are usually found in any tissue that is inflamed and infected. The etiology of LPGS is unknown at present, although immune disorders or infectious processes are suspected (see diagnosis and treatment of LPGS in cats, 4.21).

4.13 TREATMENT OF PERIODONTAL DISEASE

The first line of defense is a thorough PROPHYLAXIS, which is the cleaning of the tooth and subgingival areas. Hand instruments (scalers, curettes, explorers) and mechanical instruments (sonic, ultrasonic and rotosonic scalers) are used to clean the teeth of all traces of plaque and calculus. It is especially important to remove the plaque and calculus from the gingival pockets and periodontal pockets, and to measure the depth of the subgingival pockets of every tooth with a PERIODONTAL PROBE. Normal pocket depth in the dog and cat should be no more than 1–3 mm, depending on breed, size and age. Although any gingival recession has to be taken into consideration, pockets 4 mm or deeper usually indicate periodontal disease and should be recorded on the dental chart, and the condition treated appropriately. Bleeding from pockets is generally unavoidable during prophylaxis, and should not be used as a reason to discontinue the treatment.

After removal of the plaque and calculus, the teeth should be polished with a rubber prophy cup and medium grit pumice to smooth the tooth surface and inhibit the accumulation of further plaque. The pet owner should be instructed to check regularly for signs of plaque and calculus accumulation and to start brushing their pet's teeth. *The single most important factor in preventing the progression of periodontal disease is regular home dental care,* just as in humans. Most animals will allow their teeth to be cleaned with a small animal toothbrush (e.g., CET animal toothbrush) and an animal toothpaste (e.g., CET animal toothpaste), (see home dental care procedure, 4.20).

If the disease has progressed, the following steps should be taken:

1. Removal of all plaque and calculus.
2. Extraction of all loose teeth that do not have adequate support.
3. Splinting of all loose teeth that *can* be retained with ligature wire, fiberglass, acrylic and composite.
4. Periodontal surgery to reduce all deep pockets.

Sometimes the sequelae of periodontal disease are MUCOSAL LESIONS or ULCERATIONS OF THE BUCCAL MUCOSA (Photo 94). These ulcerations are usually due to long standing contact with calculus and infected gingival areas. Generally these heal spontaneously following prophylactic treatment.

Periodontitis in cats can be treated by thorough prophylaxis, polishing, gingivectomy if necessary, complete extraction of loose and badly destroyed teeth, and medication with antibiotics and corticosteroids. "Neck" lesions should be restored if possible.

PERIODONTAL SURGERY is performed either to eliminate or reduce pockets, remove diseased subgingival tissue and correct unfavorable gingival contours. The PROCEDURES that can be used in PERIODONTAL SURGERY include:

1. Gingival curettage, gingivoplasty and gingivectomy (Fig. 61).
2. Gingival flap operations:
   a) Free gingival graft (see *HARVEY*, Veterinary Dentistry).
   b) Open gingival flap (Fig. 62), (Photos 2, 10, 30, 31).
   c) Modified Widman flap (see *CARRANZA*, Clinical Periodontology).
   d) Reverse bevel flap (see *HARVEY*, Veterinary Dentistry).
3. Mucogingival flap operations:
   a) Apically repositioned flap (Fig. 64).
   b) Coronally repositioned flap (Fig. 65).
   c) Double reverse flap (Photo 12).
   d) Lateral sliding flap (Fig. 63).
   e) Mucogingival flap (Photo 14).
4. Mucosal flap operations:
   a) Frenectomy (removal of the frenulum).
   b) Frenotomy (cutting of the frenulum).
   c) Mucosal flap (Figs. 140 C and D).
5. Alveoloplasty and osteoplasty (Photo 27).
6. Bone graft (see *HARVEY*, Veterinary Dentistry).
7. Treatment for furcation involvement:
   a) Furcaplasty (reshaping of the furcation).
   b) Root amputation.
   c) Tooth section and hemisection (Photos 7, 9).

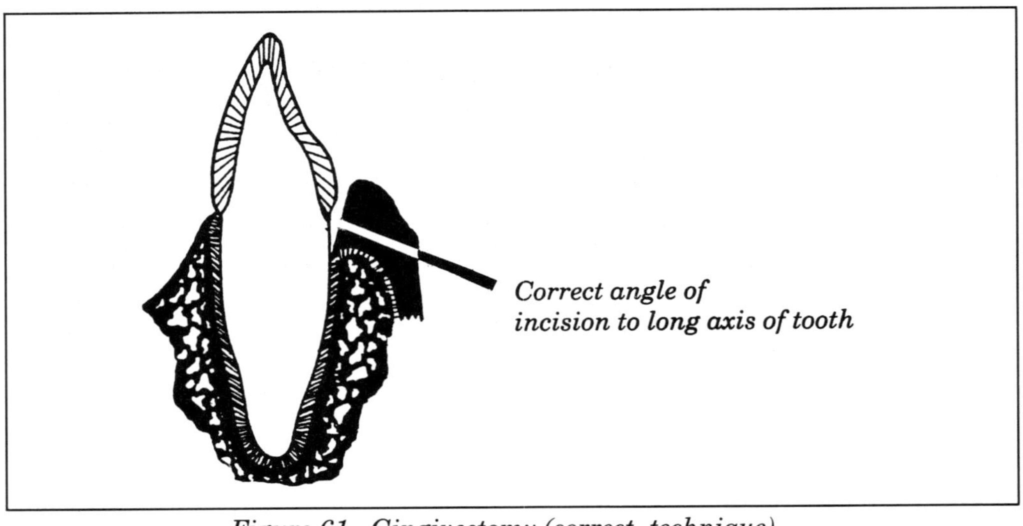

Figure 61. Gingivectomy (correct technique).

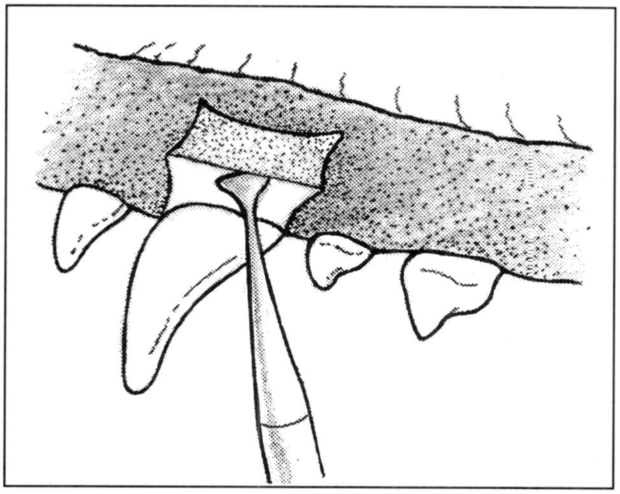

Figure 62. Open gingival flap with subgingival curettage.

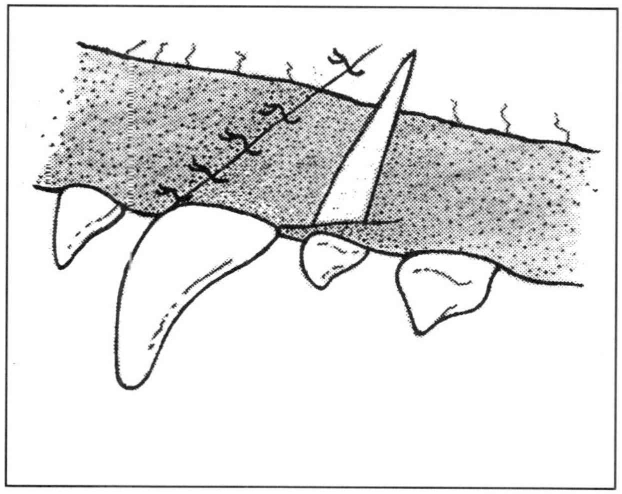

Figure 63. Lateral sliding flap.

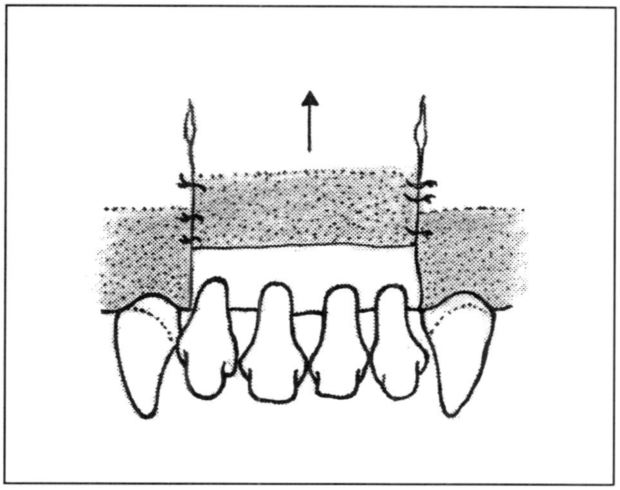

Figure 64. Apically repositioned flap.

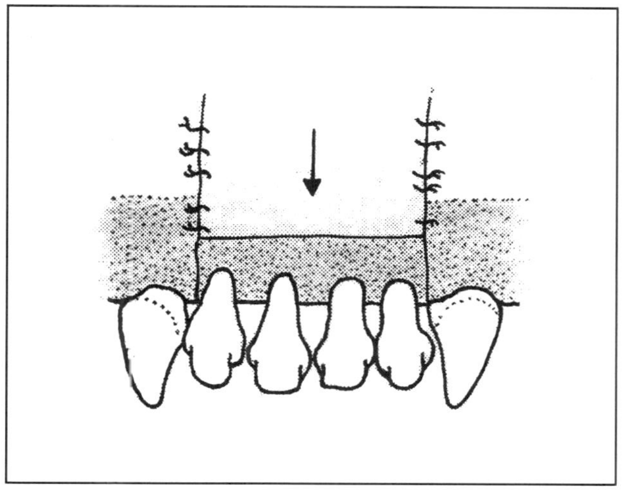

Figure 65. Coronally repositioned flap.

Although all of these procedures can be used in veterinary dentistry, the most commonly used procedure, apart from *gingival curettage*, is *gingivectomy*.

GINGIVECTOMY is the surgical removal of gingival tissue, usually with a scalpel, electrosurgery unit or fine scissors (Fig. 61). GINGIVOPLASTY is the surgical reshaping of the gingival tissue, usually with a scalpel or a bur. Gingivectomy is used to:

1. Remove excessively inflamed, infected and hyperplastic gingiva.
2. Remove EPULI and PAPILLOMAS.
3. Restore the physiologic functional gingival contour.
4. Improve oral hygiene by reducing or removing all pockets and pseudopockets. The remaining gingiva should be self–cleaning. This breaks the cycle of periodontitis and bone loss.

The GINGIVECTOMY procedure can be performed with an ELECTROSURGERY (ELECTROCAUTERY) unit, a sharp pointed scalpel or fine scissors. The incision should not be *too deep* as this will expose the alveolar bone, or *too shallow* as this will not be successful. In order to obtain an accurate incision line, the pocket depth can be marked on the gingiva with a felt–tipped pen. Several marks are made on the gingiva at the depth to be cut and then joined up, indicating the incision line.

The reduction of periodontal pockets and as much inflamed tissue as possible are of paramount importance. The goal of gingivectomy is to leave a hygienic, self–cleaning gingival margin. The cosmetics of the result are of secondary interest. However, a surgical reduction of the pathological pockets alone is not enough. The most important aspect of periodontal treatment is the creation of a clean, bacteria–free root surface to permit some reattachment of the periodontium. This is achieved by careful curettage, root planing, polishing, rinsing and disinfection.

Any residual concretion and debris are flushed out of the gingival sulcus with water or with CHLORHEXIDINE solution, which also serves to reduce the bacterial count. The effectiveness of a gingivectomy is significantly and solely dependent upon the care and attention with which the operation is performed. Incomplete gingivectomy results in only a short term reduction of the inflammation. Manual curettage can be tiring and time consuming, sometimes requiring one to two hours for the entire procedure, especially if loose teeth have to be extracted, sectioned or splinted. This is difficult work, and the time required and fees charged should not be underestimated.

The removal of resistant hard calculus and concretion can be greatly simplified by the use of a ROTO–PRO BUR. This instrument rapidly removes these deposits and at the same time provides some smoothing effect on the tooth and root surface. Unlike ultrasonic scalers, Roto–Pro burs can be used subgingivally, but must be used carefully as they can damage the softer cementum and dentin (see scalers, 3.8).

In severe cases of gingivitis and periodontal disease, antibiotic therapy is recommended three to five days before scaling and curettage, and five to ten days postoperatively, because of the likelihood of BACTERIAL "SEEDING" or the release of bacteria into the bloodstream via the gingival tissues. Broad spectrum ANTIBIOTICS that have proven successful against aerobes and anaerobes in these cases are TETRACYCLINE (except under six months of age or pregnant), AMOXICILLIN potentiated with CLAVULANIC ACID, CLINDAMYCIN HCl (especially good if there is concurrent osteomyelitis), ENROFLOXACIN and, against anaerobes and flagellates, METRONIDAZOLE.

The dog should be kept on a soft food diet for one to two weeks following the operation to prevent irritation of the healing tissues. Gingival packing compounds (GINGIVAL SPLINTS), as used in human dentistry, are not usually recommended as they can be licked or rubbed off and swallowed. As a follow up to periodontal treatment it is wise to have the owner rinse the mouth daily with ANTISEPTIC ORAL MOUTHWASHES such as CHLORHEXIDINE (although the taste may be bitter) or apply ANTISEPTIC GELS to the gingivae (e.g., CET CHX 0.12% Chlorhexidine Gel for animals). Daily home dental care with an animal toothbrush and toothpaste will greatly help to reduce recurrence of the problem.

4.14 PROPHYLAXIS

Periodontal disease patients require prolonged treatment, during which a carefully controlled recall program must be used to ensure the success of the treatment.

The prevention of plaque and calculus accumulation is the most important factor in the control of periodontal disease. Prevention does not mean a professional prophylaxis, but daily home dental care for the pet by the owner.

4.15 PROPHYLAXIS PROCEDURE (SCALING, ROOT PLANING, AND CURETTAGE)

Thorough removal of plaque and calculus from tooth surfaces should be performed regularly, depending on amount of plaque and calculus accumulation and the degree of gingival involvement. In small breeds and older pets, this may be every six months or less. Most pets will require a dental prophylaxis every one to two years. General anesthesia is necessary in order to effectively clean the teeth subgingivally (see anesthesia, 3.22). Depending on the severity of the plaque and calculus accumulation, and the degree of periodontal disease, the cleaning procedure may involve SCALING, ROOT PLANING and CURETTAGE. *Root planing (subgingival scaling) is the most important part of prophylaxis.*

4.16 SCALING OF THE CROWN

Scaling is the procedure by which plaque, calculus and other deposits are removed from the *crown* surface. Most scaling is performed *supragingivally* using either mechanical or hand scalers. If hand scalers are used *subgingivally,* great care should be exercised to minimize damage to the more delicate cementum, dentin and gingival tissue (see scaling of the root, 4.18). Large calculus deposits should be cracked off using extraction forceps or tartar removal forceps (Figs. 30–36). This is more rapid and less damaging to the delicate hand–scaling instruments. There are several different types of instruments that can be used to scale the teeth (see scalers, 3.8), and the choice is based on personal preference. All instruments should be used with care, to avoid scratching and damaging the enamel. Some teeth have CREVICES or FISSURES where calculus can be difficult to remove. The tip of an explorer can greatly assist in cleaning these areas. The WORKING ANGLE of a HAND SCALER should be about 85 degrees.

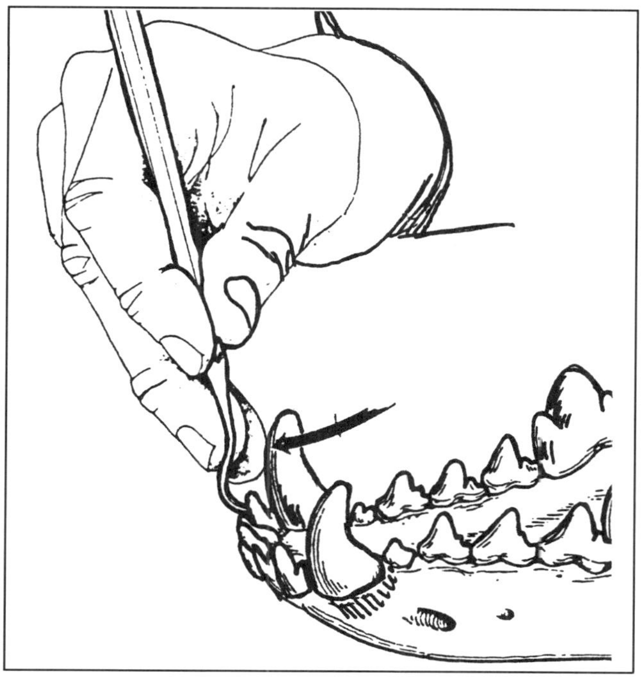

Figure 66. Correct instrument grip and finger support on adjacent tooth (arrow).

4.17 SCALING OF THE ROOT (ROOT PLANING) (SUBGINGIVAL SCALING)

Root planing (subgingival scaling) is the procedure by which subgingival calculus (concretion) and parts of the diseased cementum or dentin are removed from the *root surface*, to produce a clean, smooth surface. The root of the tooth should be scaled or curetted to the full depth of the periodontal pocket. Care should be taken not to damage the epithelial attachment at the apex of the pocket. Root planing should be performed with curettes (see curettes, 3.9), although rotosonic and sonic scalers can be used. The WORKING ANGLE of a HAND CURETTE should be between 45–85 degrees. The aim of root planing is to leave a smooth root surface. In some cases fine polishing diamonds in a high–speed handpiece can be used to produce a smooth surface.

4.18 GINGIVAL CURETTAGE (SUBGINGIVAL CURETTAGE)

Gingival curettage is the procedure of debriding or curetting the free gingiva on the inside of the periodontal pocket, in order to remove inflamed and necrotic tissue, including any involved junctional epithelium. The goal of this procedure, apart from the removal of diseased gingival tissue, is to allow some reattachment of the gingiva to the freshly cleaned root surface. Gingival curettage should always be performed in conjunction with root planing. The cutting edge of the curette (Gracey) should be turned outwards, towards the gingival tissue (see scalers, 3.8 and curettes, 3.9). Deep bleeding pockets should be reduced with electrosurgery, fine scissors or a scalpel.

4.19 POLISHING

Although this is the final procedure in a dental prophylaxis, it is very important. Any time that instruments are applied to a tooth or a root surface, whether mechanical or manual, they will cause micro–scratching of the surface. These microscopic grooves or scratches will increase the surface area of the tooth and create a surface that has a greater potential to reaccumulate plaque and calculus than a smooth surface.

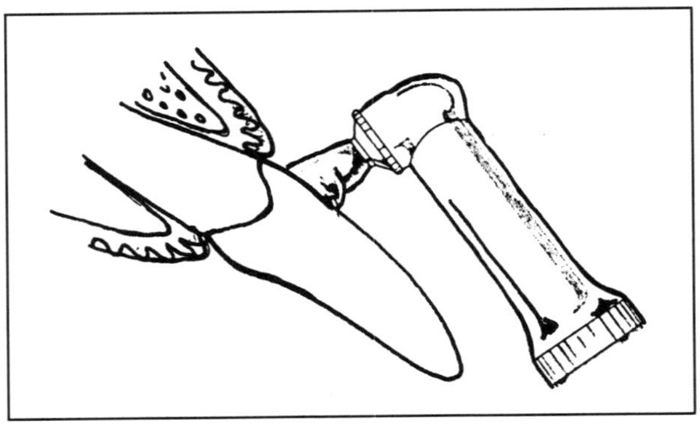

Figure 67. Polishing tooth with prophy cup and pumice.

Each tooth surface should be polished, BUCCAL (towards the cheeks) and LINGUAL (towards the tongue) as well as SUPRAGINGIVAL (above the gumline) and SUBGINGIVAL (below the gumline). Generally a medium grit prophypaste is sufficient for veterinary use. The pumice slurry left after polishing should be thoroughly rinsed from the mouth, making sure that none is left under the gumline or in the oropharynx ("down the throat"). In order to determine the effectiveness of the prophy, check after finishing by swabbing the teeth with a PLAQUE DISCLOSING SOLUTION (e.g., sodium fluorescein).

Polishing with a low–speed handpiece, contra angle and prophy cup is naturally the most efficient method. An OSCILLATING PROPHY CONTRA ANGLE ATTACHMENT (e.g., Medidenta's PROPHYMATIC) is especially useful as it prevents hair from getting caught in the spinning prophy cup shaft. If air power is not available use some type of electric driven polisher.

There are many brands and flavors of human prophypaste to choose from. There is a prophypaste developed for dogs and cats that is malt flavored and highly palatable (e.g., CET animal prophypaste).

The use of FLUORIDE pastes and pumices is somewhat controversial, however fluoride helps to strengthen the enamel in situations where it may be deemed beneficial.

4.20 HOME DENTAL CARE PROCEDURE

Foods that encourage plaque accumulation should be avoided. This includes snacks between meals, high carbohydrate foods such as left–overs and sweets. Tongue movement, during and after eating, and while panting, can help to keep the teeth clean. This means that dogs who pant a lot because they are active, have a better chance of having clean teeth than the sedentary dog. Open mouth breathing dogs (e.g., Pugs, Pomeranians) tend to have a dry oral cavity, leading to increased plaque accumulation. Although chewing dry food and rawhide chew sticks can be helpful for some surface cleaning of the teeth, there is no substitute for regular toothbrushing. BRUSHING PETS TEETH is gaining more and more acceptance by pet owners and with practice it is highly effective. For this purpose there are several ANIMAL TOOTHPASTES available. Some are based on ground bone meal, while others are bactericidal through their enzymatic action (e.g., CET animal toothpaste). They are also designed to be harmless if swallowed. Human toothpastes should not be used in pets, since if swallowed their detergent action may cause gastritis. The "tingling" sensation and taste of some human toothpastes may not be appealing to pets. The use of baking soda should also be discouraged due to the high sodium content. There is also a special double–ended ANIMAL TOOTHBRUSH (e.g., CET animal toothbrush) with brushing heads designed to fit the animal's mouth, and soft bristles for their sensitive gums. When a dog or a cat is trained to accept the toothbrush as a puppy or a kitten (start as early as six to eight weeks if possible to establish the pattern), then toothbrushing does not present much of a problem. The use of rewards, such as treats and food, will greatly assist in compliance. The dog considers it a new game and usually plays along willingly. The head of the animal is lightly held with one hand, while the other hand is used to clean with the toothbrush and paste. As an initial method to get the pet to accept toothbrushing, a gauze pad impregnated with toothpaste can be wrapped around the forefinger, and rubbed back and forth on the teeth. For optimal results, toothbrushing should be done daily.

4.21 DIAGNOSIS AND TREATMENT OF LYMPHOPLASMACYTIC GINGIVITIS – STOMATITIS COMPLEX (LPGS) IN CATS

DIAGNOSIS OF LPGS

Often by the time these cases are diagnosed, the gingiva surrounding the teeth has become chronically inflamed. Often there is a generalized, severe and usually hyperplastic gingivitis, with periodontal pockets that bleed readily when probed (Photo 25). The mandible will sometimes "chatter" when the tissues or lesions are probed, even under general anesthesia, due to the nervous tissue sensitivity. The fact that the gingiva around the incisors and canine teeth is also often inflamed, is a clue to diagnosing this condition.

There is usually a concurrent stomatitis, especially in the caudal part of the mouth, the pharyngeal area, the PALATINE FAUCES (area between palate and pharynx) and the buccal mucosa caudal to the last teeth. Taking dental radiographs of the maxilla and mandible is very important in determining the extent of the destruction of the periodontium. The degree of horizontal alveolar bone loss may be moderate to severe, and is an excellent guide in giving a prognosis. If the horizontal bone loss exposes one third or more of the roots, this should be indication enough to help you in your decision to suggest extraction of these teeth. Horizontal bone loss will never get better, and will usually be progressive.

Although many cats with this condition seem to tolerate the chronic pain and eat normally, they will usually be sensitive when the mouth is touched. They will often resist being petted (sometimes even biting the owner), and become withdrawn and hide. As the condition worsens, the cat will have more difficulty eating, lose weight and become less friendly.

In order to differentiate this condition from a moderate to severe gingivitis or periodontal disease, a simple guide is to perform a thorough prophylaxis and start antibiotic and antiinflammatory therapy. If possible, instruct the owner on how to gently swab the mouth with an antiseptic solution. After two to three weeks stop the antibiotics and phase out the antiinflammatory therapy, and see if the condition returns. Generally with the LPGS complex, the gingivitis and stomatitis will return rapidly or never completely resolve.

Biopsies and cultures are necessary to differentiate these lesions from other conditions such as eosinophilic granuloma complex. However, in classic LPGS cases, biopsies and cultures are often not necessary, since the cells and bacteria found in LPGS are similar to those in gingivitis and periodontitis. Although antibiotic and cortisone therapy will often improve the condition as long as they are given, diagnosis can be made by recurrence of the inflammation soon after therapy is discontinued.

Treatment of LPGS

To date there is no curative treatment for this condition, although tooth extraction in the worst areas contributes the best chance of alleviating the symptoms in the severe, chronic cases.

Initially a *thorough* prophylaxis must be performed. It is extremely important to do this thoroughly, treating each tooth as a separate unit, carrying out scaling, root planing and gingival curettage. The proper instruments and a sensitive touch are necessary to do this effectively. An air–driven Roto–Pro scaler is very useful to help perform this task. Once the teeth are all cleaned and polished, being sure to flush away any debris and prophy paste with copious amounts of water, the cat is sent home with a two– or three–week course of antibiotics and cortisone. Broad spectrum antibiotics such as TETRACYCLINE, AMOXICILLIN WITH CLAVULANIC ACID, CLINDAMYCIN HCl (especially where there is evidence of horizontal bone loss) and ENROFLOXACIN will help control most of the pathogenic bacteria. Short–acting STEROIDS such as PREDNISOLONE, or long–acting steroids such as TRIAMCINOLONE, along with antibiotic therapy, or later steroids alone, will help to reduce the inflammation for some time in mild to moderate cases. METRONIDAZOLE (e.g., Flagyl) therapy has also proven beneficial against anaerobes and flagellates. MEGESTROL ACETATE, although not officially approved for cat use, may help in some cases. However, it should be stressed to the owner that these medications will not cure the problem if it is a true LPGS case. Medications may cause undesirable side effects and this condition will eventually recur when drug therapy is discontinued.

It is important to bear in mind that most pet owners are not very good at administering medications orally, especially to a cat with a sore mouth. Do not just give a bottle of pills and say "here, give these to your cat." For treating this condition it may be easier for the cat owner to give a liquid preparation with an eye dropper. Show them how to administer the medication and suggest wrapping the cat in a large towel for easier restraint. For drugs such as tetracycline and clindamycin HCl, which have a bitter taste, suggest adding a few drops of clam juice to the medication. Tablets can be crushed and dissolved in water and administered with an eye dropper or a used 3 cc syringe.

Any teeth that are severely damaged, broken or have only root remnants left should be either carefully extracted or atomized (see atomization, 5.4). The gingiva around the extracted tooth or root remnant should be retracted with a fine periosteal elevator and any irregularities of the alveolar socket and margins, shaped and smoothed with a small round bur (ALVEOLOPLASTY). Dental radiography of the area should be performed at this time in order to evaluate the extent of supporting bone loss and to confirm extraction of all root remnants.

If the condition continues, with all the typical symptoms, and there is no relief of pain, swelling and bleeding, then more frequent prophylaxis under anesthesia (every three to six months) should be suggested, plus periodic medication therapy, and daily swabbing with an antiseptic mouth wash (e.g., CET Oral Hygiene Spray). If this does not help and the case is severe or is getting worse, and the cat is debilitated and having difficulty eating, a full–mouth tooth extraction is the only long–term solution to this painful condition. Although most clients are reluctant to consider this initially, the benefits of a pain–free mouth, a fatter cat and a happier personality should be stressed. Explain to the client that to date there is no other method that has such a good chance of success. Elimination of the chronic gingivitis and pain is successful in about 70–80 percent of these cases. Cats without any teeth manage to eat soft food normally, even "gumming" hard food sometimes.

It is important when performing a full–mouth extraction to be sure that all the roots are completely extracted, atomizing root tip remnants if necessary, and using dental radiographs to confirm root removal. A small root remnant will often result in persistence of the gingival inflammation in that area. Careful *alveoloplasty* should be performed as well as remodeling of any rough or infected alveolar crest bone between the sockets (OSTEOPLASTY) (Photo 27). Do not hesitate to reflect a gingival flap along the entire length of the gingival tissue in the extraction site if necessary. This *thorough alveoloplasty* and *osteoplasty* followed by careful suturing of the gums (if possible) can be the key to success. If, after all this, healing is not complete in some areas, it is often necessary to go back and perform further alveoloplasty and osteoplasty. It is thought that any remaining chronically infected bone or sharp edges of bone may be causing the gingival tissue on the surface not to heal properly. These can be difficult cases to treat successfully, thus if you do not have the equipment or the expertise, do not hesitate to refer them to a more experienced veterinary dentist.

Recent treatment studies (*LYON* and *SHIPP*) with a SOFT TISSUE LASER (Gallium–Arsenide), which creates an apparent bio–stimulating healing effect (Photo 26), have shown some promise, but more research is needed. New non–steroidal anti–inflammatory drugs are also being tested and may show promise in aiding in the control of symptoms. However, until researchers can find the cause of this complex problem, relief can only be aimed at treating the symptoms and not the cause.

CHAPTER 5

EXODONTICS (EXTRACTION OF TEETH)

5.1 EXTRACTION

EXTRACTION of teeth is indicated with:

1. Retained deciduous teeth.
2. Extensive caries.
3. Advanced mobility from periodontal disease or from trauma.
4. Fractured teeth that cannot be restored or be saved.
5. Feline teeth with irreparable "neck" lesions.
6. Teeth in a bony fracture site.
7. Impacted teeth.
8. Supernumerary teeth.
9. Malpositioned teeth that interfere with the occlusion.
10. Infected and fractured teeth, where treatment is not possible.

Since many clients do not understand why teeth have to be extracted, and can get very upset and want to blame you, it is wise for medico–legal purposes to always have the owner's permission in writing at the time of admission, that "extractions will be at the discretion of the veterinarian."

Many teeth, especially those with periodontal disease, can be removed with an elevator alone. The sharp end of the elevator is initially used with a circular motion around the tooth to cut the periodontal ligament and to loosen the tooth. The elevator is then pushed as deeply as possible into the space between the tooth to be extracted and its neighbor, and the tooth is levered out. *Ideally*, to avoid fracture, a tooth should never be "pulled," it should be "pushed." If the elevator is worked carefully around the root and the periodontal ligaments are severed, pushing into the socket with the elevator should push the tooth out. In practice this will only be possible with some teeth. If this is not successful, a scalpel or a dental elevator should be used to sever the gingiva around the teeth, freeing the tissue at the epithelial attachment. The elevator can then be used with a rotational motion, under the cingulum of the tooth to be extracted, and above the cingulum of the neighboring tooth, to lever the tooth out (Fig. 68) (Photo 8). Multi–rooted teeth must be levered out from mesial (rostral) and distal (caudal) surfaces alternately. Widely separated teeth can be extracted with this method if the elevator is set at an angle and supported with the other hand. The straight elevator is the single most useful extraction instrument, and its use should be thoroughly practiced.

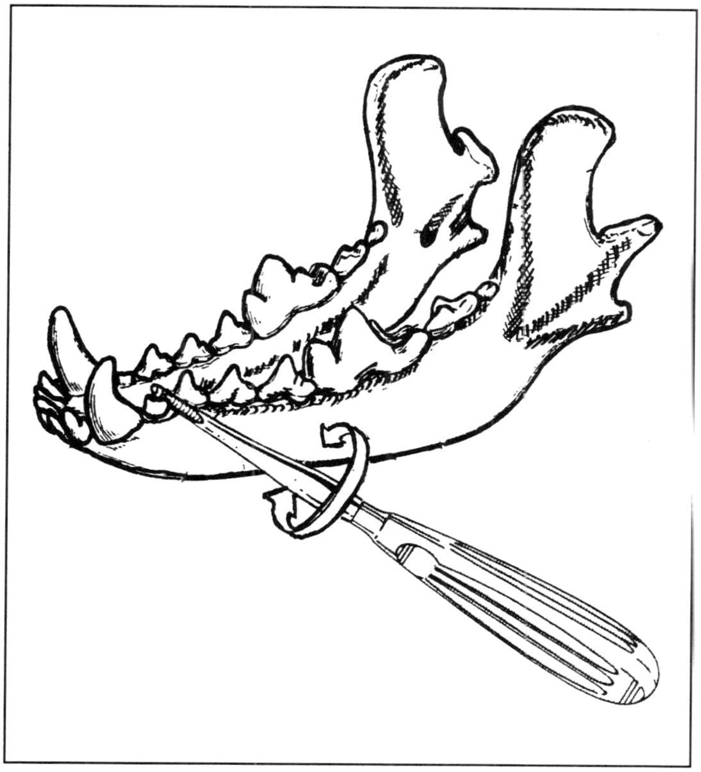

Figure 68. Extraction technique with elevator.

(Place tip of elevator under the cingulum and rotate carefully, counterbalancing the elevator on the adjacent tooth.)

The use of extraction forceps demands considerable expertise if the tooth is to be removed intact. The appropriate forceps should be selected for the position and size of the tooth. The beaks of the forceps should be curved to fit exactly with the curvature of the tooth to be extracted, otherwise the tooth may splinter or break when force is applied. The tooth should be grasped as far down on the root as possible. Prior to using extraction forceps to remove a tooth, an elevator should be used to separate the periodontal ligament as much as possible, causing a SUBLUXATION of the root. This greatly reduces the chance of breaking off the crown. The root should be as loose as possible, before attempting final luxation and extraction with the extraction forceps.

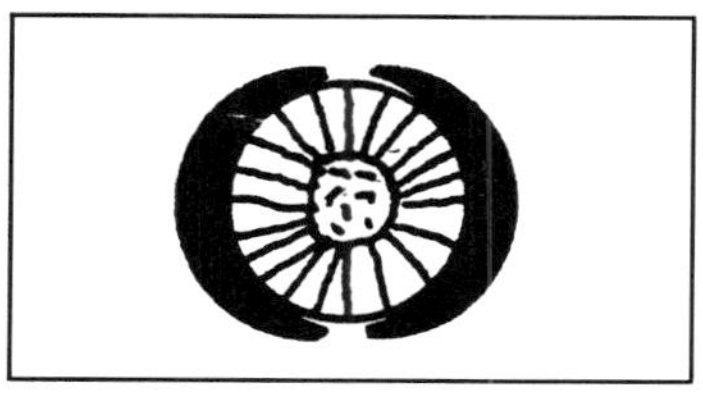

Figure 69. Correct fit of forceps. Flat contact with the tooth surface.

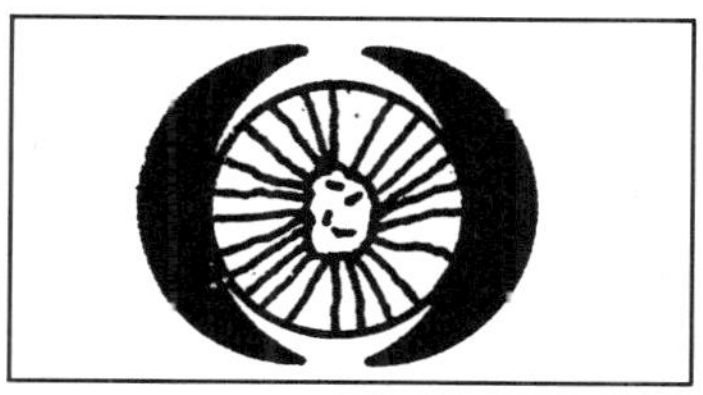

Figure 70. Incorrect fit of forceps. Contact in center. Danger of fracture.

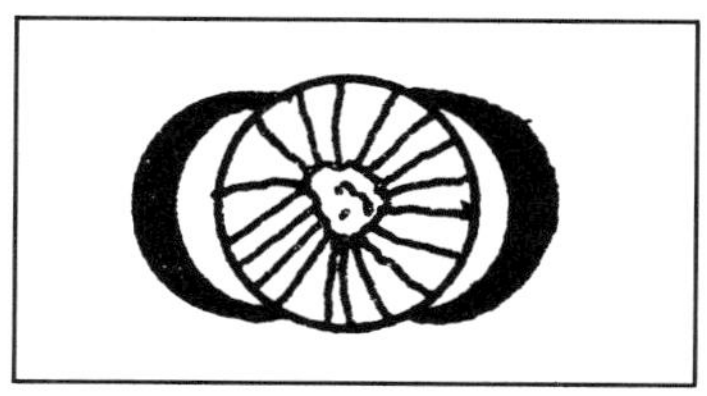

Figure 71. Incorrect fit of forceps. Contact at edge. Danger of fracture.

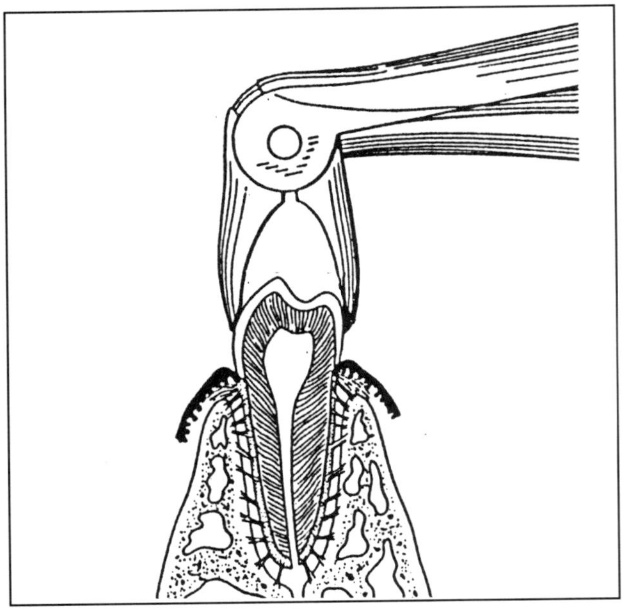

Figure 72. Incorrect grasp of forceps on the crown of the tooth.

Danger of fracture.

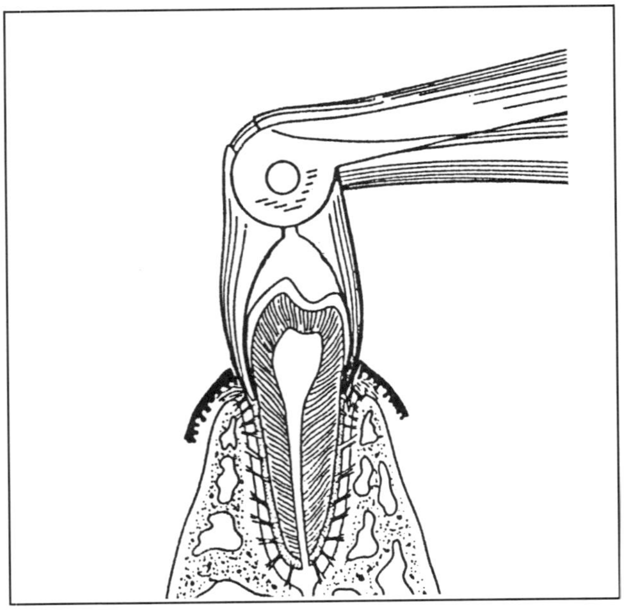

Figure 73.Correct grasp of forceps on the crown of the tooth.

(Grasp is deep into the socket.)

The thumb and finger of the hand should be used to support the alveolar bone buccal and lingual to the tooth to be extracted, and the rest of the hand used to support the jaw. The tooth is then firmly gripped with the extraction forceps and slowly moved lingually and buccally, further subluxating the tooth. SINGLE–ROOTED TEETH, or a separated tooth root, can be gently rotated and carefully removed. Incisor teeth should be loosened only by subluxation, since the curved root tends to fracture easily. DOUBLE–ROOTED TEETH can sometimes be removed intact, although cutting them in half (hemisection) through the bifurcation is preferable. Each half is then removed as a single–rooted tooth.

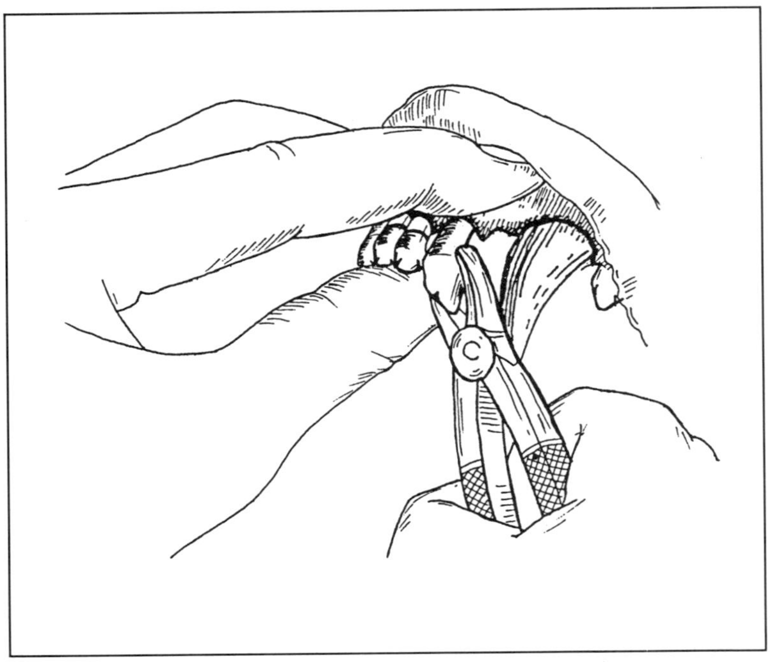

Figure 74. Correct use of extraction forceps.

(The jaw should be steadied close to the tooth being extracted.)

TRIPLE–ROOTED TEETH are easily *sectioned* into three pieces through the furcation (Photo 7), and the roots subluxated and removed separately. The *canine teeth* of dogs and cats (including *retained deciduous canines*) are more difficult to remove, unless they are already seriously periodontally damaged or are mobile. Their removal is best achieved with a gingival flap and osteotomy (see gingival flap and osteotomy, 10.11) (Photo 2). The most difficult teeth to remove are often the premolars and molars of cats. Unless the roots are already loose due to infection or trauma, these teeth will usually fracture if conventional extraction techniques are used. It is almost impossible to pass elevators into the alveolus of feline premolar and molar teeth to sever the periodontal ligament. In order to get a purchase point to begin subluxation, a fine tapered bur in a high–speed handpiece should be used to cut some of the crown and root material around the gingival margin (Photo 9). Once access has been made into the alveolus, fine elevators can be introduced to begin loosening the tooth. Should the crown break off, the fine tapered bur can be used to create a new access deeper into the alveolus. If the remaining part of the root becomes difficult to remove with elevators or fine extraction forceps, such as Stieglitz extraction forceps (Photo 10), the fractured root can be atomized (see atomization, 5.4). When the tooth has been successfully extracted, any bone splinters are removed, and the alveolus curetted with a sharp spoon excavator or a high–speed bur, to remove any debris and help to encourage blood flow. This blood will produce a clot that will later aid in the production of new bone.

5.2 ROOT AMPUTATION, TOOTH SECTION AND HEMISECTION

Sometimes multirooted teeth, usually the *larger* premolars and molars, have only partial damage from periodontal disease, caries, "neck" lesions and trauma. If possible, the good part of the tooth can be saved and the damaged part can be removed. Double–rooted teeth can be HEMISECTIONED salvaging the crown and root of one half. The *mesio–palatal* root of the triple–rooted maxillary fourth premolar is small and can be SECTIONED if it is damaged, leaving the other two roots and their crowns. Sometimes the *mesio–palatal* and *mesio–buccal* roots of this tooth are periodontally involved, but the *disto–buccal* root and its crown can be saved. The two mesial roots and their related crowns can be SECTIONED and removed, leaving only the distal crown and root.

In order to perform these procedures, a high–speed handpiece and a bur, such as a crosscut tapered fissure, are necessary. Copious amounts of water must be used when sectioning vital teeth to prevent thermal damage. Sectioning of a tooth should be made in line with the furcation. The FURCATION is the anatomical area of a multirooted tooth where the roots divide. It is known as a BIFURCATION in a double–rooted tooth, and a TRIFURCATION in a triple–rooted tooth. When sectioning a vital tooth, any remaining sharp edges should be trimmed with a diamond bur. The exposed pulp of vital teeth must always be sealed (see vital pulpotomy, 7.12) or be removed (see instrumentation, 7.13). When the damage to the tooth is PERIAPICAL (around the tip of the root), apical root AMPUTATION of non–vital endodontically treated teeth can also be performed (see apicoectomy, 10.12).

Although all teeth have their relative importance, the shearing carnassials and the grinding molars are the most important teeth for cutting and grinding food. Efforts should be implemented to salvage the entire tooth or the main functioning parts of these teeth if possible.

5.3 REMOVAL OF ROOT REMNANTS

If a tooth fractures below the alveolar crest margin during extraction, it is almost impossible to get a good grasp on the remaining piece of root with extraction forceps. In many cases the remaining piece can be removed with a sharp elevator. The technique involves using the sharp end of the elevator to separate the periodontal fibers, and luxate the root fragment enough to be able to lever it out of the socket. It is wise to have many different sizes and shapes of elevators and root–tip picks on hand, to cover all eventualities (see extraction instruments, 3.14). A fine tapered bur can be used to cut the periodontal fibers (and sometimes part of the root and alveolar bone), creating a purchase point and allowing the elevator to be set deeper into the socket.

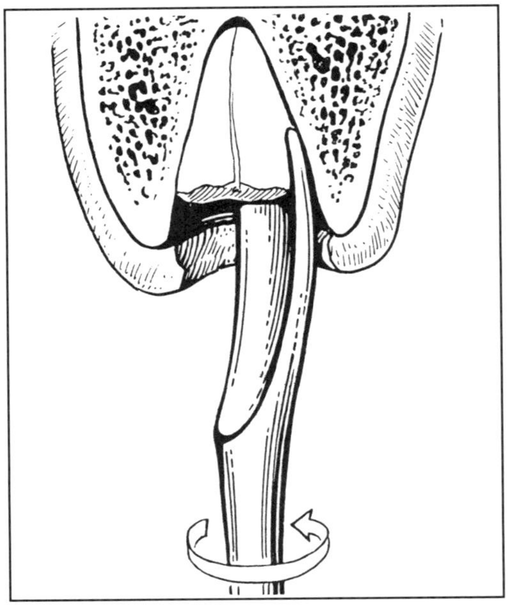

Figure 75. Careful rotation of the elevator to loosen the root tip. Drilling of alveolar bone may be necessary to gain access to the socket.

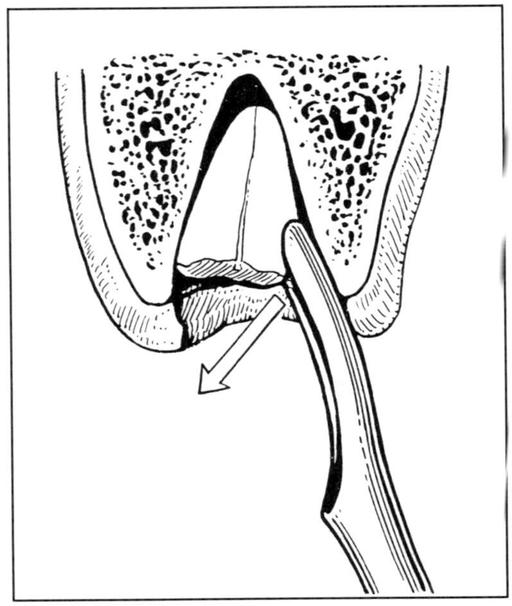

Figure 76. The loose root tip can now be levered out.

5.4 ATOMIZATION

"Atomization" is the destruction or the removal of remaining ROOT FRAGMENTS by drilling. These root fragments, left when the root breaks as it is being removed, are often unavoidable when extracting small teeth, especially in cats. These fragments can be impossible to remove with fine root–tip elevators. As a last resort they can be "drilled out" (atomized) with a small round bur in a high–speed handpiece. Some of the lamina dura of the alveolar bone may be removed at the same time, but this usually does not cause a problem, providing that the surrounding bone is solid and sufficient. However, since violation of the lamina dura exposes cancellous alveolar bone, a short course of antibiotics should be prescribed post operatively to prevent infection of the bone. Care must be exercised not to perforate the nasal sinus or the mandibular canal, or to cause thermal necrosis of bony structures.

Atomization is a skilled procedure and requires a lot of practice to be accurate. Since it is often difficult to tell visually that all the root has been removed, a dental radiograph should be taken to confirm complete removal. However, as you are drilling, you can often see a difference in color between the root tip and the surrounding bone (tooth material is whiter) and feel the difference when drilling tooth versus bone (tooth feels harder).

There comes a time when you can do more damage by trying to remove every last piece of root, than by leaving it in place. In these cases, it is safer to leave a small fragment. However, all attempts to remove root fragments should be made, within reason. Leaving a root fragment is analogous to shooting a person with an arrow, then breaking off the shaft and leaving the tip.

After the extraction of a permanent tooth some owners may require documentation as to the cause of the tooth loss, since the selection of animals to be used for breeding and show may be dependent upon a complete dentition. It is wise to check before extracting teeth, to determine whether the animal is intended for breeding and show purposes. If this is the case, a dental radiograph of the tooth in the socket before extraction or the empty socket after extraction should be kept as proof of the original existence of the tooth. As mentioned before, consent to perform the extraction of any damaged teeth should always be put in writing on the admitting form and signed by the owner. This should be done before dental procedures are started, in order to prevent client misunderstanding and possible medico–legal complications. If problems with the teeth are only found after the animal has been anesthetized, and you have not discussed what you recommend for treatment, call the owners in order to get their consent, and quote them an approximate fee.

5.5 CROWN REDUCTION

Surgical crown reduction is a procedure that involves partial removal of the tooth crown.

"Crown reduction" covers *odontoplasty* (see odontoplasty, 9.34), *crown preparation* for a cast metal crown (see crowns, 8.4) and *crown height reduction* for disarming the canine teeth (see crown reduction, 7.15).

The procedure for disarming involves removing part of a tooth (Exodontics), performing a vital pulpotomy (Endodontics) and restoring the crown (Restoration).

For the purposes of this text the subject of crown reduction is well described under Endodontics, Chapter 7 (see crown reduction, 7.15).

CHAPTER 6

RESTORATION OF DAMAGED TEETH

Restoration is the repairing of teeth to their original shape following damage by trauma, "neck" lesions, enamel hypoplasia, caries and other causes. *Conservative* repairs are made with amalgam, composite and glass ionomer, whereas more *complicated* repairs are made with prosthetic devices such as cast crowns, bridges and sometimes veneers (see Prosthodontics, Chapter 8).

6.1 CAVITY PREPARATION

When preparing CAVITIES, ENAMEL LESIONS and ENAMEL DEFECTS, the following principles should be remembered:

1. All the carious or the damaged tooth structure should be removed, without weakening the rest of the tooth.
2. Any unsupported dentin and enamel should be removed.
3. The preparation ideally should leave the enamel rods at 90 degrees to the tooth surface.
4. As much tooth structure as possible should be preserved.
5. The shape of the preparation should be designed with the type of restorative material in mind.

Cavity preparation is dependent on the type of restorative material that will be used. There are only three basic types of materials that are used for conservative restorations. These are *amalgam, composite* and *glass ionomer*, although there are many variations.

A cavity that is to be restored with *amalgam* requires a dentinal UNDERCUT all the way around the base of the cavity, in order to provide the mechanical retention necessary to keep it in place. This is not necessary if an amalgam bonding agent, such as Amalgambond (Parkell), is used under the amalgam. The undercut should only be in the dentin, and not in the enamel. No enamel should be left unsupported by dentin. The walls of the preparation should create a 90–degree angle at the surface of the tooth (Photo 28).

A cavity that is to be restored with *composite* does not always require dentinal undercuts as described with amalgam. After acid–etching there is usually adequate retention provided by the microscopic mechanical interlocking of the composite resin in the enamel (and dentin, depending on acid–etch technique) (see acid–etch technique, 6.6). Adhesion to the dentin may also be achieved by dentinal adhesives. Since undercutting prior to a composite restoration is currently controversial, dentinal undercuts are acceptable when using composite restorations, depending on the situation. Any unnecessary undermining of the enamel should be avoided if possible, since it only weakens the structure of the tooth in that area. The walls of the preparation should create a 90-degree angle at the surface of the tooth.

It is often suggested that the external margin of the enamel should be bevelled to increase the surface area of the enamel to be acid–etched, however this will also create a fine lip of composite that will be prone to wear and fracture. Although not related to cavity preparation, additional retention for some composite restorations can be achieved with the use of small parapulpal pins incorporated into the restoration (see pins, 12.14) (Photo 35).

A cavity that is to be restored with *glass ionomer* requires little or no cavity preparation, since it CHEMICALLY BONDS to both the dentin and enamel. Gentle use of a Roto–Pro bur is often useful in cleaning the lesion, any sharp edges, and the surrounding area. In some cases a dentin conditioner is beneficial for removing the smear layer when one has been created (see glass ionomers, 12.8).

6.2 CLASSIFICATION OF CAVITIES/DEFECTS

BLACK'S CLASSIFICATION of dental caries in the human is suitable for identifying cavities, lesions, defects and fractures of teeth in animals, although it does not meet all the criteria of animal teeth. The following six classes describe the location and type of lesions found in animal teeth:

Class I lesions are located on the *occlusal surfaces* of the premolars and molars, the *occlusal* two thirds of the *buccal surfaces* of the molars, the *lingual surfaces* of the maxillary incisors and occasionally the *lingual surfaces* of the maxillary molars. Although rarely seen in dogs and cats, cavities are sometimes found on the occlusal surfaces of the maxillary and mandibular molars in dogs (usually the first molar).

Class II lesions are located on the *proximal surfaces* of the premolars and molars. Although rarely seen in dogs and cats, cavities are sometimes found between the maxillary fourth premolar and the first molar, and between the mandibular first and second molars in dogs.

Class III lesions are located on the *proximal surfaces* of the incisors and canine teeth, which *do not* involve the *incisal angle*. These lesions are rarely seen in dogs and cats.

Class IV lesions (fractures) are located on the *proximal surfaces* of the incisors (and canine teeth), which *do* involve the *incisal angle*. These fractures commonly involve the incisor teeth of dogs. Since the canine teeth do not have a true incisal edge, this class does not really apply to canine teeth.

Class V lesions are located in the gingival third of the *labial, buccal* and *lingual surfaces* of the teeth. They are the second most common type of lesions seen in veterinary dentistry. Although they sometimes occur in dogs they are mostly found in cats as "neck" lesions.

Class VI lesions (fractures) are found on the *incisal edges, cusp tips* and *smooth surfaces* of the teeth. They are not a true Black classification. These are the most common types of lesions (fracture) seen in veterinary dentistry. In dogs they are seen as fractured tips of the canine teeth, fractured cusps of the premolars and molars, lateral (buccal) slab fractures of the maxillary fourth premolar (Photo 50), and occasionally the maxillary first molar and fractured *incisal edges* of the incisor teeth. In cats, these lesions (fractures) are seen as fractured tips of the canine teeth.

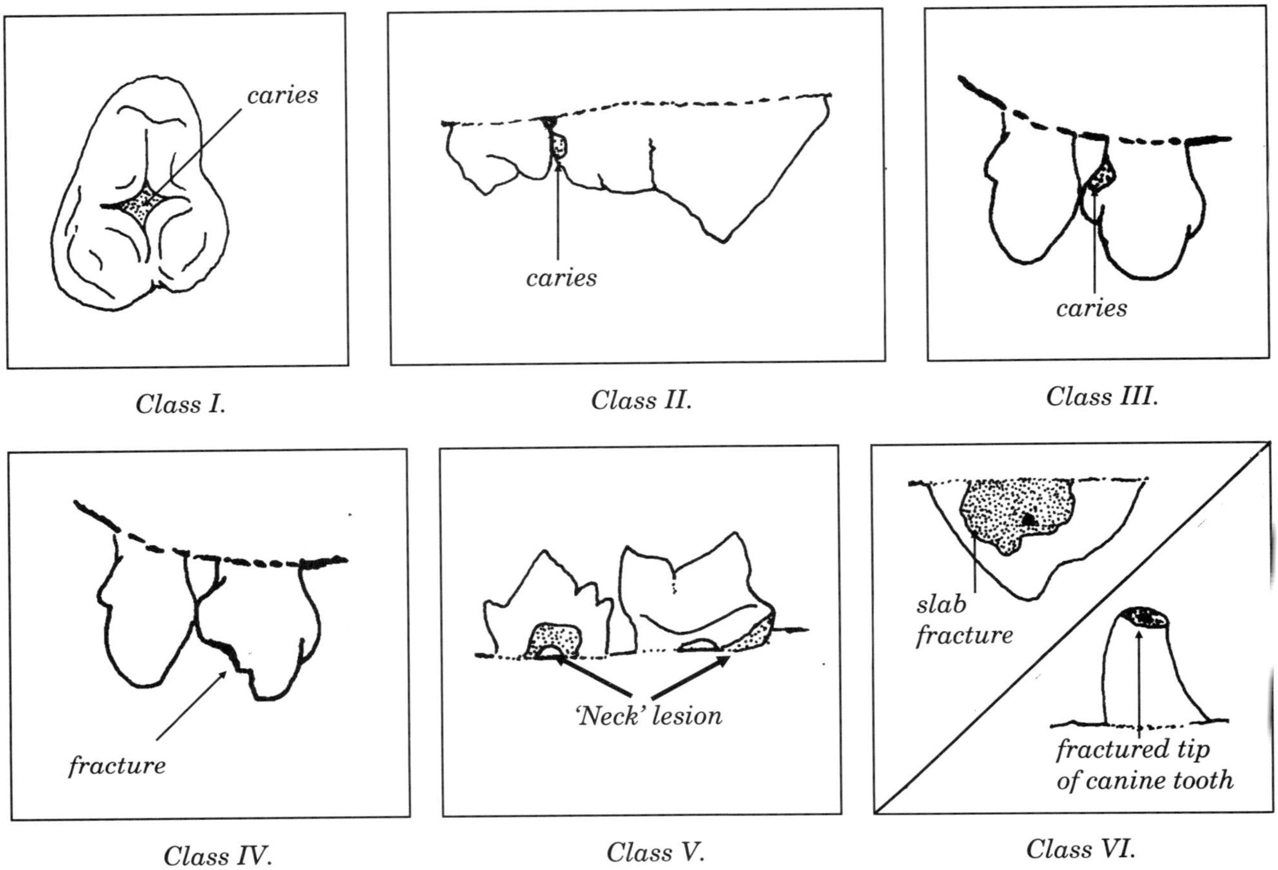

Figure 77. Classification of cavities and defects in animals.

6.3 CARIES (CAVITIES) — DOG

CARIES is defined as a bacterio–chemical degradation of the enamel and dentin, leading to its demineralization and destruction. A vital part of the etiology of caries is the existence of plaque. PLAQUE is a substance that forms on the surface of the tooth when mucin separates from the saliva and combines with food debris. It also sheds epithelial cells and, above all, bacteria. Organic acids, primarily lactic acid, are formed by bacterial action on the carbohydrate content of the plaque, which can lower the pH *under* the plaque to between 4.5 and 5.0. Once the *inorganic* part of the enamel (and cementum) has become demineralized, the organic part of the enamel (and cementum) is then destroyed by proteolytic enzymes. After the enamel is penetrated, caries spreads much faster through the less resistant dentin, undermining the surrounding enamel and leading to a cavity.

Dogs do not suffer from carious lesions to the same extent as humans, and true caries in the cat has not been confirmed by histological studies. In cats, lesions that look like Class V carious lesions are called "neck" lesions (see "neck" lesions – cat, 6.9). The reason that dogs do not often get caries is related to the shape of the teeth, the shorter life span of dogs compared to humans, and the high protein, low carbohydrate diet of dogs. Carnivorous teeth are generally conically shaped, widely spaced, have flat surfaces, have none or few of the pits and fissures of human teeth and as such are self–cleaning to a large extent. Also human teeth are required to give longer service, sometimes 80 years or more. Since the enamel of both humans and dogs is similar in hardness, the teeth of pets with a life expectancy of around 10–15 years survive better.

A research study showed that only about 6 percent of dogs' teeth were carious, and most of the lesions were so small that treatment was not indicated. The majority of the lesions were found in the central fossa of the maxillary molars, where the mandibular molars make occlusal contact. It is argued that the contact with the opposing tooth wears or splinters the enamel of the fossa, allowing the caries to penetrate the softer dentin beneath. Another theory states that there is a spot in the fossa of some maxillary molars where the embryologic development of enamel is incomplete or absent, thus allowing bacteria to invade and cause caries. Carious lesions can also be found in the central fossa of the mandibular molars (Photo 28).

The caries itself can be recognized as a brown or a black discoloration of the surface of the tooth, which is softer than the surrounding enamel and feels "sticky" when a dental explorer is inserted. Care should be taken to avoid confusion with the brown discoloration of TERTIARY (REPARATIVE) DENTIN following chronic ABRASION (ATTRITION) of the teeth (Photos 6, 34). This BROWN DISCOLORATION OF THE ABRADED TOOTH SURFACE comes from pigments in the diet that combine with saliva and flow into the microscopic tubules of the reparative dentin. There are more tubules in reparative dentin than there are in primary dentin. Reparative dentin is rapidly laid down as attrition occurs, trapping these pigments in the process. If the surface is hard and unbroken, it does not generally require treatment.

Some dogs wear down the enamel and dentin on the distal surfaces of the canine teeth. This condition is often referred to as CAGE–BITER SYNDROME or CHAIN LINK FENCE SYNDROME. The attrition produced weakens the tooth and should be repaired with a composite restoration and parapulpal pins (Photo 35), a full cast metal crown or a cast ceramic INLAY (e.g., In–ceram).

The composition of SALIVA is not conducive to cariogenic flora, because of its high urea content, and its alkaline pH (7.5) that neutralizes the bacterial acids. Caries presents itself typically as a small defect in the surface of the enamel. Once the enamel is penetrated, caries spreads much faster through the softer dentin, undermining the surrounding enamel. Even the smallest carious defect on the enamel surface can, therefore, conceal a large lesion under the enamel.

All UNSUPPORTED ENAMEL should be removed with a *high–speed* handpiece using a diamond or a tungsten carbide bur to gain access to the cavity. A large round bur in a *low–speed* handpiece, or a spoon excavator, should then be used to remove the softer dentin. CARIOUS DENTIN is softer than healthy dentin, has a light brown or a black color and tends to collect in the blades of the bur. Healthy dentin is hard, yellowish in color and comes out as dust. Additionally, healthy dentin cannot be removed with hand instruments such as spoon excavators. To make the cavity preparation retentive, the dentin walls should be parallel or slightly undercut, depending on the type of restorative material to be used (Photo 28).

6.4 LINERS AND BASES

A *liner* protects the pulp from irritation and reduces the sensitivity of freshly cut dentin. It is generally used in deep cavities when the pulp is less than 0.5 mm from the base of the cavity. A *base* is essentially a replacement for dentin that has been removed and is placed over the liner if the cavity is deep, or directly on top of the dentin when the pulp is greater than 0.5 mm from the base of the cavity. Bases help to protect the pulp and sensitive dentin from thermal, mechanical and chemical trauma.

The most commonly used liner is CALCIUM HYDROXIDE (CaOH) (although correctly this should be Ca(OH)). Calcium hydroxide stimulates the ODONTOBLASTS that begin or increase their production of peritubular dentin, producing a layer of REPARATIVE or TERTIARY DENTIN that further protects the pulp. There are many liners and bases on the market and some liners can be used as bases, or some bases can be used as liners (see cavity liners, varnishes and bases, 12.1).

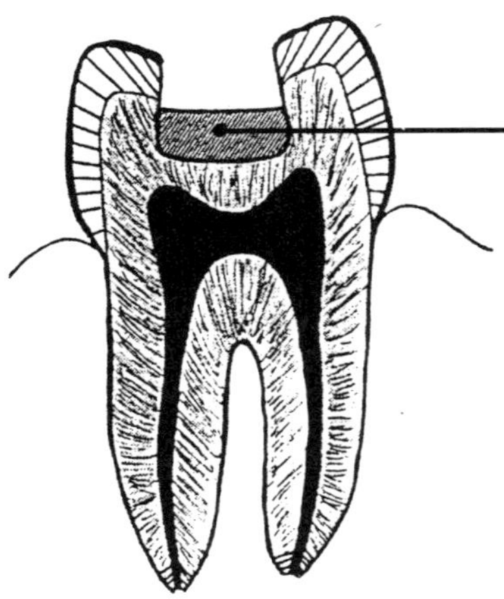

Figure 78. Cavity liner / base.

In very *shallow cavities*, liners and bases are not necessary. In *deeper cavities*, the complete depth of dentin should be replaced with a base material (see cavity cement bases, 12.4). This is not only to protect the dentin from thermal and chemical trauma, but also to protect the pulp contents from the mechanical trauma resulting from the pressure of placing the restorative material. In *very deep cavities* a liner of calcium hydroxide should be placed under the base.

Shallow fillings that are to be restored with amalgam, and fillings that have a base of zinc oxyphosphate cement can be additionally protected with a CAVITY VARNISH (see cavity varnishes, 12.3). These varnishes are copal/ether based. They protect the pulp from the acid content of the cement or the mercury in the amalgam by sealing the dentinal tubules. Do not get the varnish on the enamel edges of the cavity preparation if possible. Since this is often unavoidable, be sure to remove the varnish when it is dry. Varnish left on the ENAMEL EDGES will wash out later leaving a micro–space between the enamel and restorative material. This will lead to future problems and possible failure of the filling.

6.5 PULP CAPPING (INDIRECT AND DIRECT)

If the caries is so deep that the pulp chamber has been exposed, or if exposure is imminent, the pulp can be protected by PULP CAPPING.

INDIRECT PULP CAPPING

Indirect pulp capping is performed when the pulp chamber has not actually been exposed, but the cavity is so deep that the pulp must be protected. Often a PINK COLORED PULPAL BLUSH can be seen through the thin dentin covering the pulp. Pulp capping is achieved by covering the pulp or the pulpal area with a liner of calcium hydroxide. Several proprietary calcium hydroxide liners are available. "Dycal" or "Kerr life" are probably the best known and easiest to use, and are especially useful for *indirect pulp capping* of deep cavities. These pastes are supplied in two tubes as a base and a catalyst. The contents are mixed together in equal amounts and transferred to the floor of the cavity with a special small round–ended instrument.

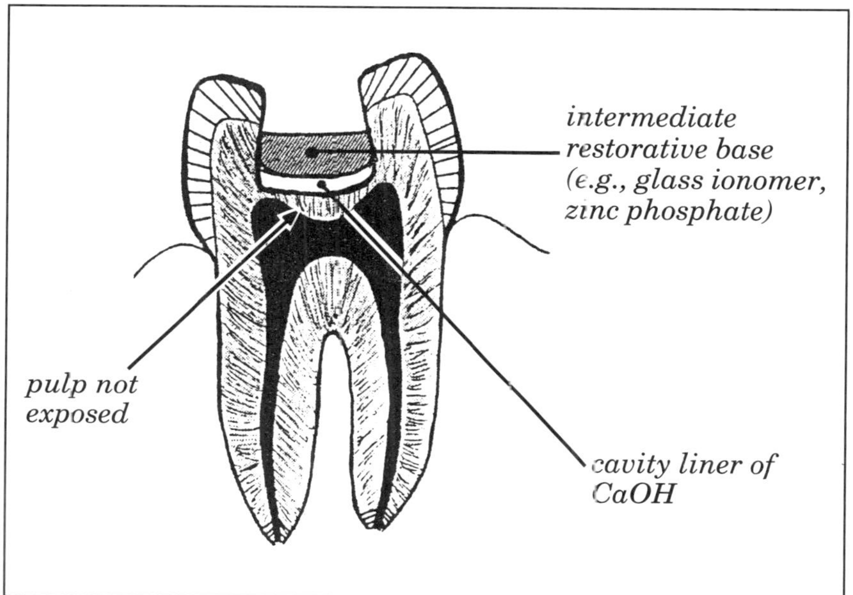

Figure 79. Indirect pulp capping (pulp not exposed but near surface).

DIRECT PULP CAPPING

If the pulp has been recently exposed, even if the exposure is only a pinhole, DIRECT PULP CAPPING can be performed in order to stop the bleeding and to save the pulp. In some cases a more aggressive approach may be required (see vital pulpotomy 7.12). The best material for pulp capping is *concentrated* calcium hydroxide such as HYPOCAL or CALCIUM HYDROXIDE PASTE. As mentioned before, calcium hydroxide stimulates the odontoblasts to lay down reparative (or tertiary) dentin that eventually covers the exposure site. One problem is that the pulp is very delicate. Attempts to dry the cavity with an air syringe may damage the pulp if the blast of air is too strong. Hypocal will not adhere to a moist surface. Exposed pulp should be treated with a mild antiseptic such as HYDROGEN PEROXIDE, rapidly dried with a gentle stream of air or a cotton pledget before Hypocal is applied. A concentrated CaOH liner, such as Hypocal, is soft and does not protect the pulp from mechanical pressures. An *intermediate* layer of restorative base material (e.g., IRM, glass ionomer) should always be placed over the CaOH liner before the *final* restorative material (Photo 61).

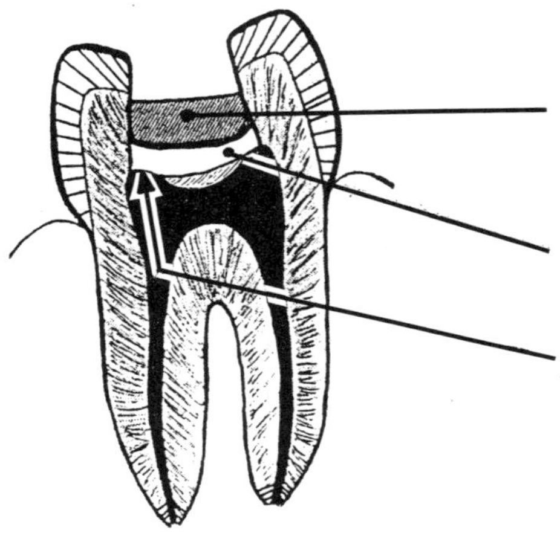

Figure 80. Direct pulp capping (pulp exposed).

6.6 ACID–ETCH TECHNIQUE

Retention of composite filling materials is provided by the acid–etch technique. The acid is provided as a gel or a liquid either in a plastic syringe or bottle, along with an application nozzle. The tooth to be acid–etched is cleaned with pumice (which should not contain either fluoride or silicone), washed with water and then dried. Liners and bases should be used, as necessary, to protect the pulp and dentin. The enamel is etched by applying a gel or a liquid of 35–40 percent PHOSPHORIC ACID. This ETCHING removes a part of the prismatic structure of the enamel, leaving microscopic pits up to a depth of 10 microns (Photo 39). The pits provide mechanical retention of the liquid bonding resin that is applied next.

Etching is recommended for up to one minute, after which the acid is washed off thoroughly with water for at least 20 seconds. Care should be taken to ensure that no concentrated acid is left in contact with the mucous membranes of the mouth, or allowed to contact the eyes. Some of the newer etching materials (e.g., Chamelon's "MIRAGE") use 2.5% nitric acid. This "etches" the dentin as well as the enamel and does not have to be rinsed off. Since the largest part of the tooth to be restored is often dentin (such as slab fractures and enamel hypoplasia), this is an important consideration. After washing off the phosphoric acid, the tooth surface is dried with a stream of air. Care should be taken to avoid physical contact with the etched area, since moisture and oils from your fingers will reduce adhesion, and saliva from the animal's mouth can cause remineralization of the enamel.

When the etched surface is dry, it has a chalky–white or a frosted appearance. A layer of adhesive liquid ACRYLIC RESIN is then applied to the tooth surface and light–cured or left to self–cure, depending on the material used. The resin flows into the tubules or the holes created by the etching, leaving a hard film mechanically locked on to the tooth surface. Next the COMPOSITE FILLING material (either self–cure or light–cure) can be placed. This is similar to the resin in chemical structure, but contains an inert filler to give it bulk and strength. It bonds directly to the resin through a molecular bonding process called POLYMERIZATION (see composite fillings, 6.8).

The acid–etch technique is also useful in the cementation of orthodontic appliances, such as expansion screws, brackets, splints, wires and other devices.

6.7 AMALGAM FILLINGS

After correct cavity preparation (see cavity preparation, 6.1), a liner of calcium hydroxide (CaOH) is placed if the cavity is deep, followed by an intermediate restorative material such as reinforced zinc oxide–eugenol (e.g., IRM), zinc oxyphosphate cement or a glass ionomer. This prevents compression of the CaOH liner that would cause pressure on the pulp. After these have hardened the cavity walls are cleaned again with a bur and, if necessary, the undercuts are reshaped. The cavity is now ready for the final filling with amalgam.

Amalgam used to be mixed by hand. A prepackaged amalgam capsule mixed in an amalgamator (electric mechanical mixer) is much more convenient, safer and accurate. The amalgam is condensed firmly into the floor of the cavity with a condenser or a plugger. Care must be taken that all the corners are filled. The filling is built up in layers, each layer being firmly packed onto the layer below until the amalgam is above the cavity margins. The excess amalgam is then carefully carved down until it approximates the shape of the missing tooth material. Finally the amalgam is burnished smooth with a round or an oval–shaped BURNISHER to create a smooth transition from enamel to amalgam (Photo 29).

Theoretically the amalgam should be polished after 24 hours, but since this would necessitate another anesthetic, it is not practical to do this. If an animal is anesthetized at a later date, it is a good idea to polish old amalgam fillings. This will reduce the chances of secondary carious lesions developing between the amalgam and the enamel, as well as removing any plaque accumulation.

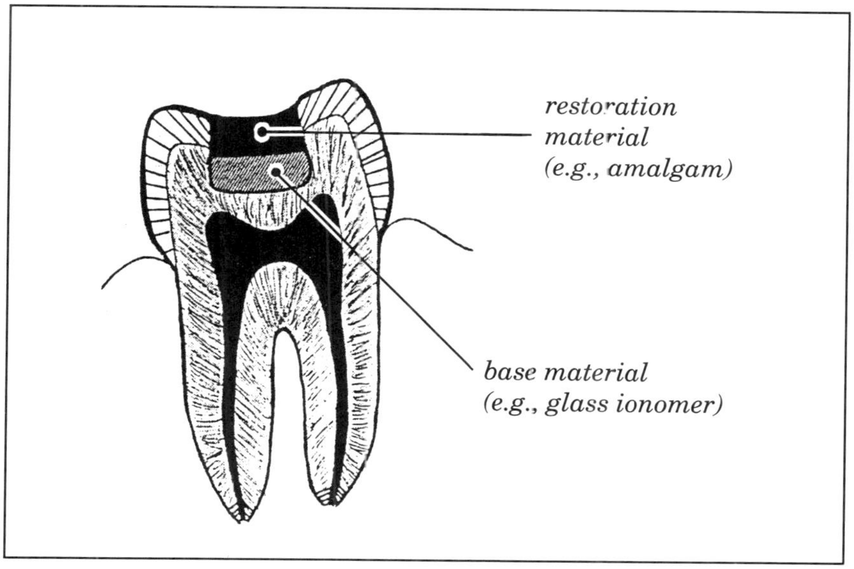

Figure 81. Restoration without pulp capping.

6.8 COMPOSITE FILLINGS

Composite fillings have cosmetic advantages, as well as an ability to mechanically lock directly to the enamel tubules following etching. Composites are usually satisfactory for non–occlusal surfaces (Photos 36, 45, 48). Teeth with enamel hypoplasia, and which are not subject to occlusal or to shearing forces, can be restored with composite. The disadvantages of composite include a poor retention under occlusal forces and a poorer resistance to wear than amalgam.

After correct cavity preparation (see cavity preparation, 6.1), the cavity should be carefully dried, since composite is more susceptible to moisture than amalgam. A liner of calcium hydroxide is placed if the cavity is deep, followed by an intermediate restorative base layer, such as a glass ionomer. Reinforced zinc oxide–eugenol (e.g., IRM) should not be used as a base directly under composites (see cavity cement bases, 12.4). The base does not need to be thick, since composite insulates well. Varnish, as long as it is not copal based, can also be used to seal the dentin under composite in shallow cavities. Any varnish that gets on to the enamel edges of the preparation should be removed with a bur, before acid–etch bonding of the composite.

The composite is supplied either as a SELF–CURING (COLD–CURING, AUTO–CURING, CHEMICAL–CURING, CHEMICALLY ACTIVATED) ACRYLIC, which comes as two pastes that must be mixed together in order to POLYMERIZE, or as a LIGHT–CURING (PHOTO–CURING, LIGHT–ACTIVATED) ACRYLIC, which cures with the blue component of WHITE LIGHT. The advantage of the light–curing variety is its increased working time. Its only disadvantage is the cost of the curing–light and the depth to which the composite can be cured (up to about 2 mm in depth). Both types of composite are available in a variety of SHADES to closely match the color of the tooth to be filled. Although a standard shade is adequate for veterinary use, the advanced veterinary dentist should use a SHADE GUIDE and shaded composites (see composite, 12.7).

When using a self–cure composite, the two pastes are mixed, then transferred rapidly to the cavity preparation or to the tooth surface defect. The site is overfilled, and the composite is compressed into place using a plastic or a mylar strip ("Scotch" tape or adhesive tape with the sticky side outward also works well "as a last resort"). After the composite has cured, the FLASH (excess material around the margins) should be removed with a high–speed carbide or a diamond bur. The margins are then polished flat with a fine diamond bur, white stone or sanding disc. The self–curing materials should be stored in a refrigerator to extend their shelf life. If they are used while still cold they will have a longer working time, which can be useful for the inexperienced practitioner.

6.9 "NECK" LESIONS – CAT

"Neck" lesions (also known as FELINE CERVICAL LINE LESIONS, CERVICAL LINE EROSIONS, OSTEOCLASTIC RESORPTIVE LESIONS, FELINE SUBGINGIVAL RESORPTIVE LESIONS, EXTERNAL and INTERNAL ODONTOCLASTIC RESORPTIVE (ROOT) LESIONS, DENTAL RESORPTIVE LESIONS and IDIOPATHIC BUCCOCERVICAL EROSIONS) are defects found in the teeth of cats, usually over five years of age. Although commonly classified as Class V defects, this is not really correct, since Black's classification for humans refers to caries (see classification of cavities/defects, 6.2). These enamel and dentin defects are formed just above and below the gumline, or at the "neck" of the tooth, most commonly in the maxillary and mandibular premolars and the especially around the distal root of the mandibular molars (Photo 24).

"Neck" lesions are not caries (or cavities) although they may look like a cavity. Caries is defined as a bacterio–chemical degradation of the enamel, leading to demineralization of the enamel (see caries, 6.3). "Neck" lesions, although previously thought to be caries, are presently considered to be resorptive defects of unknown etiology. The odontoclasts in the periodontal ligament cause an ODONTOCLASTIC RESORPTIVE PROCESS, with some evidence of repairs with reparative dentin. Histologically "neck" lesions show no demineralization of the enamel, which is the classic finding of caries, and the defects are lined with odontoclast filled lacunae. True caries has not been demonstrated by histological studies in the cat.

"Neck" lesions are seen as small, crater–like defects in the enamel that can expose the pulp. They are very painful when probed, even provoking a pain response on an anesthetized animal. They are progressive, and often lead to loss of the tooth crown. When this occurs, the remaining root can irritate the gingiva, cause periapical necrosis or even a fistula. They generally appear on the buccal surface of the premolars and molars. Multiple lesions at different stages of development are not uncommon, and small, unremarkable lesions can be found on the root surface all the way down to the apex of the root.

The "neck" lesions are often hidden under calculus deposits or under hyperplastic gingiva. It is strongly recommended that during every routine examination and every operation, (e.g., castration and spay), the teeth of cats are checked for "neck" lesions. If there is any doubt about the extent of the "neck" lesion, a dental radiograph should be taken prior to treatment, since there is often deep–root involvement and bone destruction, including apical granulomas.

6.10 GLASS IONOMER FILLINGS FOR TREATMENT OF "NECK" LESIONS

In cases of small or single lesions, the teeth should be radiographed, thoroughly cleaned, any hyperplastic gingiva removed by gingivectomy or by electrocautery and the defects filled with glass ionomer cement. Important teeth, such as the carnassials, can have root canal therapy to avoid extraction. If only one root is badly involved in the double–rooted tooth it can be HEMISECTIONED (cut in half) or in triple–rooted teeth, the damaged part SECTIONED and any remaining root(s) endodontically treated. A large part of the success in treating "neck" lesions depends on good access of the lesions and a dry operating field, since gingival hemorrhage is often a problem.

In order to *access* small marginal lesions, GINGIVAL RETRACTION CORD can be packed into the gingival sulcus. If the gingiva is bleeding or a gingival flap has been made, HEMOSTATIC GINGIVAL RETRACTION CORD should be placed under the gingival margin. To access large subgingival lesions, it is usually necessary to make a small gingival flap (Photo 31). Hemostatic retraction cord usually controls the hemorrhage, and a small gingival retractor or a suture can be used to hold the flap away from the site (Photo 32).

In "neck" lesions, GLASS IONOMER cement placement has the advantage of requiring little or no cavity preparation since it bonds directly to the dentin and can be placed subgingivally. If the pink color of the pulp can be seen through the dentin, indirect pulp capping should be performed, prior to placement of the glass ionomer (see pulp capping, 6.5). Since little or no excavation of the lesion is required, the chance of damaging the pulp is dramatically reduced. However, gentle cleaning with a Roto–Pro bur is sometimes useful in cleaning the tooth defect. The lesion should be *lightly* air–dried before placing the glass ionomer cement. The cement (powder and liquid) should be mixed according to instructions and applied, without bubbles, to the defect.

Removal of the smear layer on the tooth surface is still controversial, but is probably a good idea (see glass ionomers, 12.8). This is done by applying a conditioner of 10% polyacrylic acid on the exposed tooth surface for about 10 seconds and then rinsing it off with water.

The capsule glass ionomers systems (e.g., Ketac–Fil and Chelon–Silver) provide for perfect mechanical mixing using an amalgamator and allow placement of the glass ionomer directly from the capsule through a special syringe–like plastic tip built into the end of the capsule. Light–cured glass ionomers (e.g., Vitrebond) are also very useful since they flow readily to the edges of the lesion when they are applied. Occasional long–term failure of the thicker encapsulated glass ionomer materials may be due to the difficulty of making a good marginal seal. Because light–curing only takes 20–30 seconds, the risk of blood being incorporated into the filling is minimized. When the glass ionomer has hardened, it should be shaped with a high–speed fine finishing bur (or a perio Roto–Pro bur), and polished with either a fine sanding or polishing disc, or a hand sanding strip, to help reduce the formation of new plaque.

Composite and amalgam can be used in some restorations, but are not very retentive or practical to use. A new product called Geristore (Denmat) shows promise in restoring "neck" lesions. It is a combination of a glass ionomer (providing fluoride release) and a composite (providing strength). It flows readily and it bonds to dentin and enamel.

Since "neck" lesions occur with or without periodontitis, other unknown, predisposing factors must exist. Autoimmune responses, immune deficiencies, infectious processes such as viruses, nutritional (calcium/phosphorus) imbalances, metabolic imbalances and other factors are under investigation.

Severely damaged teeth, such as teeth where so much substance has been lost that the tooth will surely fracture, or has already fractured, must be extracted. Every effort should be made to retain teeth that are required for shearing and chewing, such as the maxillary fourth premolar and mandibular first molar (the carnassials), as well as those that are required for appearance or for defense, such as the canine teeth. When practical, some teeth can be restored with cast crowns, if the owner can afford it, and as long as it is not a show pet. Extraction can also prove difficult, since multirooted teeth often require sectioning and/or osteotomy. Small root remnants can, as a last resort, be drilled out with a high–speed drill (see atomization, 5.4).

Complete restoration is costly and time consuming and requires systematic, painstaking, patient work. The rapidly increasing number of household cats means an increase in demand for feline dentistry. The purchase of an air–driven handpiece is necessary for practices with a large cat clientele.

After dental treatment, regular examinations should be made. A recall system is recommended. "Neck" lesions are rarely found in dogs. If they are found, the treatment should be the same as described for cats (Photo 30).

6.11 ENAMEL HYPOPLASIA

Enamel hypoplasia is a defect in the enamel that usually occurs during tooth development. The enamel formation by the ameloblasts is disrupted, leading to inadequate or absent mineralization of this hard dental tissue. Often caused by the distemper virus at an early age, enamel hypoplasia can also be caused by trauma and inflammation of the permanent tooth bud, systemic infections, massive parasite infestations, endocrine problems and excessive fluoride in the water.

6.12 TREATMENT OF ENAMEL HYPOPLASIA

Most enamel defects can be restored conservatively using the acid–etch composite bonding technique (see acid–etch technique, 6.6). The new *dentin adhesive products* may be a beneficial adjunct to this technique. This bonding strengthens the weakened tooth structure and prevents further wear of the exposed dentin. If the teeth are either severely worn or broken, cast crowns are indicated (see cast metal crowns for enamel hypoplasia, 8.3). If the owner cannot afford or does not want complete restoration, a temporary procedure for sealing the dentinal tubules with a dentin sealing agent can be performed. This should be repeated every six months. The best sealing agents are varnishes that contain fluoride. The varnish protects the pulp from thermal irritation and the FLUORIDE strengthens the dentin by producing fluoroapatite.

CHAPTER 7

ENDODONTICS (ROOT CANAL TREATMENT)

Endodontics is the branch of dentistry concerned with morphology, physiology and pathology of the dental pulp and the periradicular areas. The practice of endodontics involves the diagnosis, prevention and treatment of diseases and injuries of the pulp and associated periradicular tissues.

7.1 PULPAL AND PERIRADICULAR DISEASE

Pulpal disease is only one of several possible causes of diseases of the PERIRADICULAR TISSUES (tissues surrounding the root). Other causes include neoplastic disorders, periodontal problems, developmental factors and trauma. Periradicular diseases of pulpal origin, which can be either acute or chronic, generally require endodontic treatment. Although the exact mechanism of resolution of periapical lesions is not known, several hypotheses have been published. The most recent hypothesis and the most feasible is that "if periapical lesions are inflammatory responses to the antigen content of the root canal system, and the epithelial proliferation is a response to these irritating materials, then when the source of irritation is removed, the immune system gradually destroys and removes the proliferating epithelial cells." Dental radiographs are required for accurate diagnosis of RADICULAR PROBLEMS (problems pertaining to the root) and surrounding tissues. Periradicular disease can spread to the adjacent soft tissues causing cellulitis and infection.

7.2 CAUSES OF PERIRADICULAR DISEASE

1. Acute periradicular disease.
   b) Acute periapical abscess.
   c) Acute periapical periodontitis (vital and non–vital).
2. Chronic periradicular disease (with areas of rarefaction).
   a) Chronic periapical abscess.

b) Chronic periapical granuloma.

c) Chronic periapical cyst. (It is impossible to distinguish among these three by radiology alone — histopathology would be required.)

3. Condensing osteitis.
4. External root resorption.
5. Diseases of the periradicular tissues of non–endodontic origin.

7.3 ACUTE PERIAPICAL ABSCESS

This is a localized collection of purulent exudate between the root and the alveolar bone at the apex of the root, usually following either infection or death of the pulp. The abscessation is the end result after traumatic pulpal exposure, damage to the supporting bone and mechanical irritation such as a partial avulsion or luxation of the tooth.

7.4 CHRONIC PERIAPICAL ABSCESS

This is a chronic, low grade infection of the periradicular bone. The source of infection is generally the root canal. In a severe or a chronic case, a fistulous tract may either develop into sinus, or through the bone and skin to the exterior. The classic ABSCESS BELOW THE EYE (Photo 51) is generally caused by proliferation of a periapical abscess of the mesio–buccal and disto–buccal roots of the maxillary fourth premolar. Abscessation of the mesio–palatal root of the maxillary fourth premolar, the distal root of the maxillary third premolar and the mesio–buccal root of the first maxillary molar, usually causes drainage via the maxillary sinus. Endodontic treatment will generally resolve the problem.

7.5 ACUTE PERIAPICAL PERIODONTITIS

This is a painful inflammation of the periodontium as a result of tooth trauma, pulp irritation or pulp infection, through the root canal into the periapical tissues.

7.6 CHRONIC PERIAPICAL GRANULOMA

This is a chronic inflammatory response at the root apex, and consists of a mass of proliferating granulation tissue. It develops some time after the pulp is dead and can be preceded by a chronic alveolar abscess.

7.7 CHRONIC PERIAPICAL CYST

This is a slowly expanding epithelial sac located at the apex of a tooth, which lines a pathological cavity in the alveolar bone. The cyst results from infection and necrosis of the pulp caused by traumatic, chemical or bacterial insult, which has stimulated the epithelial cell rests (Malassez's epithelial rests) in the periodontal ligament. On a dental radiograph the chronic periapical cyst occasionally exhibits a thin, radiopaque line around the periphery of the radiolucent area. This indicates a reaction of the bone to the slowly expanding mass. The *periapical granuloma* can look similar on a dental radiograph in many instances.

7.8 CONDENSING OSTEITIS

This is a mild irritation from the pulpal tissue that stimulates osteoclastic activity in the alveolar bone. Radiographically the dense bone has a reduced trabecular pattern.

7.9 EXTERNAL ROOT RESORPTION

This is a resorption of the cementum (and dentin) at the apex of the root. There are many causes, including trauma, inflammation, granuloma, cyst and systemic diseases.

7.10 PERIRADICULAR DISEASE OF NON–ENDODONTIC ORIGIN

These may result from systemic diseases, periodontal disease, cysts, granulomas and tumors.

7.11 TOOTH FRACTURE

Although a large percentage of dogs get fractured teeth, they will not always require root canal treatment. In older dogs the PULP CHAMBER may be so reduced in size through the deposition of secondary dentin, that no exposure of the pulp occurs. It is only necessary to round off any sharp edges, or restore the tip of these teeth with composite. Younger dogs have a greater risk of fracturing teeth. Their immature teeth have thinner dentin, thus a large proportion of tooth fractures in young dogs will involve exposure of the pulp. Because of the tendency of young dogs to become involved in accidents (through play and lack of experience), and sometimes during training or due to mistreatment, young dogs are more prone to tooth fractures.

In most cases fractured teeth with pulp exposure should be treated using conventional endodontic therapy. Exceptions include *recently* fractured teeth with an exposed bleeding pulp, which can often be treated with a vital pulpotomy (see vital pulpotomy, 7.12). The open canal provides a direct communication between the oral cavity and the alveolar bone, allowing food remnants and bacteria to enter to the canal, causing periapical abscesses and infections of the jaw.

7.12 VITAL PULPOTOMY

Recently fractured teeth, where the exposed pulp may not yet be grossly infected, can be saved by a VITAL PULPOTOMY, which is the removal of the damaged coronal part of the pulp. This is especially true in young animals with large pulp canals and a high resistance to infection. The odontoblasts are capable of producing enough reparative dentin to isolate the remaining pulp. The procedure is similar to direct pulp capping.

A sterile round bur should be used to remove the damaged coronal part of the pulp. Any bleeding should be controlled and calcium hydroxide powder or concentrated calcium hydroxide paste placed over the exposed pulp. A base filler, such as a glass ionomer, should then be placed over the CaOH followed by a final restoration such as light–cured composite or amalgam. Any sharp edges on the fractured part of the crown should be contoured and a radiograph taken of the tooth.

Three months later a follow–up radiograph should be taken and compared with the initial radiograph. If the treatment has been successful, a reduction in the size of the pulp chamber should be seen and it may even be possible to see a DENTIN BRIDGE (REPARATIVE or TERTIARY DENTIN) sealing off the coronal pulp completely. If reparative dentin is not formed within about 50 days, there will be none.

If the treatment has not been successful, symptoms of pain will manifest themselves, such as slow and careful eating, a direct painful reaction to biting and/or howling or whimpering if the jaws are held closed. In severe cases there is often swelling of the gingival tissues and fistulas may occur.

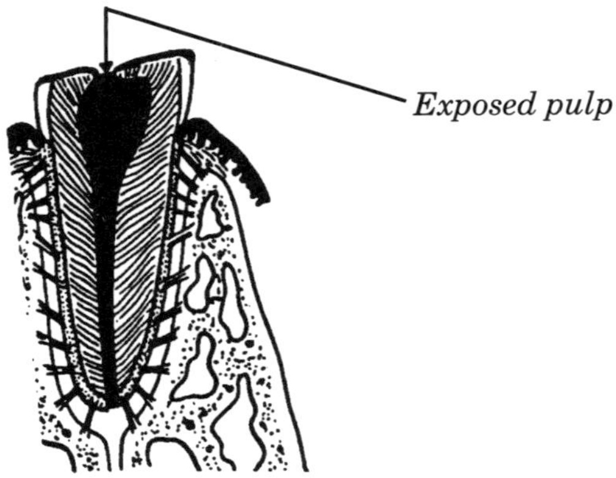

Figure 82. Fracture of the crown exposing the pulp.

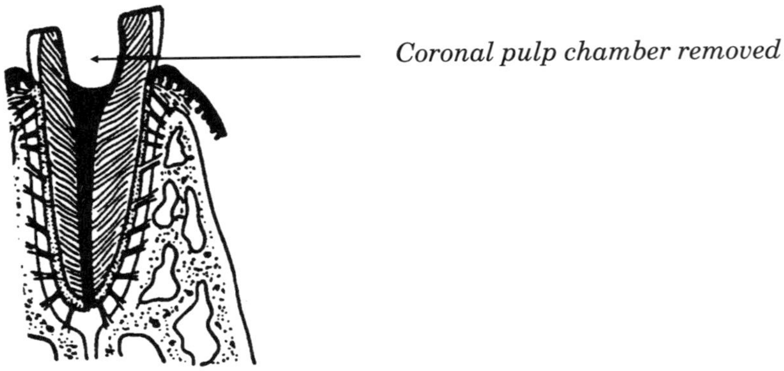

Figure 83. Coronal pulp removed with a sterile round bur.

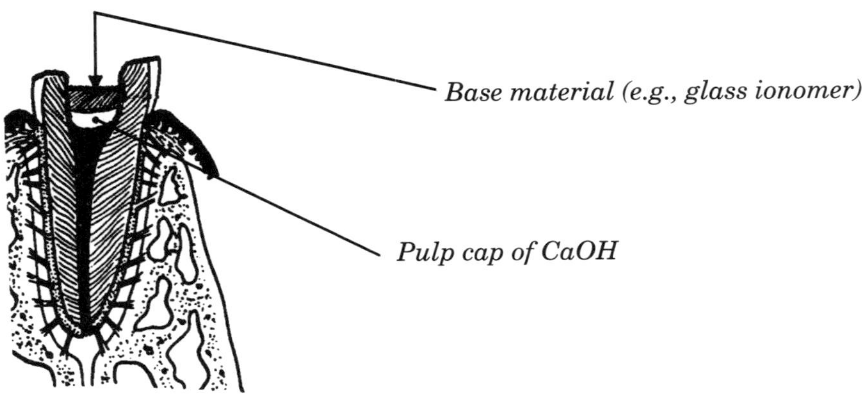

Figure 84. Calcium hydroxide pulp cap covered with sealing base material, after hemorrhage is controlled with hemostatic agents.

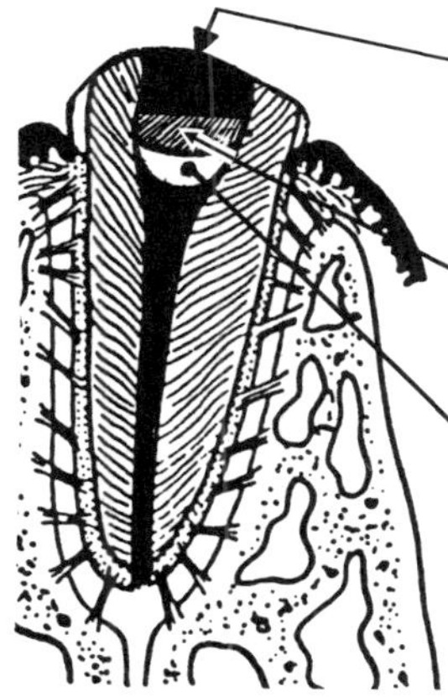

Figure 85. Amalgam filling, sealing base and pulp cap. Sharp edges of the tooth are contoured.

It is often difficult to decide between vital pulpotomy and root canal therapy. Generally speaking, when the fracture is fresh (ideally within a few hours, but sometimes up to a few days) and if the remaining pulp is actually bleeding, or starts to bleed when lightly probed, then vital pulpotomy can be attempted. If there is no bleeding, but there is a black color to the pulp contents, or a smell of necrosis can be detected, complete endodontic therapy should be performed.

Animals seem to have a greater resistance than humans to early infections occurring in exposed root canals. Successful pulpotomies have been achieved in animals up to two weeks after exposure of the pulp, although the risk of abscessation is high. Direct pulp capping, where the exposed vital pulp of the tooth is capped and sealed, is basically an endodontic procedure. This has been covered in Chapter 6 (see pulp capping, 6.5).

7.13 ROOT CANAL PREPARATION (INSTRUMENTATION)

Root canal preparation (or instrumentation) is the complete removal of the vital pulp (PULPECTOMY), the remains of the pulp and the infected dentin. Before endodontic treatment is started, a radiograph of the tooth must always be taken to determine the size, length and curvature of the canal, and to check for fractures of the root and any internal or external abnormalities.

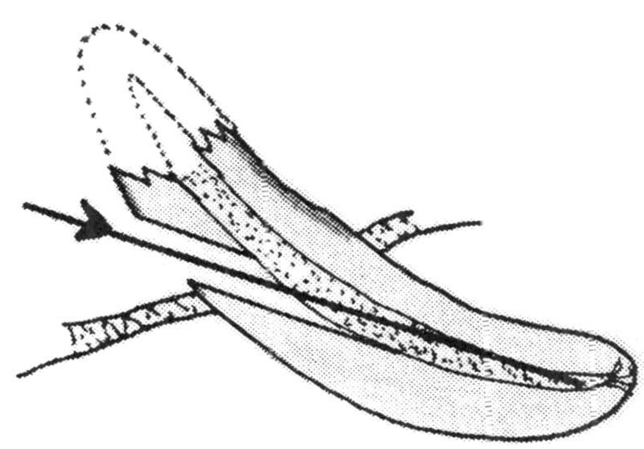

Figure 86. Additional access hole just coronal to the gingival margin (arrow).

The initial step is to provide as direct a line of access as possible to the apical portion of the canal. The coronal access hole can be opened up with round or tapered carbide or diamond burs, and the coronal one third of the canal flared with a Gates–Glidden bur. Next a small (#10 or #15) endo reamer or endo file is inserted as far as possible to establish entry into the root canal. A radiograph with the reamer or the file in place should then be taken to confirm that the canal has been entered correctly and that the apex has been reached.

After this, a BARBED BROACH is used to remove any remaining living tissue. It is inserted as far into the root canal as possible without binding, and slowly removed with a twisting movement. A vital pulp can often be removed in one piece by this method (Photo 40), but a necrotic pulp may require several attempts, and even then pieces may remain. If the pulp was necrotic, all tissue must be removed from the pulp chamber and walls. This can be achieved by a combination of flushing, reaming and filing (INSTRUMENTATION). *Reamers* and *K–files* are used to clean and shape the root canal and *Hedstrom files* to file, smooth and widen the root canal. The surfaces of a root canal are irregular and interspersed with recesses, crevices and fissures, which have resulted from the deposition of secondary dentin.

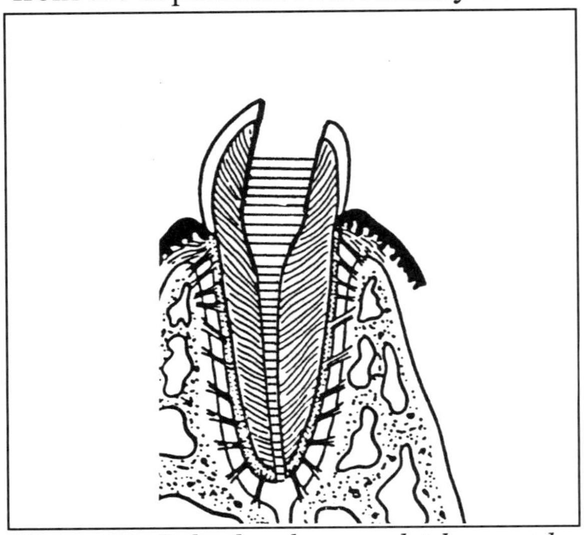

Figure 87. Pulp chamber completely opened to achieve straight access.

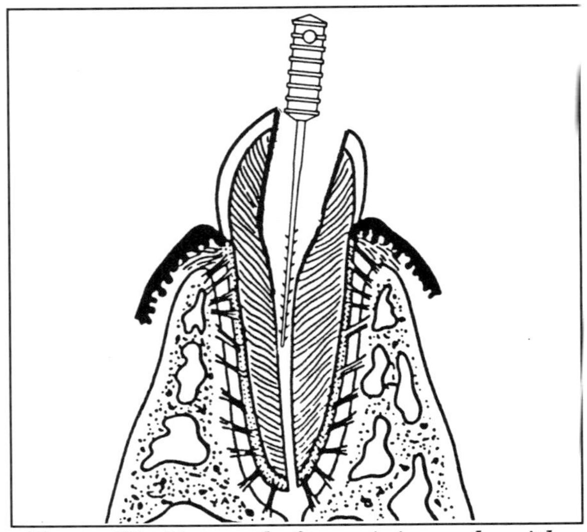

Figure 88. Removal of remaining pulp with a barbed broach.

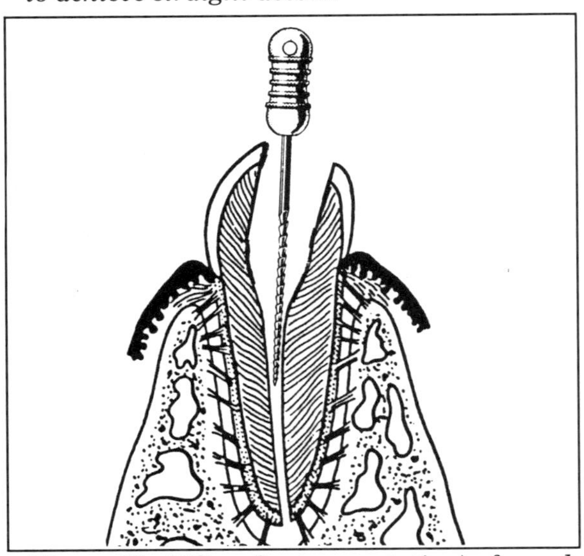

Figure 89. Filing (instrumentation) of canal walls with a Hedstrom file.

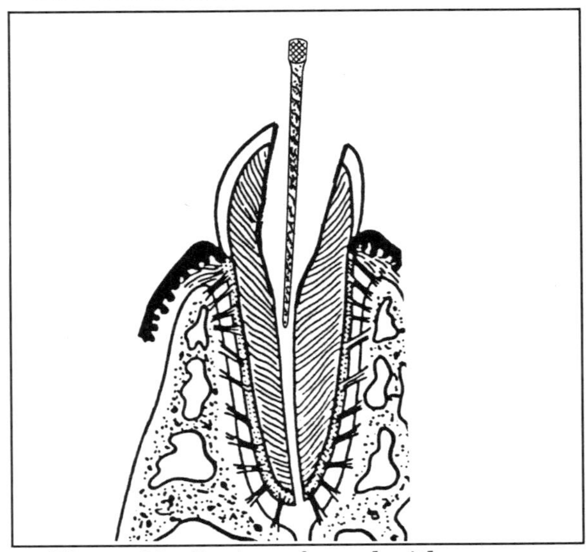

Figure 90. Drying of canal with a paper point after irrigation.

After the root canal has been entered successfully and the pulp removed with a barbed broach (or a Hedstrom file), the next step is to pass a small file or a reamer to the root apex. When the tip of the file is within 1–2 mm of the radiographic apex, the WORKING LENGTH of the file can be established (Photo 52). This is the distance from the tip of the file to a fixed point at the coronal access point, and can be marked by using a rubber stop on the shaft of the file. The working length should be confirmed by a radiograph, measured on a millimeter ruler and recorded.

Root canals need to be cleaned and widened for four reasons:

1. To mechanically remove microorganisms from the canal surface.
2. To remove tags of pulpal tissue and odontoblasts that cling to the canal wall that will undergo necrosis and provide an environment for bacterial growth.
3. To increase the capacity of the root canal to permit irrigating solutions to reach the apical third of the root canal for effective debridement.
4. To shape the root canal to receive gutta–percha, because the wider the canal, the easier to fill, especially if it is narrow to start with.

The PRINCIPLES OF INSTRUMENTATION are as follows:

1. *Always* work files in a canal with an irrigant.
2. Irrigate frequently and copiously. This is *mandatory* between each instrument size change.
3. Always explore with smaller files in order to gauge the canal size and configuration. *Never* attempt canal enlargement until final corrected working lengths are established.
4. Progressively enlarge, using successively larger files. *Never* skip an intermediate size.
5. Loosen debris and remove dentin from the walls on the outstroke only (filing) or with a 1/4 to 1/2 rotating action (reaming).
6. Avoid having instruments bind on insertion. Insert files by teasing them to length with a "twiddling" action. TWIDDLING is a back and forth rotation of the file between the thumb and forefinger while continually working it apically. Careful file insertion (twiddling) followed by filing on the outstroke will help avoid packing of debris in the apical region.
7. REAMING is the action used for the apical preparation and cleaning. The remainder, or the step–back portion of the preparation, is by *circumferential filing*.
8. *Reaming* is accomplished by twiddling the instrument, then working it back and forth, 1/4 – 1/2 a turn, until it can be freely rotated continuously in a clockwise direction.
9. FILING is a planing or filing motion that is accomplished with a pull stroke. The file is twiddled until it locks slightly, and then withdrawn while pushing the tip alternately against the walls.
10. *Filing* is accomplished with files only and not with reamers.
11. After each insertion and filing, remove the file and clean the flutes of debris, using alcohol–soaked gauze or cotton, then reinsert to file the next wall.

12. Return to the working length frequently with small files to remove any debris that has become packed in the apical region. This is known as RECAPITULATION and should be done *at least* once between each instrument size change. Do not file the walls or enlarge the canal during recapitulation.
13. Do not *overprepare* the canal walls near the furcation of multirooted teeth, since the dentin tends to be thinner at this point.
14. Never try to force or continue rotating a file that binds. This tends to untwist, weaken and break the file.

During instrumentation, frequent IRRIGATION of the root canal should be completed at least once between each instrument size change, using 1 ml or more of the irrigation solutions. The first irrigant should be 2.5–5.25 percent SODIUM HYPOCHLORITE (which destroys microorganisms, dissolves necrotic tissue and lubricates the canal), followed by 3% HYDROGEN PEROXIDE (the effervescent reaction forces debris and microorganisms out of the canal. The oxygen liberated assists in destroying anaerobic microorganisms). Hydrogen peroxide should *never* be used last, at the end of instrumentation, because if it remains in the canal it can react with pulp debris and blood to produce gas. Any gas trapped within the tooth will cause continuous pain. Ideally the final rinse should be sterile saline. These irrigating solutions should be administered using sterile irrigating syringes and needles (25– or 27–gauge), preferably with blunt ends and a hole on the side near the tip.

The most important part of instrumentation is the APICAL PREPARATION. The apical 1–2 mm of the canal should be enlarged only one or two sizes larger than the first file that demonstrates any binding, establishing the WORKING LENGTH of the file. Use care not to overprepare the apical region, particularly in a curved canal. The largest instrument that binds slightly at the working length is called the MASTER APICAL FILE (MAF). When apical preparation is complete, the tapering is created by shortening the working length of each successively larger instrument by 0.5–1.0 mm and by peripheral or circumferential filing. This is called the STEP–BACK TECHNIQUE. After each step–back file, return to the working length with the MAF or a smaller file (recapitulation) to loosen any debris that has been forced towards the apex.

Large files up to #60 or #70 (or even up to #140 in very wide canals) may be necessary when stepping back more coronally, to give adequate debridement and provide a sufficient taper to the canal.

In order to evaluate if instrumentation is complete, press the MAF tip against each wall on the outstroke. All the walls should feel smooth and free from irregularities. A selected *spreader* should pass easily to within one to two millimeters of the working length. The dentinal shavings should be clean. On a radiograph the preparation should show a continuous taper in an apical direction. During instrumentation it is also useful to take radiographs periodically to monitor your progress.

The final size of file that fits the apical third of the canal without binding (MAF) should be recorded and used as a reference for selecting the size of the PRIMARY (MASTER) GUTTA–PERCHA POINT to be used for obturation or filling (see obturation, 7.14). The master gutta–percha point should be the same size as the MAF. To determine the fit of the master gutta–percha point, it should be inserted to exactly the working length and a "tug–back" be elicited on withdrawal.

Following instrumentation the canal is flushed with saline and dried with tapered ABSORBENT PAPER POINTS (Photo 42). The paper points should be inserted to the entire length of the canal and continually renewed until the tip of the point is dry. It is possible to experience excessive bleeding caused by the mechanical irritation of the apical (and periapical) tissues. This is especially true in young animals where the apical opening is large. Normally a paper point left at the apex for a few minutes will stop the bleeding, or reduce it so that a second paper point will succeed in stopping the bleeding. A higher concentration of hydrogen peroxide (10–30 percent) will often have a more positive effect. Epinephrine at a dilution of 1:30,000 or 1:50,000 can also be used as a HEMOSTATIC AGENT, as can 4% liquid cocaine. In extreme cases, the paper point must be left in the tooth for a day or two, although this is to be avoided if at all possible, because of the necessity for a second general anesthetic. When the root canal is clean and dry, then the canal can be filled (see, obturation, 7.14).

Root canal therapy can be prone to ENDODONTIC COMPLICATIONS, such as broken files, reamers and lentulo spiral fillers, perforated roots and chambers, and canals that are impossible to instrument.

If possible, a BROKEN FILE or a BROKEN REAMER should be removed by drilling parallel to it (a tapered Roto–Pro bur can be very effective), and then retrieving it with another file, hemostat or a special extraction instrument. If retrieval is impossible, and the root apex has not been sealed, then an apicoectomy (see apicoectomy, 10.12) should be performed to attempt removal of the file followed by sealing of the apex. If the apex is sealed, or sealing can be obtained around the broken file, then the broken instrument can be left in the canal. The root canal is then filled as much as possible, although the chances of success may be jeopardized.

BROKEN LENTULO SPIRAL FILLERS are often easily removed by spinning another lentulo down the canal in a reverse direction. If this does not work, treat it as described for broken files and reamers.

PERFORATIONS of the ROOT APEX should be sealed via apicoectomy. PERFORATIONS elsewhere in the ROOT CANAL should be immediately filled with calcium hydroxide before continuing with the root canal procedure. The prognosis for teeth with perforations is often good, but periradicular inflammation and infection should always be anticipated. Antibiotics and occasionally steroids are recommended and frequent rechecks are necessary.

If, following filling of a perforation, signs of a periapical abscess occur, such as swelling, tenderness and pain, then an apicoectomy should be performed and the infected periapical tissue removed. If apicoectomy is not feasible or not successful, the involved root or the entire tooth should be removed.

Some ROOT CANALS are IMPOSSIBLE TO FIND OR INSTRUMENT, such as the mesio–palatal root of the maxillary fourth premolar of small and old dogs. In multirooted teeth, all root canals must be treated. *Never* leave one canal untreated. Therefore, the best solution for treatment of roots that cannot be instrumented is either to section the root and remove it or seal the apex via apicoectomy. In some cases MUMMIFICATION of the pulp may be attempted. To perform mummification, as much of the canal as possible is opened and the accessible pulp removed. The canal is filled with the mummifying agent, which is sealed in place with amalgam or with composite. The MUMMIFYING AGENT, such as FORMOCRESOL, contains FORMALDEHYDE that penetrates the pulp remnants and eliminates microorganisms. However, if the root apex is not completely sealed, the formaldehyde may irritate the periapical tissues leading to periapical inflammation. This procedure should be completed with caution. Follow–up radiographic examination is recommended three months after the procedure.

Root canal treatment of canine teeth, especially in larger dogs, can create further difficulties because of the length and curvature of these teeth. Files up to 60 mm in length are now available, which helps in solving at least one of these problems. The canine teeth of older dogs have narrow curved canals making it difficult to reach the apex. In the 1930s, *BODINGBAUER* (Austria) suggested making an additional ACCESSORY HOLE in the canine tooth just coronal to the gingiva using a round carbide, diamond or other bur in order to improve access. This opening should be directed towards the apex. The apical portion of the root canal can then be prepared through this hole. The chamber of the pulp cavity should be prepared through a coronal access of the tooth. The SECONDARY ACCESS HOLE further weakens the tooth structure and should not be made if the root apex can be reached through the CORONAL ACCESS HOLE (Photo 41).

Root canal treatment of the maxillary fourth premolar requires a triple root canal procedure. In order to access these canals, two or three access holes must be prepared. The most difficult root to access is the mesio–palatal root. Access to this root can be made either through the occlusal surface (Photo 46) or TRANSCORONALLY through the access hole made for the mesio–buccal root (Photo 47). As straight a line of access as possible should be made to all roots.

Although root canal procedures are most commonly performed on the canine teeth and the maxillary fourth premolars in dogs, all teeth can potentially receive endodontic treatment (Photo 49), providing they are large enough.

7.14 ROOT CANAL FILLING (OBTURATION)

The object of obturation is to create a seal throughout the entire length of the root canal system, from its coronal opening to its apical termination. The CORONAL SEAL is as important as the APICAL SEAL for long–term success.

The most common obturating materials are a combination of paste–type (e.g., ZOE, AH–26) and semi–solid type (e.g., gutta–percha). Although there are a large number of materials to choose from there are only a few that are widely used. Some of the obturating materials contain medication (see root canal filling materials, 12.12).

The major advantage of the semi–solid obturation materials is length control and a reasonable ability to create an adequate seal. Gutta–percha is the most widely used semi–solid material, although some people still use solid silver points. Gutta–percha points (or cones) are available in "*standardized*" and "*conventional*" shapes. Standardized points have the same size and taper as standardized instruments. The conventional points have a tapering tip of one size and a body of another size. Conventional points are intended to be used as ACCESSORY POINTS in conjunction with a CENTRAL PRIMARY or MASTER STANDARDIZED POINTS.

Standardized points are usually preferred in veterinary medicine, although personal choice is usually influenced by the method of canal preparation.

Although gutta–percha points can fill the canal fairly well, they do not usually give a complete seal, either apically or laterally. In order to achieve a complete seal a sealing cement is used in combination with gutta–percha (Photo 44). These cements are the paste–type obturating materials mentioned earlier (see root canal filling materials, 12.12). Various techniques are used to place the sealing cement. It can be placed in the canal using paper points, as a coating on the primary and subsequent gutta–percha points, injected into the canal with a syringe or placed into the canal with a lentulo spiral filler. The most common method used in veterinary medicine is with a lentulo spiral filler (Photo 43).

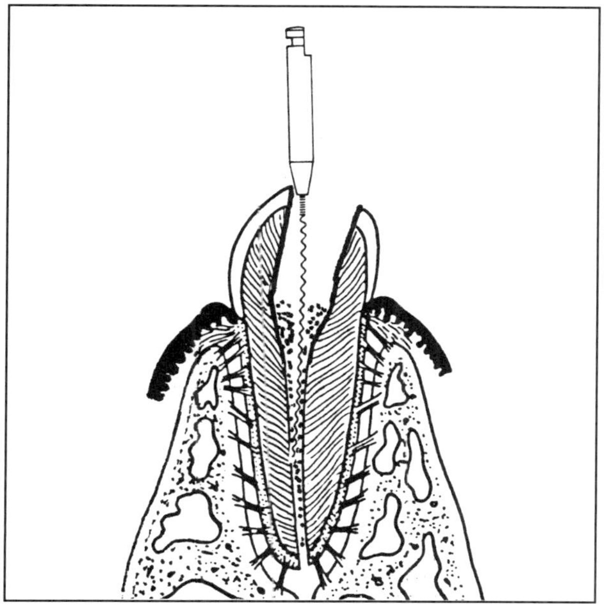

Figure 91. Filling (obturation) of canal with sealant, using a lentulo spiral filler.

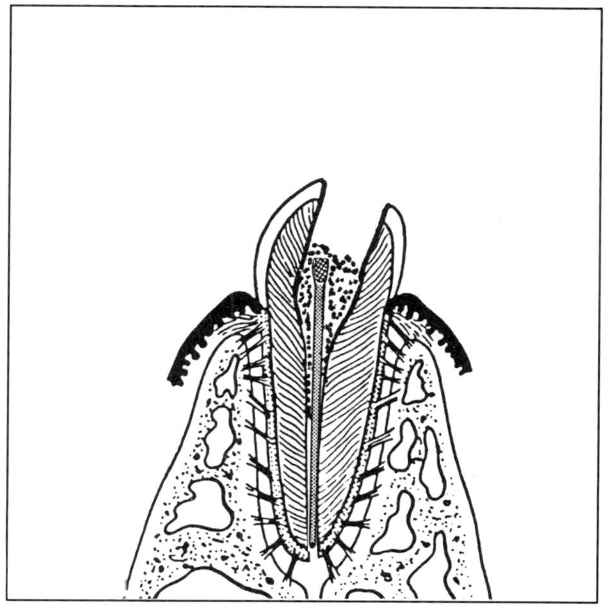

Figure 92. Insertion of gutta–percha point to obturate the canal.

The lentulo spiral filler, in a low–speed handpiece, is coated with the sealing cement and inserted into the canal. The low–speed handpiece should be used at its lowest speed to spin the material to the apex. The handpiece must be rotating in a clockwise direction to introduce the material. If the spiral filler is withdrawn while it is spinning clockwise, it will not withdraw the paste. Care must be taken that the tip of the spiral filler does not bind at the apex and break off. The lentulo spiral filler works best in a canal *only slightly larger* than the spiral filler itself, and in very wide canals it may not work well. In wide canals only the apex may be filled by this method. The rest of the canal has to be filled using a disposable syringe with the smallest needle that allows passage of the paste. The needle is inserted as far as possible into the canal, and then backed out slowly using continuous pressure on the plunger to ensure complete filling.

One or more gutta–percha points are pushed into the sealing cement and laterally condensed to ensure complete diameter filling. A radiograph must be taken either after the primary gutta–percha point has been inserted or after condensation of the subsequent points to confirm that the canal is properly filled to within one to two millimeters of the radiographic apex of the tooth. The most popular method of SEATING semi–solid points is *lateral condensation* followed by *vertical condensation*.

LATERAL CONDENSATION is the spreading of the gutta–percha point in a lateral direction in the canal using a SPREADER (a long tapered and pointed instrument). This spreading creates room for the next point to be placed alongside, although not to the same length as the first. A number of points are inserted this way until the entire diameter of the canal is filled with gutta–percha. A rotary instrument called a McSPADDEN COMPACTOR can be used for condensation. This instrument generates frictional heat that plasticizes the gutta–percha and forces it laterally to obturate the canal in three dimensions. When lateral condensation is completed, the protruding ends of the points are removed with a heated instrument, such as an old Beaver tail carver. The tip should be made *red hot*.

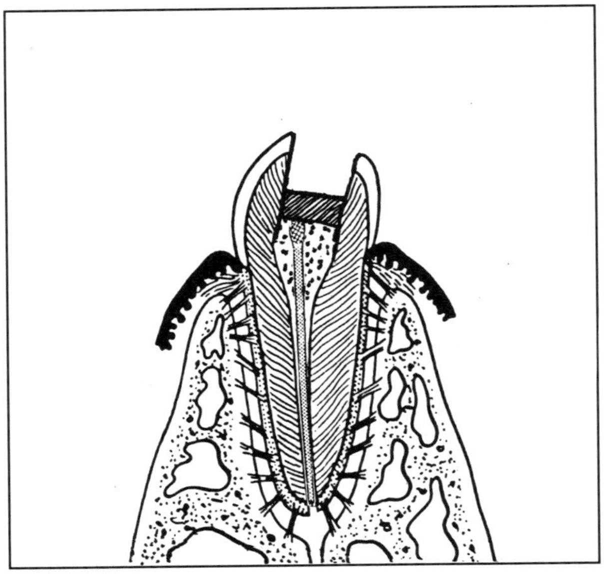

Figure 93. Applying base above gutta–percha and sealing cement surface.

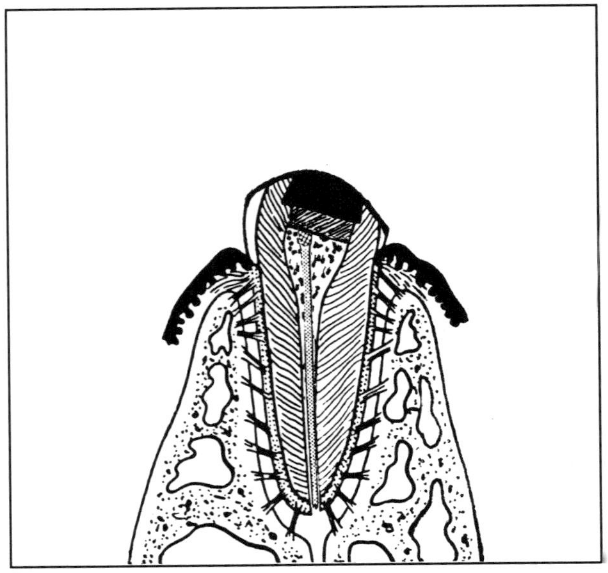

Figure 94. Finishing with restorative material and contouring the tooth.

VERTICAL CONDENSATION is then performed, using a long, straight and blunt instrument called a PLUGGER or CONDENSER. This technique condenses the gutta–percha towards the apex. Care must be exercised not to push the gutta–percha through the tip of the apex. After the canal is adequately filled with gutta–percha and condensed, the remaining coronal ends of the gutta–percha points have to be removed with a heated instrument. Gutta–percha should be removed from four to six millimeters below the access opening. The remaining access opening of the canal is restored with a base and restorative. Any unsupported enamel, or sharp edges of the access preparation should also be removed.

7.15 SURGICAL ENDODONTICS

Occasionally due to the errors in instrumentation and/or obturation, periradicular problems, failure of root canal treatment or due to the morphology of the canal apex, endodontic treatment of the apex of the tooth has to be performed surgically. This procedure, called an apicoectomy or sometimes referred to as "surgical endodontics" is covered in Chapter 10 (see apicoectomy, 10.12).

7.16 CROWN REDUCTION (DISARMING OF CANINE TEETH)

One problem that veterinarians are often confronted with is what to recommend for a pet that bites people or other animals. This is a behavioral problem usually, although some breeds are genetically predisposed to aggressive behavior. Neutering a pet and behavior modification by a professional trainer/behaviorist, although important, are really not the total answers. Nobody can guarantee, even after this has been done, that some day, in the heat of the moment, the pet will not bite, sometimes with disastrous or even fatal results.

However, one thing that a veterinarian can offer, either initially or as a last resort, is disarming the pet (crown reduction). This means reducing the crown length of the canine teeth (or fangs) to the length of the neighboring incisor teeth. Canine teeth are used in nature to grasp and tear an animal's prey or aggressor. In the domestic pet these teeth are not really necessary, except in the case of police and guard dogs. Even if somebody wants a pet for protection, usually the sight of a dog or its barking will deter most people.

Therefore disarming a biting pet has become an acceptable and effective alternative to giving up the pet, having it put to sleep, or extracting the canine teeth. Extraction of the canine teeth is not a good alternative. Normal, well–developed canine teeth can be extremely difficult to extract and usually require a mucogingival flap and osteotomy, as well as much time and patience. There is also a great risk of perforation of the nasal sinus and fracturing the anterior jaw. Also, the remaining sockets are prone to collect food and debris causing further problems. The bases of the mandibular canine teeth help to keep the tongue in the mouth. If the tongue hangs out of the mouth to one side, it will be subject to self–inflicted trauma, not to mention an unaesthetic appearance and increased drooling. The bases of the maxillary canine teeth help to keep the upper lips out of the mouth. If the base of one or both of these teeth is missing, the lips may turn in and become traumatized during chewing.

The finished product should be one that if the pet bites, the reduced crown length and flattened tip will cause minimal damage. *It should be stressed to the client that this procedure does not guarantee that the pet will not bite in the future.* If the pet does bite, the damage caused will be a less severe crushing damage rather than a more severe tearing damage.

Dogs with a reduced crown length of the canine teeth often lose their aggressive behavior because psychologically they become aware that they can no longer, as in nature, act aggressively to become the "leader of the pack." Theoretically people around a biting dog often emit "pheromones," substances secreted outside the body invoking a specific reaction of behavior such as *fear*, dominance, love and hate, which the dog senses and reacts to. With the fear gone, the dog no longer senses it, and backs down. In one family of five dogs, who were constantly fighting and causing extensive damage, all fighting ceased after the crowns of the canine teeth of all the dogs were reduced.

Although the crown reduction is not a guarantee that a dog (or cat) will not bite or cause harm, it is the canine teeth that inflict most of the damage when a dog (or cat) bites. It is worth giving the pet owner the choice and the pet a chance.

7.17 CROWN REDUCTION PROCEDURE ON CANINE TEETH

The procedure of disarming the canine teeth is called crown reduction (correctly termed a SURGICAL CROWN HEIGHT REDUCTION). The procedure involves cutting down the four canine teeth to the level of the surrounding teeth (i.e., incisors and anterior premolars). A vital pulpotomy and restoration are part of the procedure. After the animal is anesthetized and the teeth cleaned if necessary, the mouth is sprayed with an antiseptic solution such as chlorhexidine. Although a RUBBER DAM (a sheet of rubber fitted over the tooth being treated in order to reduce contamination) would be ideal, it is not usually necessary, since there is plenty of working space and asepsis can be achieved by technique. Ideally a dental radiograph should be taken to rule out any fractures of the tooth or surrounding bone and to evaluate the size and length of the pulp canal. A preoperative injection of an antibiotic is given to help minimize the effects of accidentally introducing infection.

The crowns of all four canine teeth are then amputated with a DOUBLE–SIDED DIAMOND DISC on a low–speed handpiece with water coolant. For small animals, such as cats, a straight or a tapered diamond bur on a high–speed handpiece with water coolant can be used. The level to which the cut is made is about level with or just below the incisor crown height (Photo 60). This means that about two thirds to three quarters of the crown length is removed.

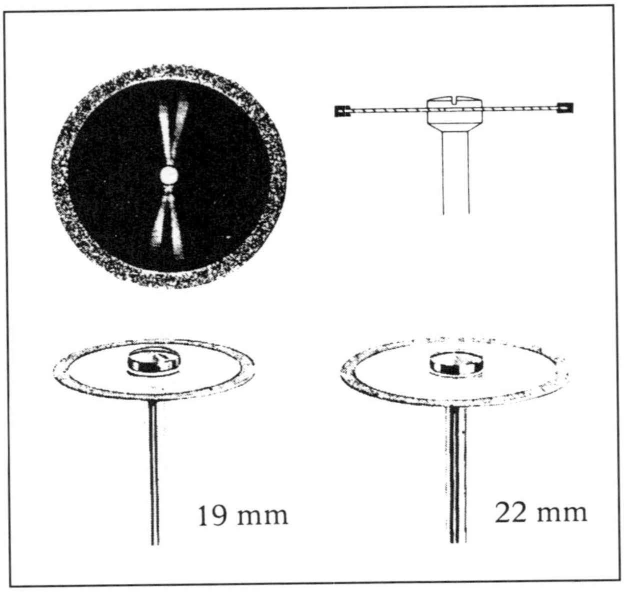

Figure 95. Diamond disc for cutting teeth.

(Beware — dangerous instrument. May cut finger or shatter in face.)

An important word of caution at this time is that a diamond disc is a very dangerous instrument. If it locks up or catches, it can fly out and severely damage fingers or the pet's oral tissues. It can also break and parts will fly out in the plane of rotation and injure your face or eyes. Safety glasses are highly recommended. Holding the handpiece with two hands will afford safer control and more precise cutting. The angle of the cut should be in a horizontal line with the incisors and premolars.

In most cases, the pulp of the tooth will be exposed immediately and usually bleeds. However, before any attempt to stop the bleeding is made, the vital pulpotomy must be completed. This is done with a sterile, sharp, round bur, a size just smaller than the pulp chamber, and must be used in a high–speed handpiece. At high speed, the pulp is cut without tearing.

Although the pulp within the remaining stump of the crown can be removed down to the level of the gingiva, it is only necessary to remove enough pulp to place all the filling materials. These are an initial layer of calcium hydroxide, an intermediate layer such as a glass ionomer and a final restorative material such as composite.

In order to stop the bleeding, a tiny cotton pledget, soaked in epinephrine (1:30,000 or 1:50,000) or other hemostatic agents, is packed gently into the pulp canal. This procedure may have to be repeated several times to stop the bleeding. The blunt end of sterile paper points can also be used. Healthy pulp will usually stop bleeding after a few minutes. If there is still some seepage that will not respond to the hemostatic agent, the first of the filling materials, calcium hydroxide, can be gently packed into the cavity. However, under these circumstances, powdered CaOH should be used, since it will absorb the blood and usually stop the seepage. When there is no further bleeding, hard setting concentrated CaOH, such as "HYPOCAL" or CaOH paste, is placed on top of the powdered CaOH. The thickness of these layers should be about 1 mm each.

Calcium hydroxide is always used as the initial layer, because it stimulates the odontoblasts to produce a bridge of reparative dentin, thus sealing the sensitive exposed pulp.

Due to the small size of the working area, there is bound to be some calcium hydroxide on the walls of the pulp chamber or even filling most of the exposed pulp chamber. This must be cleaned out with a small inverted cone bur to make room for the next or INTERMEDIATE RESTORATIVE LAYER, which provides strength over the sensitive and easily compressible pulp.

Although many materials can be used for this layer, such as reinforced zinc oxide–eugenol (e.g., IRM), zinc oxyphosphate and glass ionomers, the most effective and rapid is a light–cured glass ionomer (e.g., Vitrebond). The thickness of this layer should be about two millimeters. The glass ionomer bonds with the dentin, releases fluoride, and desensitizes to the dentin. However, the most important reason to use a light–cured glass ionomer is that you don't have to wait for it to dry, which saves unnecessary anesthesia time. The remaining coronal part of the pulp chamber (1–2 mm) is then drilled out with an inverted cone bur to aid in the retention of the final restorative material (Photo 61).

Although traditionally amalgam has always been used as a final restorative in these cases, the disadvantage is that an "amalgam tattoo" will occur later and does not look esthetically pleasing. The AMALGAM TATTOO that develops, appears six months to one year later as a black stain in the surrounding dentin. It often spreads throughout the entire cut surface of the reduced crown, and is due to the corrosive products of amalgam leaching out into the dentin. This may be prevented by applying an amalgam adhesive bonding agent, such as Amalgambond (Parkell), over the dentin in the cavity preparation. This bonding agent is a two–part self–curing system that is applied with a brush. Amalgam Bond also bonds the amalgam to the dentin, giving additional retention to the amalgam restoration. In very large dogs or those with a strong bite (such as Pit Bull terriers), amalgam is the best final restorative material. The amalgam is placed, condensed and contoured level with the flat reduced crown of the tooth (see amalgam fillings, 6.7).

A better esthetic result, which also protects the exposed dentin on the cut surface of the crown, can be obtained by using a light–cured composite (numerous brands are available). For maximum retention it is best to CHAMFER the enamel 1–2 mm around the coronal edges of the cut "stump" of the crown, before placing the composite (Photo 62). Since the largest part of the cut surface to restore is dentin, a relatively new etching compound such as Chamelon's "Mirage" should be used. This is 2.5% nitric acid and is designed to etch the dentin as well as the enamel. These etching products are also good for etching enamel hypoplasia lesions and lateral slab fractures of the maxillary fourth premolars prior to restoration. DENTIN ADHESIVES may also prove beneficial in these cases, but are currently controversial.

The etching is followed by a dentin primer and composite adhesive (resin). After the composite has been placed and light–cured, the edges and coronal surfaces are contoured with a finishing bur in a high–speed handpiece. The restorative material is then sanded with a sanding disc and polished with a polishing pad in a low–speed handpiece, leaving a "flattened dome–like" crown (Photo 63).

Be sure to use a fine spray of water when sanding, to prevent any heat build up. Running your fingers or an explorer over the edges will tell you if it is finished smoothly and properly.

Sometimes there will be sharp points on the tips of the incisors. These can also be removed with a diamond bur, smoothed with a sanding disc and then polished.

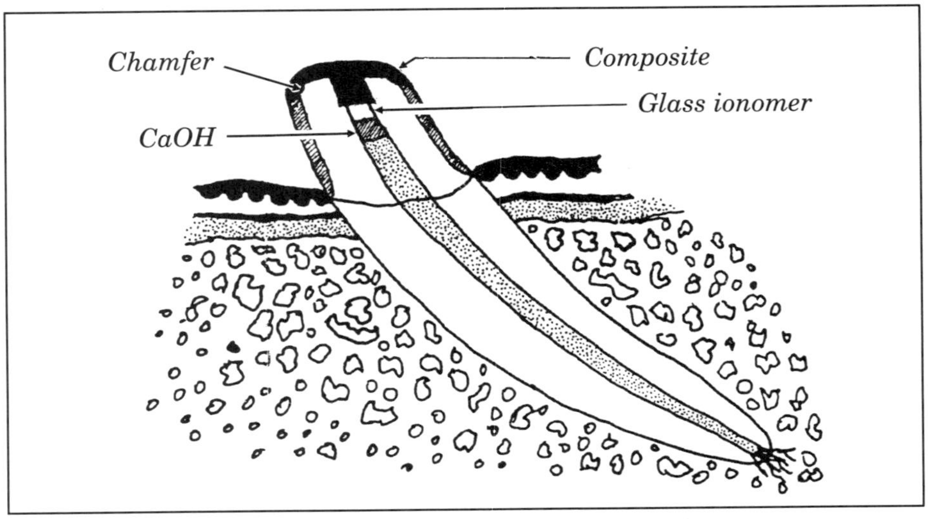

Figure 96. Diagrammatic section showing the layers of the direct pulp capping materials.

Caution should be used when performing a crown reduction procedure on dogs under one to one and a half years of age, because the pulp chamber can be very wide. This may create difficulties in retaining the final restoration, since it may fall out or be pushed in. Small cast metal caps should be considered to protect the stump. The owner should be advised that because the walls of the tooth will not be very strong until the pulp canal has matured, at one and a half or two years of age, there is a risk of fracturing the stump. An alternative to vital pulpotomy is to perform a complete root canal procedure, after the crown has been reduced, sealing the apex and then filling the entire cavity with amalgam, metal–reinforced glass ionomers or titanium–filled composite. Of course this will not allow closure of the pulp cavity with secondary dentin, but in turn these materials will provide strength to the remaining tooth structure.

In some old dogs, there may be only a small pulp chamber, with little or no pulp exposure. In these cases a pulpotomy should still be performed as described above.

7.18 CROWN REDUCTION OF RODENTS

The most common dental problem seen in rodents is malocclusion, although periodontal disease, caries and stomatitis can be found. The incisors of all rodents and the molars of some, such as guinea pigs and chinchilla, are open–rooted and have continuous eruption and constant wear in normal occlusion. Any malocclusion will allow uncontrolled overgrowth of the misaligned teeth. Another factor contributing to constant wear on the incisors is the lack of enamel on the lingual surface of the tooth. Enamel is found only on the *labial*, *mesial* and *distal* surfaces of the incisors. On the *lingual* surface there is only dentin, although there can be a thin layer of enamel (and sometimes cementum). Constant wearing of these teeth in normal scissor–like occlusion creates a sharp, chisel–like edge on the labial surface of the incisors.

Malocclusions occur for different reasons, including genetics, trauma, diet, loss of teeth and bad dental and chewing habits. Symptoms of affected animals include obviously overgrown teeth, such as the incisors, drooling and wet hair around the mouth, swelling of the jaw, inappetence and weight loss. Maloccluded mandibular cheek teeth tend to overgrow and form sharp points *lingually* and on the maxillary cheek teeth *buccally*. Maloccluded incisor teeth tend to overgrow straight or deviate sideways. Unless realignment can be achieved, which is usually impossible, treatment is to reduce the crown on a regular basis, every one to two months or as necessary, using straight carbide or diamond burs, nail clippers, rongeurs, rasps or files (Photo 59). Care must be taken not to crush or splinter teeth with hand instruments, as damage can lead to infection and abscesses, not to mention being painful. If the pulp is exposed during crown reduction, calcium hydroxide and an intermediate restorative material, such as IRM, should be placed over the pulp. Removal of an open–rooted tooth should only be done if absolutely necessary, since the root often takes up 80 percent of the total length of the tooth, which will be difficult to accomplish and will also create an overgrowth of the opposing tooth.

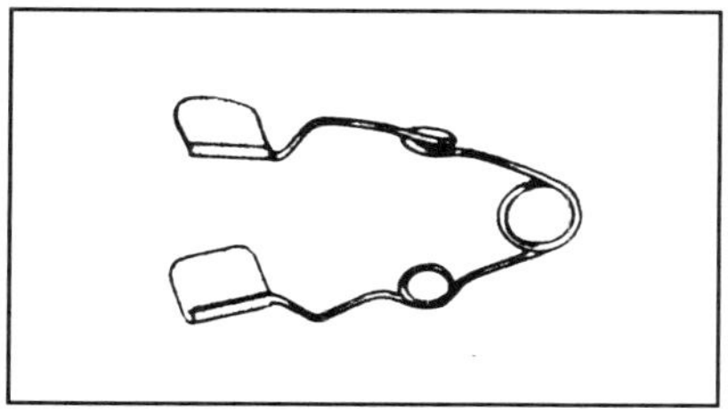

Figure 97. Rodent cheek expander (small).

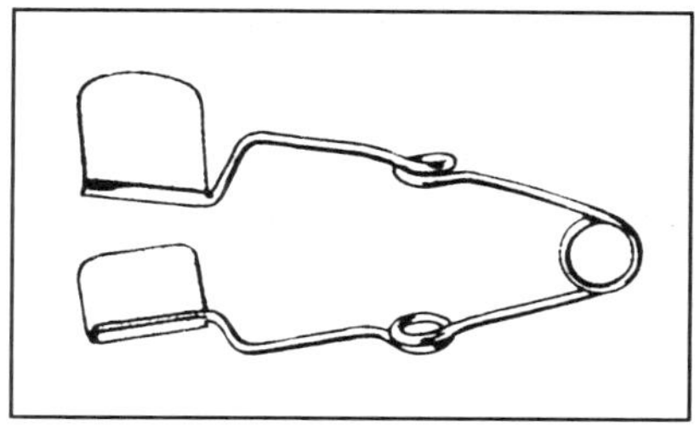

Figure 98. Rodent cheek expander (large).

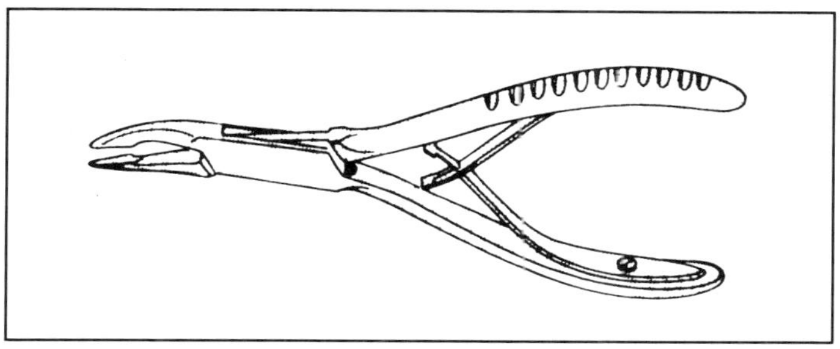

Figure 99. Rongeur (small) for clipping rodent teeth.

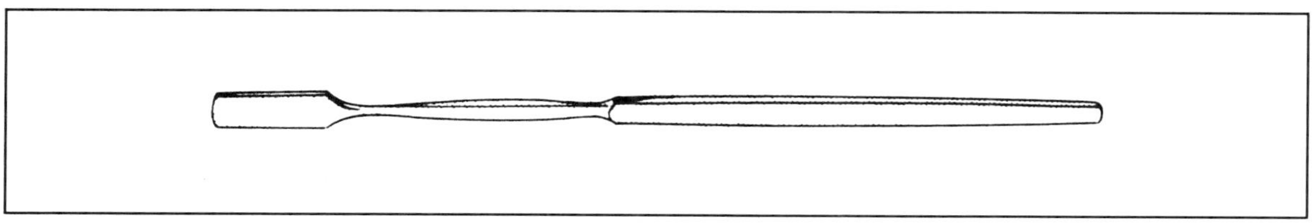

Figure 100. Tongue spatula.

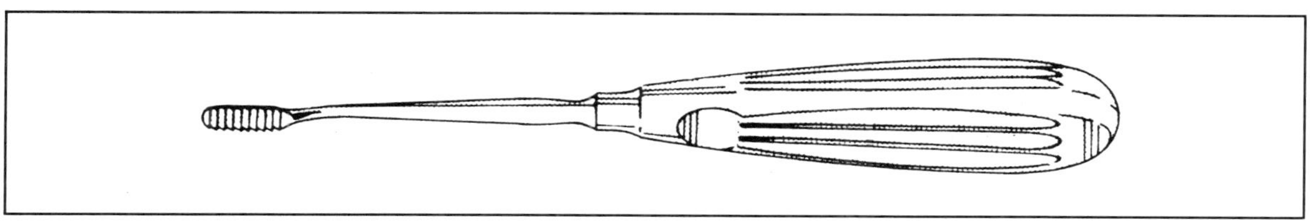

Figure 101. Rasp (to smooth surface).

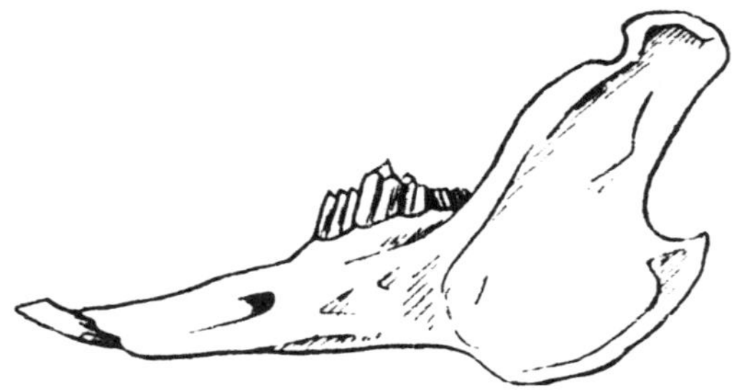

Figure 102. Molar overgrowth on a rabbit.

Generally the crowns of the incisors of rodents can be reduced with the animal awake, but to work on the premolars and molars, sedation or anesthesia is usually necessary. Ketamine, diazepam, xylazine and isoflurane can all be used with care. Access to the cheek teeth can be made easier with the use of various instruments, such as special rodent mouth gags, cheek expanders, tongue depressors and spatulas. Although these instruments will allow forcible access to the cheek teeth of an unanesthetized animal, this can be painful, cruel and even lead to heart failure. Some form of chemical restraint is generally best.

Although gas anesthesia, such as isoflurane, is the safest method, rabbits (and rodents) are very difficult to intubate. To avoid any unnecessary trauma that may occur in attempts to pass an endotracheal tube, an alternative technique is suggested. After initial induction or sedation, pass the endotracheal tube so that the tip lies at about the level of the epiglottis. Although this is not the ideal method, enough anesthetic gas will be inhaled by the animal to maintain anesthesia.

If this technique is used, a face mask should be worn by the operator and any assistant. A fan can be placed near by to blow the escaping gas away from the area. Because of the risks to personnel of inhaling the escaping gas, this method should only be used as a last resort and for short procedures.

CHAPTER 8

PROSTHODONTICS (PROSTHETICS)

Prosthodontics (or prosthetics) is the restoration and maintenance of oral functions by replacement of missing teeth and contiguous tissues with artificial substitutes. The branch of prosthodontics most commonly used in veterinary medicine is the replacement of a damaged tooth crown with an artificial (usually cast metal) crown.

Generally the demand is for the replacement of the crown of a *single* damaged tooth. The most commonly involved teeth are the canine teeth, maxillary fourth premolars, and sometimes the incisors. The journals and texts contain descriptions of how almost every type of human prosthetic device has been used on animals. The long term prognosis is dependent upon the biting and oral habits of the pet and varies from average to good.

CROWN RETENTION can be divided into:

HIGH RETENTION

1. Cross–pinned crown.
2. Stainless steel crown on vital, full length tooth crown (e.g., enamel hypoplasia teeth).

ACCEPTABLE RETENTION

1. Crown and post unit (there may be difficulty in getting an accurate impression of the post).
2. Crowns on large "stumps" and older dogs (where the thick dentin layer allows parallel preparation of the remaining "stump," sacrificing some dentin material).

POOR RETENTION

1. Composite build–up.
2. Crown on reduced "stump."

3. Crown on juvenile “stump” without adequate core build–up.
4. Jacket crown (breakage or loss if poor fit).
5. Porcelain bonded crown (loss of facing).
6. Plastic crown (abrasion).

The following is an attempt to systematically present successful solutions to the most common prosthetic problems. In each case consideration should be given to the condition of the other teeth, the age of the animal, the usefulness of the prosthesis and, last but not least, the financial limitations of the owner.

8.1 COMPOSITE CROWN RESTORATIONS

Composite crown restoration is strictly speaking a *conservative restorative treatment*. The principles of composite restoration have been discussed (see composite fillings, 6.8). Composite is useful to restore the fractured tips of the canine teeth in small dogs. The composite is either built up on the fractured tip, or a strip–off crown form can be used. Additional retention of the composite can be achieved by incorporating pins or posts into the preparation. Small parapulpal pins (e.g., TMS pins), can be inserted into the dentin in vital and non–vital teeth, and pulpal posts can be inserted into the pulp canal of non–vital, endodontically treated teeth. Pins and posts are recommended for additional retention of composite on oblique crown tip fractures.

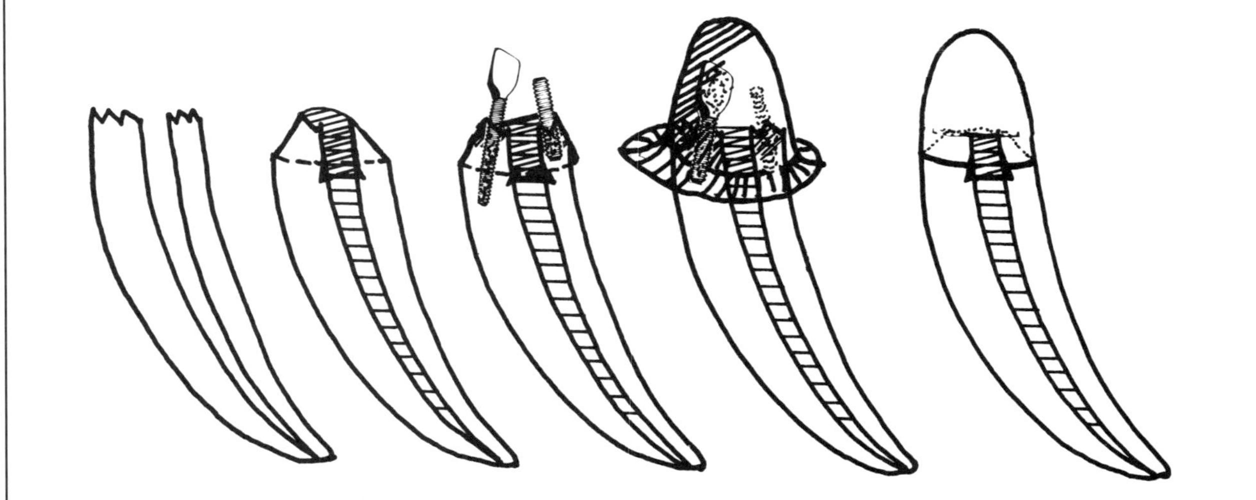

Figure 103 A–E. Crown build–up with composite, using strip–off crown form.

103 A. Fractured canine tooth after instrumentation.
103 B. Canal filled and sealed.
103 C. Parapulpal pins placed in dentin.
103 D. Placement of composite in strip–off crown form.
103 E. The finished preparation, shorter and rounder than the normal tooth.

For a crown with small fracture of the tip that is perpendicular to the tooth, and with no pulp exposure, it is wise *not* to restore the tip to its original height, because the composite can easily break off. Just restore the tip with a thin "dome" of composite and contour it with a bur and sanding disc. Another option is to smooth the fractured tooth surface with a bur and sanding disc, without placing any composite. The exposed dentin tubules will eventually acquire a brown stain. This is secondary dentin that will form to help protect the exposed primary dentin.

Composite is not as durable as a cast metal crown. Although a good esthetic result can as be obtained, composite restorations of the tip of a tooth are especially susceptible to shear forces. For this reason, composite crown restorations are recommended more for small pet dogs than for working dogs, such as police or guard dogs. As a guide, only pet dogs under 40 pounds of weight should be treated with composite crown restorations.

8.2 CAST METAL CROWNS (CAPS)

A cast metal CROWN (or CAP) is a FIXED PROSTHETIC DEVICE, which is placed over the damaged crown of the tooth or over a core build–up. Many different combinations of metal are available (see metals for crowns, 12.17). Cast metal crowns are indicated for the restoration of:

1. Fractured tooth crowns.
2. Teeth with severe enamel hypoplasia.

8.3 CAST METAL CROWNS FOR FRACTURED TEETH

The prognosis for retaining cast metal crowns on *fractured teeth* is not always good. Constant abuse of the teeth leads to the loss of the crown, sometimes shortly after fitting. Since the costs for cast crown restorations are high, it is important to warn the owner of the possible risk of crown loss before beginning the procedure. Acknowledgement of this risk by the client should be recorded on your diagnostic dental chart.

It is important to take a good history to discover the cause of the tooth fracture. Accidental tooth fractures, since they are unlikely to be repeated, have a better prognosis than tooth injuries caused by habitual dog fighting and chain link fence chewing. It is inadvisable to place too much reliance in the *strength* of a cast crown. A tooth with a cast crown should always be considered weaker than a natural tooth and is only as strong as the tooth structure it covers. The accuracy of the fit is also very important.

Another consideration when recommending cast crown restorations concerns which tooth is involved. Fractured incisors, premolars and molars are often better treated by conservative restoration or extraction, since domestic dogs can live perfectly comfortably with partially restored or even missing teeth. However, try to retain the carnassial teeth and the maxillary first molars since these are the important teeth used in shearing and chewing. The mandibular canine teeth present an especially good case for crown restoration since:

1. Extraction of periodontally sound mandibular canine teeth is difficult and usually requires a mucogingival flap and osteotomy. There is also an associated risk of iatrogenic and spontaneous fracture of the mandible.
2. The mandibular canine teeth provide a guide for the tongue. Their loss allows the tongue to slip to one side where it can be bitten, often traumatizing the tongue and its nerve supply (lingual nerve).

Fractured carnassial teeth (maxillary P4, mandibular M1) are generally restored with amalgam, light–cured composites and some glass ionomers. Usually it is only the buccal enamel that has split off and can be repaired with a simple filling. Although restoration of the carnassial teeth can be made with a cast metal crown, the procedure is more difficult because:

1. The shape of the carnassial teeth is far more complicated than that of the canine teeth and requires more skill and experience to prepare for a cast crown.
2. The steep occlusion must meet the facets of the antagonist accurately. Very accurate impressions of the teeth and the bite are necessary.
3. The forces developed by these teeth are so great that the slightest inaccuracy during the preparation and casting will lead to failure of the crown.

Notwithstanding the fact that some teeth are more difficult to prepare, cast crowns are by far the most satisfactory method of restoring a fractured tooth. Gold crowns can be used, but their high cost and softer composition make them less suitable than crowns made of other metals, such as chrome–cobalt–molybdenum alloy, stainless steel (Photo 67) and silver–palladium alloy (see metals for crowns, 12.17). Although full cast crowns are generally used, partial and half crowns can be made depending on the situation (Photo 75).

Before the tooth impression can be made for crown fabrication, it is usually necessary to repair the remaining crown or "stump" of the damaged tooth. In order to give the remaining "stump" of the tooth the strength and shape necessary to retain the crown, a core build–up, or a post and core build–up may be necessary (see post and core build–up for fractured canine teeth, 8.6).

An important factor in preparing the "stump" of the crown for a metal crown, is to leave a good diameter of tooth material at the gingival margin. If the entire circumferential edge of the cast crown overlaps the prepared axial walls of the tooth at the gingival margin by 1.5 mm or more, it will act much like the metal ferrule band around a wooden mallet, creating a "FERRULE" EFFECT. The crown will hold the tooth together, reinforcing it against fracture under functional load. The crown of the tooth and core build–up just above this point should be BEVELLED. Whether this is above or below the gingival margin depends on the individual situation, but slightly above the gingival margin is generally preferable.

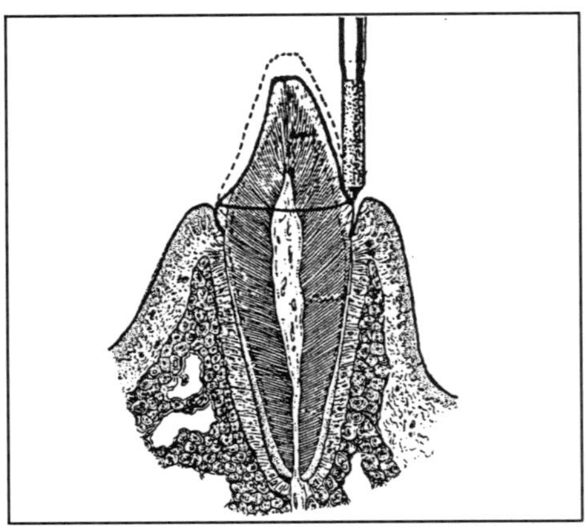

Figure 104 A.

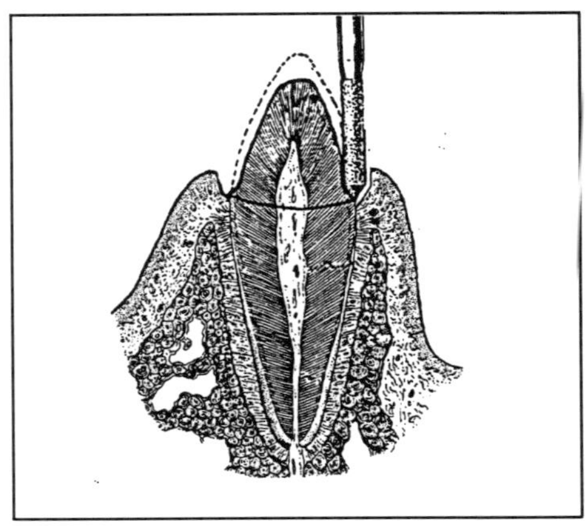

Figure 104 B.

104 A. Bevel preparation above gingival margin. (Impression technique easier and self cleaning of joint better.)

104 B. Bevel preparation below gingival margin. (Impression technique more difficult due to hemorrhage. Food debris more likely to be retained due to irregularity at crown–tooth margin.)

Occasionally lost or missing incisors can be replaced with a bridge. A BRIDGE is a fixed or stationary prosthesis, replacing one or more lost or missing teeth. It is supported or held in place by the adjacent teeth or ABUTMENTS. The part of the bridge that replaces the lost crown and occupies the space it previously occupied is called the PONTIC. Bridge restorations can be expensive, and generally have a poor prognosis. Irritation of the gingiva under the bridge is sometimes so unpleasant that the dog will try to remove it. The construction is inherently unstable because of the leverage forces involved and will often fail unless both canine teeth are included. A bridge from I3 to 3I for example will usually fail.

More recently core implants have been used to successfully replace missing or lost teeth. A modern IMPLANT is a cylindrical hollow titanium (or similar) post, which is implanted, after careful drilling, into the osseous tissue of the jaw. The artificial tooth or crown is attached to the implant after osseous integration has secured it (e.g., Branemark technique).

Placing of crowns on the canine teeth is the most common and rewarding prosthetic procedure in veterinary dental practice. With a little practice this operation can be economically and successfully performed.

8.4 CAST METAL CROWNS FOR TEETH WITH ENAMEL HYPOPLASIA

Enamel hypoplasia is an enamel defect due to partial failure of the enamel to develop (Photo 76). This is acquired during the development of the tooth and may be hereditary. Enamel hypoplasia is occasionally caused by trauma that affects the developing enamel without damaging the pulp or otherwise affecting tooth development. Viral infections such as canine distemper and vitamin A, C or D deficiency can also damage the developing enamel.

The prognosis for placing cast metal crowns on hypoplastic teeth is generally good. However, constant overloading forces on teeth restored with cast metal crowns, such as occurs with police and guard dogs or aggressive and mistreated dogs, can adversely affect the prognosis of these cast crowns. *GRECK* et al (1976) reported a case of enamel hypoplasia in which four cast metal crowns were placed in a Boxer dog. These cast crowns remained clinically adequate over a period of 12 years.

Simple cast crowns are made of a thimble–like construction that resembles the tooth it restores. Cast crowns for veterinary use are normally made from CHROME–COBALT–MOLYBDENUM ALLOY or from STAINLESS STEEL (nickel–chrome alloy), because they are less expensive and harder than gold. Cast crowns can be made of GOLD ALLOY, which is easier for the dental laboratory to work with, but the material cost is higher. It is worth getting estimates for different materials from the dental laboratory. Although gold is strong, stainless steel is harder and more resistant to abrasion. A few dental laboratories are now making crowns made of TITANIUM ALLOY (Photo 66). They are stronger and lighter than other metals, but may cost as much as gold alloy crowns (see metals for crowns 12.17).

Cast metal crowns are ideally suited for most enamel hypoplasia cases. The only preparation necessary is reduction of the remaining enamel with a diamond bur. The crown preparation should have a conical shape without undercuts and end at, or just above, the gingival margin (Photo 77). The occlusion should then be checked. Since hypoplastic teeth are smaller than normal, they are often out of contact with opposing teeth prior to the crown preparation. In this case, only minimal preparation is necessary to provide enough space for the thickness of the crown (about 1–2 mm). When the prepared "stump" has been cleaned and dried, an impression is made, preferably with a silicone based impression material (see impressions and stone models, 12.16). The impression is sent to a dental laboratory, which should return the finished cast crown in about five days. Next, the cast crown should be put in place to check the occlusion (Photo 78). If any part of the cast crown contacts any part of the opposing teeth before the rest of the teeth achieve contact, the cast crown must be reduced with a diamond or tungsten carbide bur until sufficient clearance is achieved. The cast crown is then carefully repolished.

Contact of the cast crown with opposing or antagonistic teeth should be avoided since it can lead to:

1. Misalignment of the temporomandibular joint with consequential arthrosis.
2. Additional stress on the muscles of mastication resulting in MYOFACIAL PAIN SYNDROME.
3. Periodontal loosening of the restored tooth or the opposing tooth.
4. Wear on the cast crown, if a softer gold alloy crown has been used.
5. Enamel abrasion on the opposing tooth(or teeth), especially if the cast crown is made of a hard metal such as stainless steel or titanium.

Before cementing the cast crown, the tooth and the inside of the cast crown should be washed with water and dried, and then rinsed with alcohol to remove any oily film. Luting cements such as glass–ionomer cements and zinc oxyphosphate cements can be used to attach the cast crown. Newer luting cements such as Panavia (Parkell) and Geristore (Denmat) are extremely strong and effective for animals' teeth. It is important to carefully follow the manufacturer's instructions for mixing. After a few minutes, when the cement has set, the flash can be removed with a scaler.

8.5 PORCELAIN, CERAMIC AND RESIN CROWNS

An excellent cosmetic effect can be attained by using tooth–colored materials, although in animals, strength is more important than cosmetics. There are several types of tooth–colored crowns available:

1. Cast metal crowns with polymerized resin facings.
2. Porcelain jacket crowns.
3. Cast metal crowns with vacuum–fired porcelain facings.
4. Porcelain jacket crowns with hardened ceramic cores.

They are not all suitable for animal use, and then only with special conditions.

CAST METAL CROWNS WITH POLYMERIZED RESIN FACINGS are not suitable for animal use since the resin (or plastic) facing can be lost or become abraded.

PORCELAIN JACKET CROWNS are also not suitable for animal use since the porcelain by itself is brittle and has the tendency to shatter, even under moderate forces.

CAST METAL CROWNS WITH VACUUM–FIRED PORCELAIN FACINGS (PORCELAIN FUSED TO METAL CROWNS) have been in use for decades in humans and are available from every dental laboratory (Photo 68). The facing, however, is not usually strong enough to withstand the sort of wear that large working dogs experience, so the cases and particular teeth should be chosen carefully. Should the facing become damaged it can be smoothed with a fine diamond or stone bur and left in place. Its function will generally be adequate, even if the esthetics suffer.

PORCELAIN JACKET CROWNS WITH HARDENED CERAMIC CORES are also suitable for small dogs and certain teeth, such as the incisors. The new generation of *type four* hard–cored all ceramic crowns (e.g., IN–CERAM), have high strength ratings and are a potentially acceptable restoration in selected cases.

The high cost of porcelain fused to metal crowns, and porcelain/ceramic crowns, plus their limited durability under high occlusal or pulling forces, emphasizes how good a simple cast metal crown can be. Porcelain and ceramic crowns are not generally recommended for maxillary fourth premolars and maxillary and mandibular molars. This is because the occlusal forces to which they will be subjected are very strong, and may result in a fracture of the porcelain.

8.6 POST AND CORE BUILD–UP FOR FRACTURED CANINE TEETH

If more than two thirds of the canine tooth crown has been broken off, it will be necessary to build a new core on the remaining tooth structure ("stump") in order to provide a stable base for a crown. To provide reinforcement and retention of the core build–up, a post or a cast dowel is necessary. This will aid in the distribution of stress, generated by torque, throughout the remaining tooth structure. The place where it is most important that a post achieves a close fit is at the coronal opening. Endodontic therapy must be performed before beginning the post and core build–up.

The choice of which type of core will provide the most durable restoration is dependent upon the size and shape of the root canal, and this in turn is dependent upon the age and size of the animal (Fig. 4). Additional support for the core build–up material is obtained by placing parapulpal pins in the dentin (see pins 12.14), and pulpal posts in the pulp cavity of endodontically treated teeth (see posts 12.15). There are several different methods of building up a core, depending on the situation presented:

1. ***Small and medium size young dogs, older large dogs with a root canal under 2 mm diameter*** (confirmed by radiograph). Drill out canal and place appropriate posts (e.g., FLEXI–POST, PARA–POST), followed by core build–up.
2. ***Large dogs with a root canal over 2 mm diameter*** (confirmed by radiograph). Preparation of the canal with cutting and tapping drills, and fitted with steel or brass bolts/posts, followed by core build–up.
3. ***Large dogs or very young dogs with very wide root canals*** (confirmed by radiograph). Pulp canal filling with amalgam, metal–filled glass ionomer (e.g., Ketac–Silver, Chelon Silver and "Miracle Mix") or titanium composite (e.g., Ti–Core). Posts or bolts can be incorporated into glass ionomers and composite.
4. ***Large dogs over about 15 months with a medium size root canal with slightly conical coronal part of the root canal*** (confirmed by radiograph). Prepare with tapered bur or drill, take an impression of the pulp cavity, fabricate an integrated cast crown and post unit (see cast crown and post unit, 8.12), or a separate cast post and cast crown.
5. ***Dogs with structural damage to the remaining crown of the tooth, but with no exposure of the pulp cavity***. Core build–up material, with or without additional support from parapulpal pins.

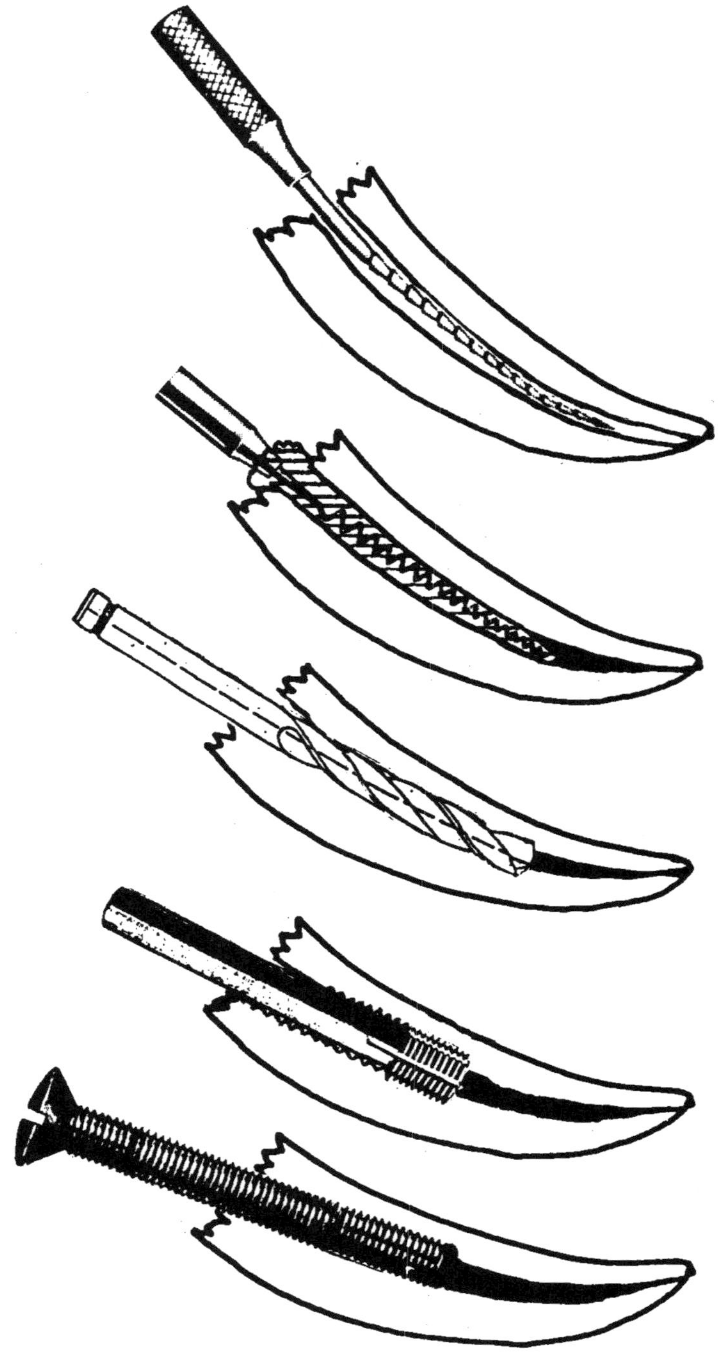

105 A

105 B

105 C

105 D

105 E

Figure 105 A–E. Threaded post preparation.

105 A. Instrumentation of canal followed by irrigation and drying.
105 B. Obturation of apex with sealer–filler paste using a lentulo spiral filler, followed by placement of gutta–percha points.
105 C. Drilling of canal to post depth. Some coronal gutta–percha will be removed.
105 D. Cutting a thread in the dentin with a tapping screw.
105 E. Cementation of appropriate screw.

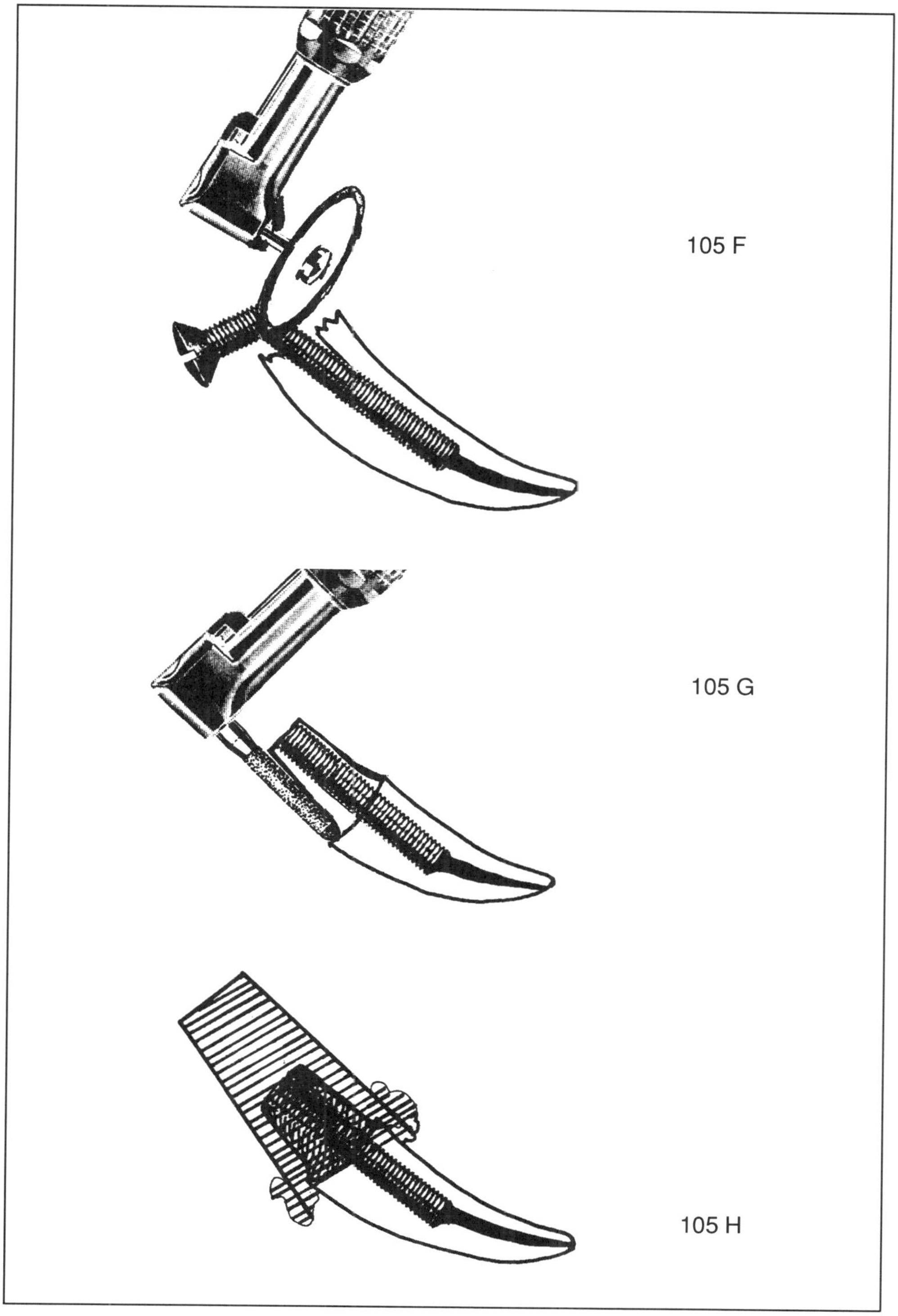

Figure 105 F–H. Threaded post preparation.

105 F. Cutting off excess screw length with diamond disc.
105 G. Circumferential beveling of core build–up with a tapered diamond bur (cut down to the gingival margin).
105 H. Taking impression with silicone impression material.

This seemingly bewildering choice is made necessary by the anatomy of the root canal. The goal of a core build–up is to provide a solid "backbone" or framework to stabilize the remaining tooth to accept the crown. This "backbone" and the remaining tooth "stump" provide a solid unit upon which a crown may be fabricated. After the tooth has been built up, the tooth material and core build–up are reduced with a diamond bur, to produce a conical preparation without undercuts, ending at, or just above, the gingival margin. An impression of the preparation is sent to the dental laboratory for fabrication of the crown. The fit of the finished crown is highly dependent upon an accurate impression. It is wise to practice taking impressions, since a poor impression will lead to a bad fit and the procedure will have to be repeated.

Passive and *active posts* used in human dentistry are effective for core build–up, but are only available up to a diameter of 2 mm and a length of 20 mm. This means that they are ineffective for long, wide canals. Although not strictly medical grade, but nonetheless effective, stainless steel tapping screws or appropriate bolts from the local hardware shop make excellent posts for large pulp cavities (see posts, 12.15). These screws and bolts should be sterilized prior to use.

8.7 POST CHANNEL PREPARATION

Prior to preparing or drilling a channel for a post, a complete endodontic filling should be in place (preferably with gutta–percha and a sealing cement material).

The gutta–percha should be removed to the required post length with a Peeso reamer drill. This helps orient the parallel–sided post drill. When drilling the canal to accept the post, it is best to start with a small diameter drill, and increase the size progressively until the desired canal size is reached, thereby reducing the risk of perforation. For example, if a 4–mm diameter screw is chosen, it is best to start with a 2–mm diameter drill. A radiograph can be taken with the drill in the root canal to confirm the drill position, as well as the thickness of enamel and dentin that is still available. The point at which the drill enters the tooth can be marked on the drill with a marking pen and used to measure the drilled depth on the radiograph. Care should be taken not to remove too much endodontic filling material. As a rule of thumb, about two thirds of the length of the root canal should be prepared to accept the post. This should be approximately the length of the original crown.

When the canal has been drilled and any necessary thread has been cut, a few drops of thin luting cement are applied to the post, which is then screwed or placed into the canal. Care must be taken to ensure that the torquing pressure does not split the tooth or force the root filling material through the apex.

The risk of creating a perforation should not be underestimated (Fig. 106 B–D). *A perforation* is a serious complication and may cause damage that will lead to eventual loss of the tooth. A PERFORATION is the accidental drilling of a hole through a wall of a tooth. Periodontal and osseous will usually be involved also. The greatest chance for perforation is in the first portion of the root, and results from too steep an angle of entrance. The curvature of the root should not be underestimated, and the position of the apex should be visualized and used as an aiming guide. Larger "stumps" will often have to be reduced mesially in order to achieve the proper access (Fig. 106 A).

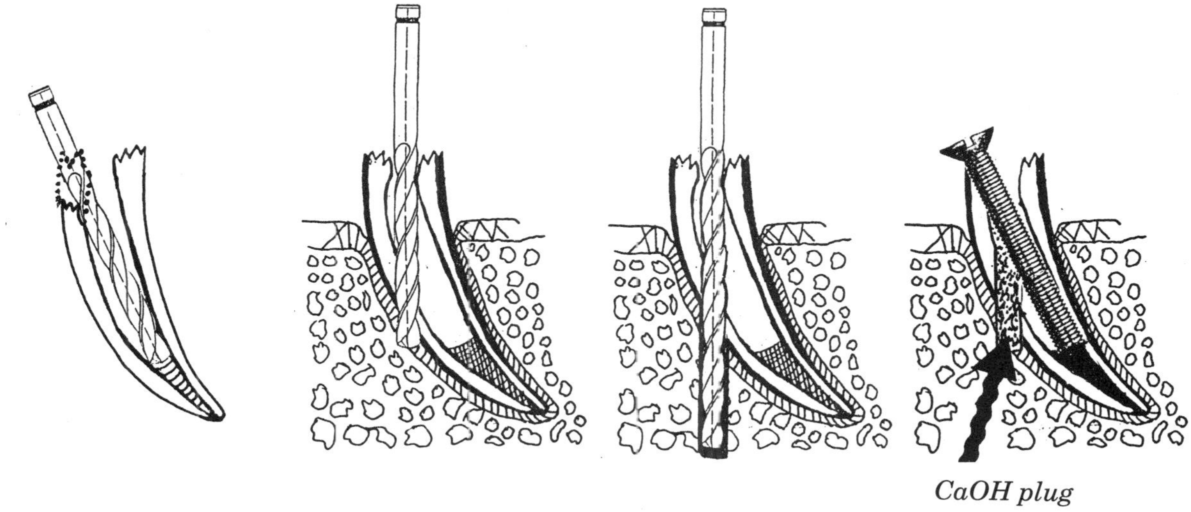

Figure 106 A–D. Post channel preparation.

106 A. Correct positioning — aim tip of pilot drill towards apex (some mesial dentin may have to be removed).
106 B. Small and shallow perforation — can be sealed with CaOH and tooth saved.
106 C. Large and deep perforation — periodontal and osseous tissues destroyed. Extraction of tooth may be necessary.
106 D. Fill perforation with CaOH paste, then place screw in correct position. (For completion of preparation see Fig. 105 F–H.)

A large perforation, and especially one that is discovered late, where the drill is already through the periodontal ligament and into the alveolar bone, will often necessitate future extraction of the tooth. However, a small perforation may be treatable. The drill must be removed immediately, and the preparation continued with the correct angulation. Immediately before the post is inserted, the perforation should be covered with a layer of calcium hydroxide paste. The calcium hydroxide stimulates osteoblastic new bone formation, which, since the calcium hydroxide is extruded into the periodontal space, can cause ankylosis between the tooth and the surrounding bone. The remaining periodontium is normally adequate for the retention and continued function of the tooth. A radiograph should be taken after four to six months to evaluate the integrity of the periodontium. If the periodontium should become infected after the operation, hemisection, apicoectomy or extraction of the tooth may be necessary.

8.8 CORE BUILD–UP WITH PULPAL POSTS

Pulpal posts or endo posts (e.g., Para–Posts) are parallel–sided steel posts with a flattened or a cylindrical head (Photo 64). Posts are available either as SERRATED or as SELF–THREADING. These posts are only of use in small teeth or in teeth with small diameter and depth of root canals.

Para–posts are available in 5 diameters — 0.9 mm, 1.0 mm, 1.25 mm, 1.5 mm, 1.75 mm. The posts are all 20 mm long.

Teeth with wide and long root canals will require custom–made posts (see posts, 12.15). Since large diameter drills are needed in order to prepare the canal for large custom–made posts, ordinary electric drill bits can be used. The shank of the drill bit must be reduced on a lathe, at a local machine shop, in order to fit the dental handpiece.

After placement of the post, the protruding post head is reduced and bent as necessary.

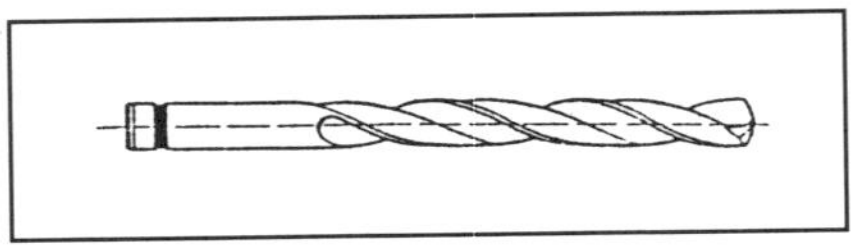

Figure 107 A. Normal drill bit.

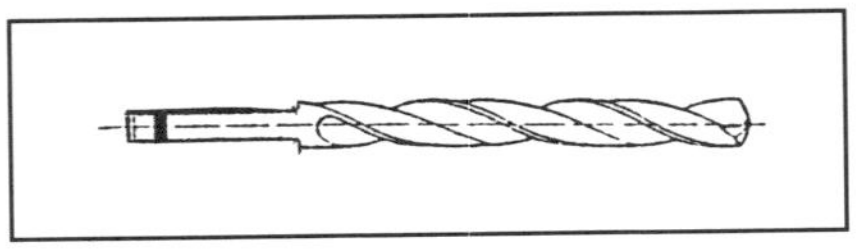

Figure 107 B. Shank turned on lathe to fit dental handpiece.

8.9 METHOD OF CORE BUILD–UP

When the post has been fully positioned into the tooth and the luting cement has set, core build–up and crown preparation can commence.

If an additional accessory hole from root canal therapy (*BODINGBAUER* method) has been made, as in a canine tooth endodontic procedure, the position of the post will need to be planned with special care. The new accessory entrance cannot be used for the post, so the actual position of the post, especially in highly curved roots, will lie somewhere between this access entrance and that of the original canal, even if a part of the remaining tooth crown must be sacrificed. The post should be placed in the middle of the remaining tooth. The additional entrance, and any space between the post and the wall of the canal, and over the post, should be filled with core build–up material. The core build–up should now be prepared for a crown. During the preparation it should be noted that retention is a major consideration. The CROWN PREPARATION should not be completely round, or forces that rotate the crown will tend to shear the cement (Photo 65). Facets, a groove or both can be cut on both sides of the core to prevent rotation. It is best to have the crown preparation end at, or just above, the gingival margin. It is not necessary to remove 1–2 mm of tooth structure over the entire crown surface (as in humans), since removing tooth tissue only weakens the underlying tooth. Where there are, or could be, occlusal contacts, sufficient tooth removal must be performed to allow for the thickness of the crown (1–2 mm), so as to prevent premature contacts. The only other removal necessary is removal of the surface curvature and the creation of straight sides, with the axial walls converging coronally at about *five* to *ten* degrees. The tooth and core build–up should be either bevelled or chamfered at the gingival margin.

The impressions can now be taken (see impressions and stone models, 12.16) and the crown can be fabricated by the dental laboratory. Since the tooth will be completely sealed a temporary crown is not necessary. Coordination with the laboratory will ensure the shortest waiting time, and give you a time schedule for fitting the crown. When received, the finished crown should be tried on and, if it fits, cemented into place.

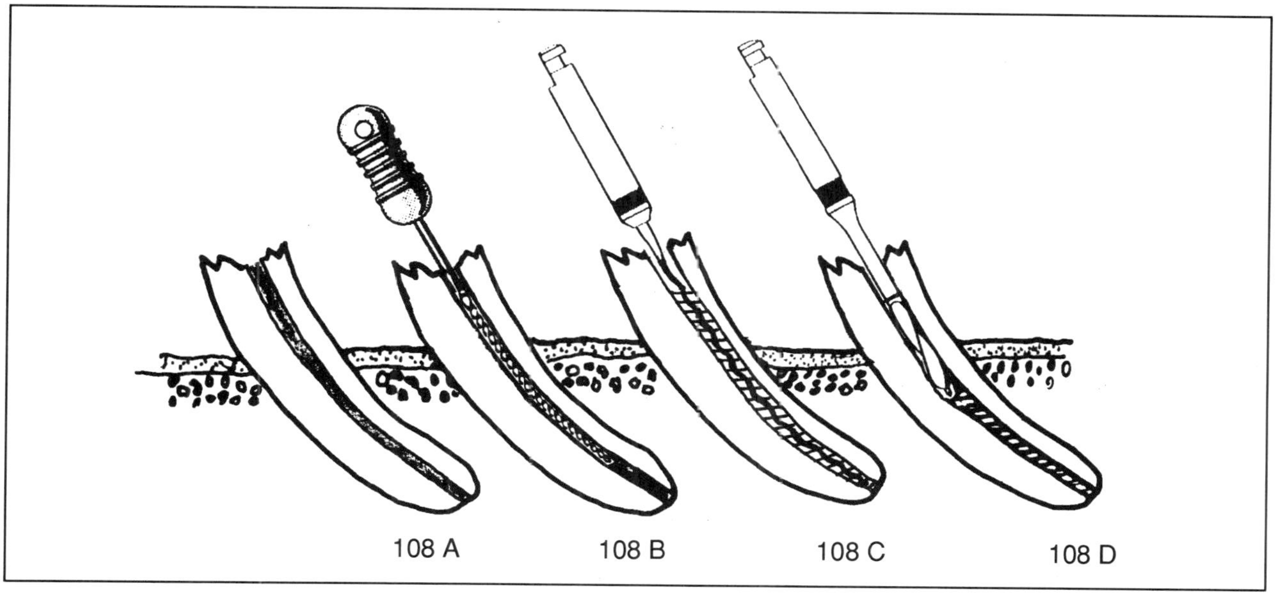

Figure 108 A–D. Preparation of a fractured canine tooth for post placement.

108 A. Canine tooth fracture with exposed pulp.
108 B. Instrumentation of canal with K–file.
108 C. Obturation of canal with sealer/filler using lentulo spiral filler.
108 D. Canal partially drilled to accept post, using matching drill.

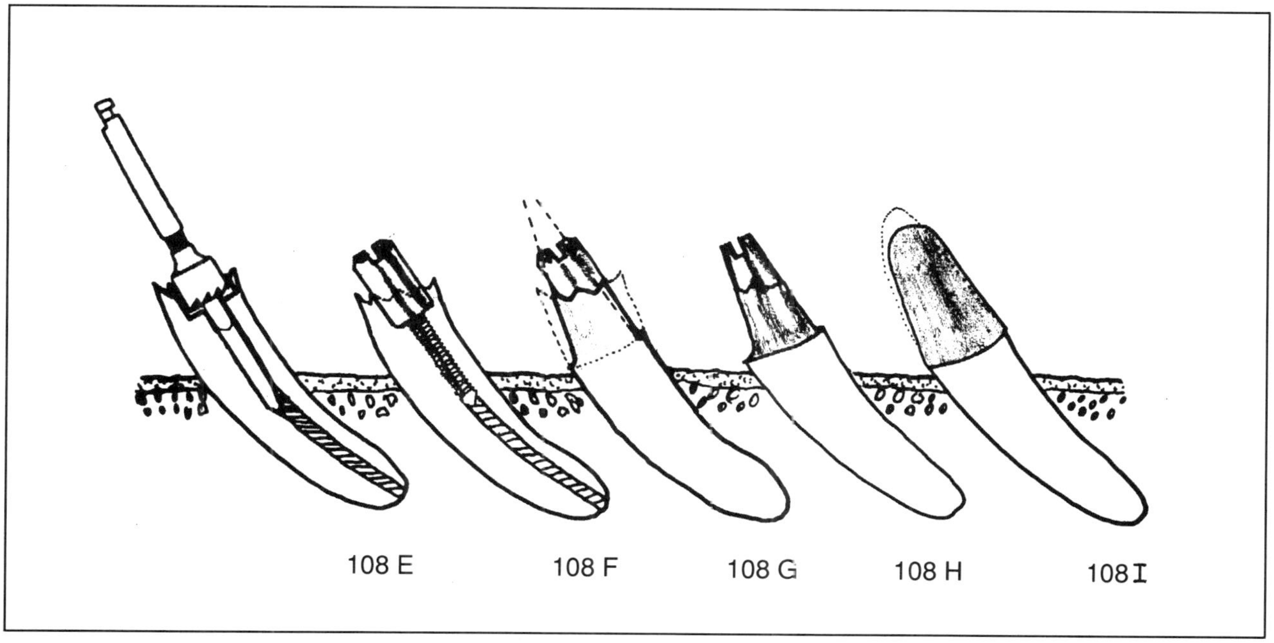

Figure 108 E–I. Preparation of a fractured canine tooth for post placement.

108 E. Preparation of coronal dentin with root facer.
108 F. Post cemented in place.
108 G. Circumferential beveling and preparation of stump.
108 H. Finished preparation with retention grove ready for impression.
108 I. Cast crown cemented in place. Crown is shorter and more rounded than original shape, to prevent fracture or loss due to the high leverage forces.

In order to reduce the leverage produced, the crowns planned for canine teeth should be shorter than the natural crown. The tip of the crown should also be more rounded to prevent any possible interference or trauma.

In the event that the animal has broken or damaged the core build–up and post during the crown fabrication period, all is not lost. If it is impossible to remove the remaining broken post, another post can usually be inserted parallel to the broken one. The core build–up can be reformed by placing some core build–up material in the cast crown and fitting it back over the post and remaining "stump." The inside of the crown should first be smeared with a thin layer of vaseline. This enables the crown to be removed for luting. Any excess flash of core build–up material must be removed from around the crown margin.

8.10 CORE BUILD–UP WITH A POST FOR JUVENILE TEETH

Fractured teeth in dogs under one to one and a half years of age have a WIDE PULP CANAL, which makes the preparation of a solid core considerably more difficult. In these large pulp canals, a good apical seal can be achieved using gutta–percha points and a sealing cement. However, standard posts or other systems cannot be used, because the largest available size is far too small for the canal. This is especially true for the canine teeth. The only contact would be at the root tip, and possibly at the coronal part of the tooth. The post would have no contact with the walls in the midsection of the root canal. Although they are not strictly medical grade, normal electric drill bits and stainless steel tapping screws, or specially threaded surgical intramedullary (I.M.) pins, can be used to get around this difficulty (Fig. 105A–H). If the post or the screw cannot be satisfactorily placed in the canal because the canal is too large, it can be incorporated into a canal filling of metal–reinforced glass ionomer or titanium–filled composite. Be sure that there is a hardened base in the root canal, over the root canal sealing cement, before the metal–reinforced glass ionomer, composite, post or screw is placed, or placement may force the sealing cement through the apex. If a post is used by itself, it is cemented into place with a luting cement. After this has set, the post or the screw is trimmed to size, bent if necessary, and the core built up (Fig. 105F–H).

8.11 CANAL AND CORE BUILD–UP WITH AMALGAM FOR JUVENILE TEETH

The post or the threaded screw method is not particularly good for the teeth of young dogs with very WIDE CANALS. Since most canine teeth have an elliptical root canal, the opening with a round drill leaves only very thin tooth walls on the buccal and lingual sides, which tend to fracture during or after placement of the screw. An excellent method for restoring these teeth is to fill the apical two thirds of the root canal and the remaining pulp chamber of the crown with amalgam.

The first point to note is that the juvenile root canal is shaped like a banana. Since the root canal should be filled, properly packed and free of bubbles, it is important to ensure adequate access. The coronal opening should be enlarged with a diamond or tungsten–carbide bur to the largest cross–section of the tooth. If the opening is too small, the amalgam cannot be properly condensed and becomes weak and shatters.

The usual amalgam plugger is too short. A better result is achieved with a simple nail or an intramedullary (I.M.) pin of the appropriate diameter. The end of the pin is cut off and filed smooth, and if desired the nail or the pin can be carefully bent to fit the curvature of the canal. A selection of curved and straight nails and pins of varying sizes should be pre–made.

The amalgam root canal filling is relatively simple and very strong.

It should be noted here that other materials can be used instead of amalgam, such as METAL REINFORCED GLASS IONOMERS (e.g., Ketac–Silver, Chelon–Silver and "Miracle–Mix") or TITANIUM REINFORCED COMPOSITE (e.g., Ti–Core). "Miracle–Mix" and Ti–Core FLEXI–FLOW can be injected into the canal with a special syringe (Centrix, "speed slot" with needle tubes).

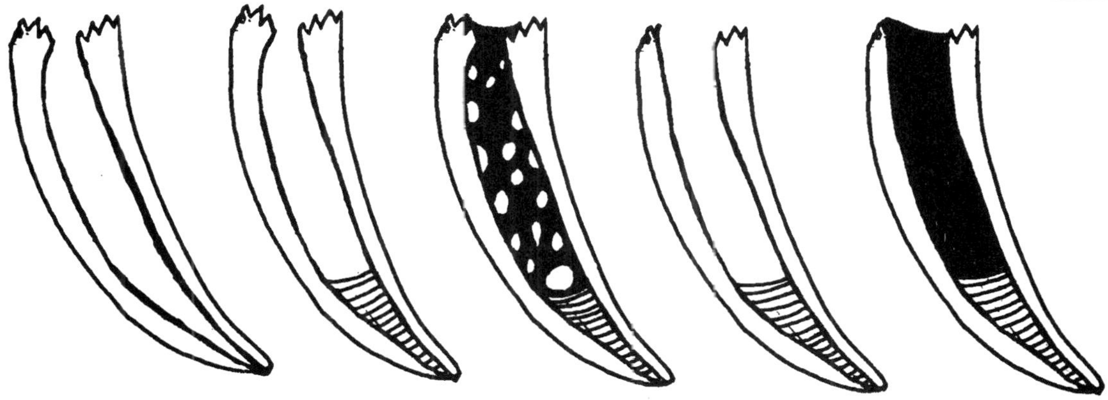

Figure 109 A–E . Filling pulp cavity of immature canine teeth with amalgam.

109 A. Fractured canine tooth of a young dog with wide pulp chamber.
109 B. Apex obturated with sealant and gutta–percha.
109 C. Incorrect condensation with amalgam, trapping air, due to narrow coronal access.
109 D. Coronal access widened for proper obturation.
109 E. Correct obturation and condensation with amalgam.

8.12 CAST METAL CROWN AND POST UNIT

An alternative method of prosthetic replacement is the INTEGRATED CAST METAL CROWN AND POST UNIT (Photo 74). After the canal has been filled with appropriate endodontic filler, the coronal two thirds is removed with a Peeso reamer drill. The canal is then widened with a tapered fissure or diamond bur to a slightly tapering form *without undercuts*. The external part of the "stump" should also be reduced, as usual, to a conical form down to the gingival margin. These two preparations must be aligned to have the same path of insertion. The most difficult part of the operation is obtaining an adequate impression of the coronal part of the canal. Additional support is required for the impression material. This is done with posts that are made of acrylic and can be purchased through a dental distributor. The acrylic posts are heated over a flame until malleable, and inserted into the root canal. They should extend about 4 mm out of the canal, and while still warm should be bent to form a hook or a ring to ensure better retention in the impression material. Homemade metal impression posts can also be made that serve the same purpose (Fig. 110B).

This "backbone" post should be roughened and coated with impression adhesive to prevent separation of the impression material. The canal is filled with light–bodied silicone rubber or polyether impression material from a syringe and the pin inserted. When the impression has hardened, it can be carefully removed. This impression material is accurately adapted to the interior of the canal, and is supported by the acrylic "backbone." This impression post is repositioned, and an impression of the rest of the tooth is made in the usual way. The impression tray should have deep vestibules to ensure that the tray does not press on the impression post, causing the impression of the canal to be deformed. The impression should be carefully removed in alignment with the long axis of the tooth. The bent end of the pin or the acrylic post holds it firmly in the impression material.

While the cast crown is being fabricated, the canal should be filled with cotton or temporary cement to prevent impaction of food. When the cast crown is finished, it should be tried in place and, if it fits properly, cemented with the appropriate cement. Since not only the inside, but also the outside of the preparation is cemented, good retention and stability can be expected.

Although the crown and post unit has its place in selected cases, a separate crown and core post are generally considered more advisable. The two–step crown and core fabrication is more accurate, since compromises often have to be made when making a single crown and post unit. If the cast crown fractures or the restoration has to be modified, a cast metal crown and post unit can be very hard to remove. When the crown is cemented separately from the core, it can improve the integrity of the remaining tooth, providing that 1.5 mm or more of the crown's gingival edge of the crown overlaps the axial wall of the tooth, creating a "ferrule" effect (see cast metal crowns for fractured teeth, 8.3).

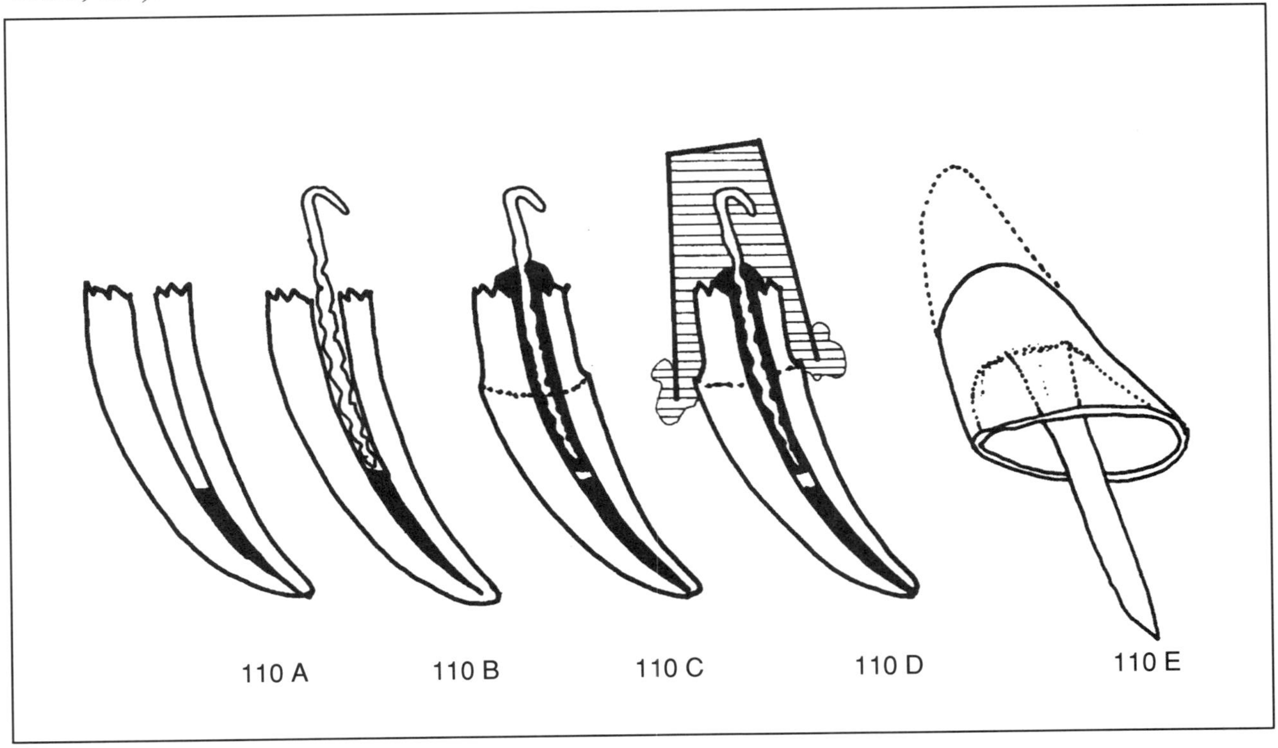

Figure 110 A–E. Taking impression for cast crown and post unit.

110 A. Apex obturated with sealant and coronal access widened.
110 B. Homemade metal impression post following contour of canal with bent tip for retention.
110 C. Impression post with impression material in canal. Stump bevelled and tapered.
110 D. Second impression incorporating previous impression of post (hook aids in retention).
110 E. Cast integrated crown and post unit ready for cementation. Crown itself is shorter and more rounded than original tooth.

8.13 CAST METAL POST AND CORE BUILD–UP

As an alternative to a cast crown–post unit, the post and core build–up can be cast in metal, separately from the crown.

Since pulpal posts are not currently available for the large pulp cavities of some dogs, a cast metal post and core can be custom made to provide a strong and accurate base for the cast crown.

Several methods are available. The canal preparation is similar to that just described for a cast crown and post unit, up to when the impression post is removed. The laboratory casts a custom–made post and core from this impression. When this is returned, it is fitted and cemented in place (under a second anesthesia). When the cement has set, the core and tooth structure are prepared for a crown impression. A third anesthesia will be necessary to fit the crown.

As an alternative to avoid this third anesthesia, the whole process can be made into a two–step procedure. After the post and core build–up has been prepared and the stump bevelled, an exact impression is made. The post and core build–up is then removed from the tooth. From the impressions and the post and core build–up, the dental laboratory will be able to design and make a cast crown, and a cast metal post and core build–up.

Before cementing the cast core and crown, minor corrections of the crown and the cast core build–up may be necessary due to inaccuracies or imperfections.

8.14 CROSS–PINNED METAL CROWN

As already mentioned, cast crowns of canine teeth, especially in guard dogs or police dogs, must be able to withstand large shearing forces (e.g., pulling on leather sleeves or cage bars). These forces tend to loosen the cast crown, which then falls out and is lost.

The most durable cast crowns are not only cemented, but also supported by a pin driven through both the core build–up and the cast crown.

The method can only be used on non–vital teeth, as the pin would otherwise penetrate the pulp cavity.

This method works best with cores of amalgam, metal–reinforced glass ionomer, metal filled composite, and reasonably well with brass posts. Since the hole can only be drilled through the core build–up when the cast crown is in place, stainless steel posts are not recommended, and are difficult to drill accurately.

CROSS–PINNING METHOD

The apical third of the fractured canine tooth should be filled with root canal filling material. The remaining two thirds of the root canal should be filled with a core material such as amalgam, metal–reinforced glass ionomer, or titanium–filled composite. The "stump" is then prepared for the cast crown and impressions are taken and sent off to the dental laboratory. The finished cast crown should be tried in place on the "stump." If there is not a good fit, the stump can be carefully reduced in order to produce a tight fit. It should be possible to push the cast crown down on the tooth until the junction of the crown and bevelled tooth touch. Ideally the cast crown should fit so tightly that it is difficult to remove, even before cementing.

The cast crown is removed, and firmly held with pliers (to avoid burning your fingers) on a wooden block. A hole is then drilled with a dental handpiece (or an electric drill) and a tungsten carbide drill bit through the buccal side of the cast crown, about 2–3 mm coronal to the margin. Any "FLASH" (jagged pieces of metal produced by drilling) produced on the inside of the cast crown should be removed with the drill or a file.

The cast crown should then be repositioned on the core and pressed down firmly. Under continuous pressure on the tip, a hole should now be drilled through the "stump," from the original hole in the cast crown to the opposite side of the cast crown (Photo 70). This hole must pass as near as possible through the middle of the "stump," through the buccal dentin, the core material, the lingual dentin, and then stop at the lingual wall of the cast crown. Do not drill through the cast crown at this point, but only mark it with the drill. If you try to drill through the steel with the cast crown in place, the pressure or the heat generated will almost certainly damage the "stump" and weaken the dentin.

In order to drill the hole on the lingual side, the cast crown is removed, held with pliers and this second hole is drilled inside by carefully drilling through the first hole and aiming at the mark on the inner lingual wall of the cast crown.

Conical tapered pins or bolts and matching reamers are available from special manufacturers or toolmakers (they are often used to secure gears in machines). The ideal conical pins have a taper from 2 mm to 3 mm in diameter, and are about 30 mm long.

After replacing the cast crown on the "stump," there should now be a parallel hole through the cast crown and "stump," without deviation. The next step is to make this hole tapered from buccal to lingual in order to accept the conical pin. This is done with a matching conical reamer and a hand chuck (Photo 71).

The conical pin is now tested in this hole and should fit perfectly with no movement at either end.

Both conical pin and cast crown are then removed, thoroughly cleaned with alcohol, dried and prepared for cementation. The "stump" and hole should also be cleaned and dried.

The inside of the cast crown is then filled with luting cement, and slowly pressed firmly onto the "stump" to allow excess cement to escape. The two holes in the crown aid in relieving some of the pressure that builds up from the cement.

Gentle tapping with a small wooden or metal mallet helps to achieve a good tight fit. The conical pin is immediately placed through the holes, and both the cast crown and conical pin lightly hammered until there is a tight fit (Photo 72).

When the cement has hardened, the protruding ends of the pin are cut off with a diamond disc, diamond bur or tungsten carbide bur. To avoid overheating, do this in stages or use a water coolant.

Finally, the junction of the cast crown and conical pin are smoothed and polished to a high gloss with silicone abrasives on a low–speed drill.

The junction of the cast crown and conical pin should barely be detectable if properly finished (Photo 73).

This method has worked well in practice and usually will not fail. It is probably the best and strongest method of attaching a cast crown. This is especially true of large breeds or working dogs, such as those used for hunting, guard and police activities, where extreme forces are exerted on these teeth.

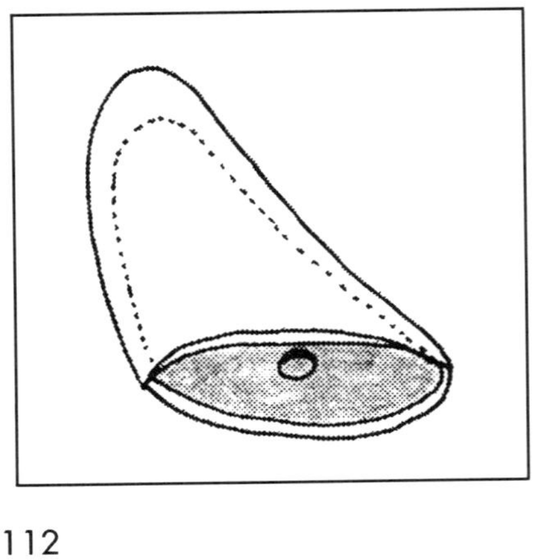

Figures 111 A–G. Transverse pinning of cast crown.

111 A. Crown fabricated with one hole on buccal side only.

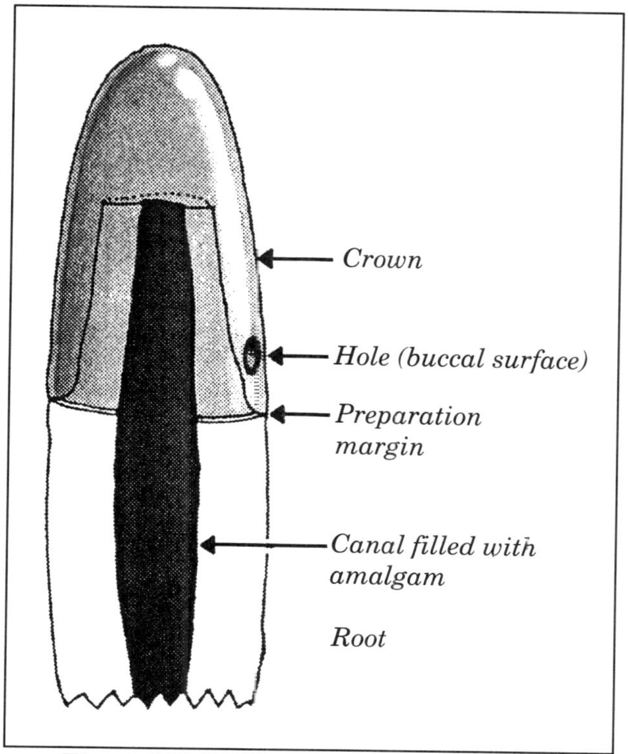

Figure 111 B. Testing crown for alignment (rostral view).

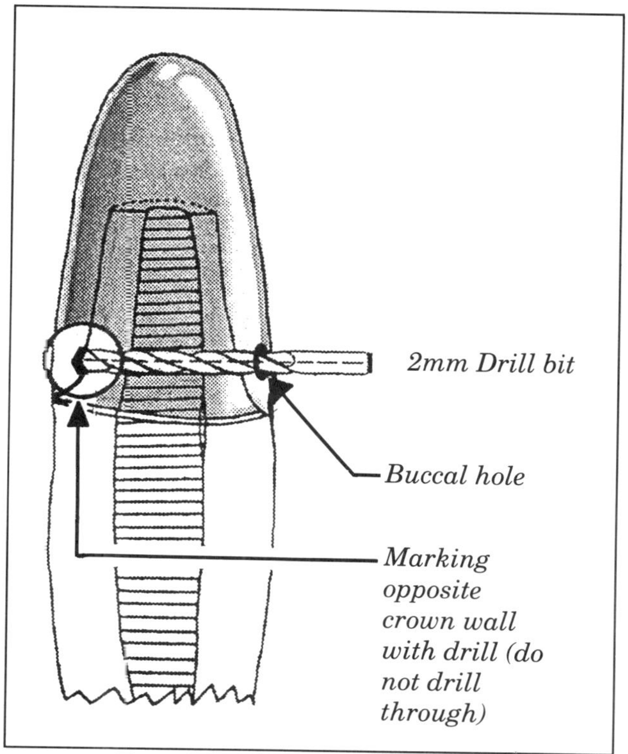

Figure 111 C. Drilling of stump.

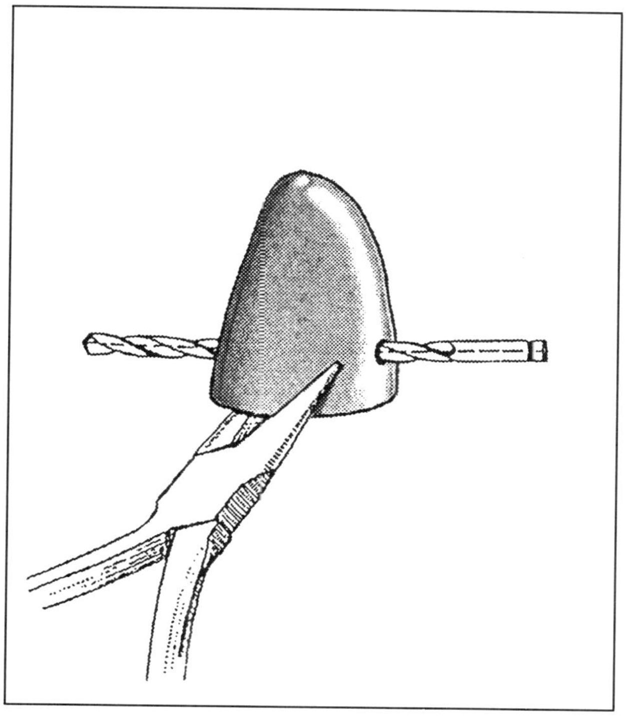

Figure 111 D. Crown removed. Opposite crown wall is drilled through when crown is outside the mouth to avoid overheating the "stump."

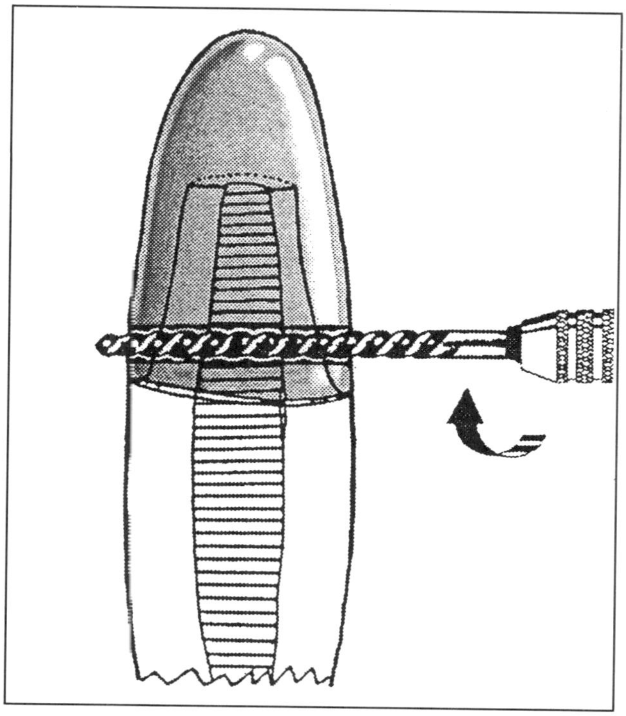

Figure 111 E. Reamer preparing conical shape to hole.

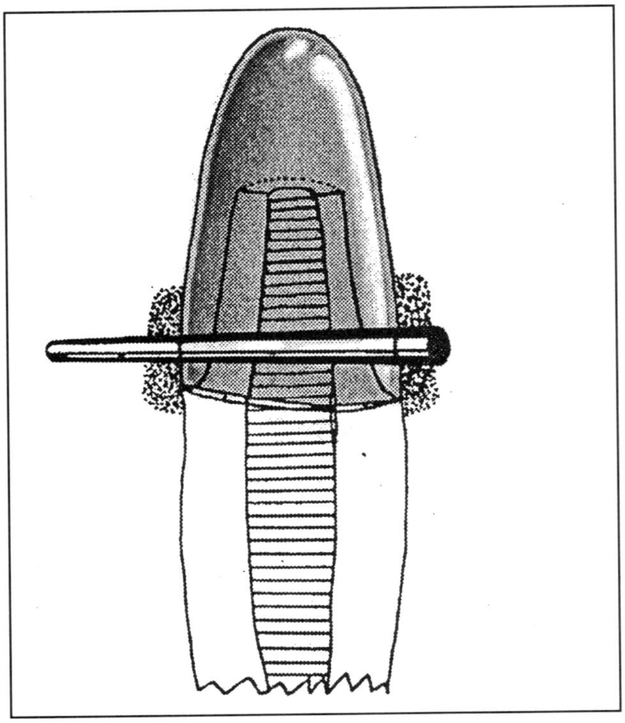

Figure 111 F. Crown and tapered pin cemented in place.

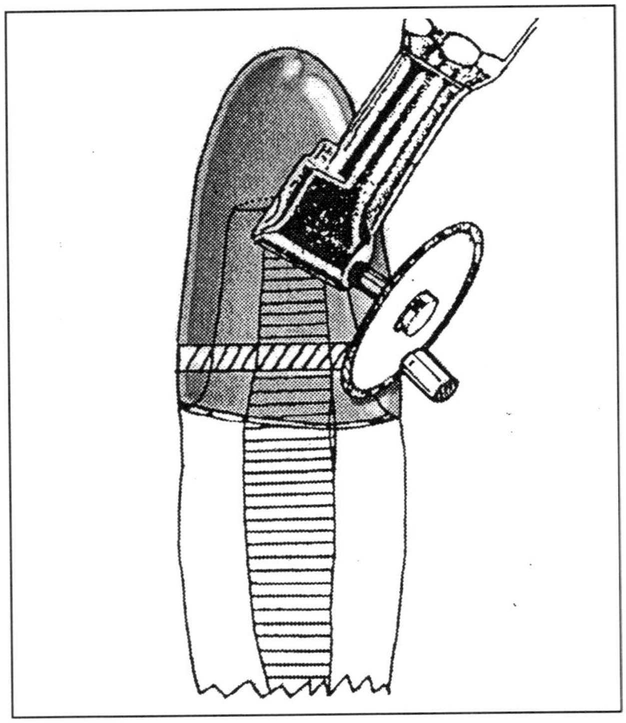

Figure 111 G. Diamond disk cutting off protruding pin. Rough edges smoothed with diamond bur, then surface polished.

8.15 IMPRESSION AND STONE MODEL TECHNIQUE

To fabricate prosthetic devices (and some orthodontic devices), impressions and stone models will be required. In order to provide the dental laboratory with an exact duplication of the crown preparation or the involved teeth, as well as the surrounding occlusion, accurate impressions must be made.

For the best results, correctly designed animal impression trays are now available (Photo 55). If a set of animal trays is not available, human trays can be used and in some instances they will have to be modified. Custom trays can be made by a dental laboratory or hand made in the hospital. For best results, a skull or a dental model (e.g., Visi–Model, Dr. Shipp's Laboratories) can be used to form the tray. A rough impression of the dentition can also be made by placing a "roll" of silicone impression material over the dental arcades. As a last resort, plastic or cardboard containers can be cut to serve as a compromise impression tray.

First, the correct size and shape of tray must be selected and tried in place in the mouth of the anesthetized patient.

For prosthetic devices an extremely accurate impression is required. Therefore elastomeric material (see impressions and stone models, 12.16) must be used, since alginate does not provide enough marginal accuracy. The best material for veterinary use is silicone. This material is available in several viscosities. For most accurate results, a base of HIGH VISCOSITY (regular) "putty–like" SILICONE material is placed in the tray. A LOW VISCOSITY (light–body) SILICONE material is then placed over this in the area of the required accurate impression. This is called a PUTTY WASH IMPRESSION TECHNIQUE.

One–step Putty Wash Impression Technique

This involves placing the high–viscosity "putty–like" silicone and the low–viscosity silicone in the tray together. The "putty–like" catalyst and base material are thoroughly mixed carefully following manufacturing instructions. It should be mixed with bare hands since some latex gloves inhibit proper polymerization. This mixed "putty–like" material is then placed in the tray. A small amount of the light–bodied, low–viscosity silicone wash material is then mixed with its catalyst. Using a spatula or a special impression syringe, the gingival sulcus at the bevelled margin is carefully filled with a bubble–free mix of light–bodied silicone, followed by a covering of the prepared "stump." Additional light–bodied material is placed on top of the "putty–like" material in the tray, in the area of the preparation site. When the two materials cure they will bond to each other. The most convenient method of mixing and applying the light–bodied silicone is the SELF–MIXING EXTRUDE DELIVERY SYSTEM. A hand–held "gun–like" CARTRIDGE DISPENSER instrument mixes the catalyst and base in a spiral nozzle as they are injected into the required area.

The tray containing both high– and low–viscosity silicone is immediately placed in the mouth. When this is set, about three to five minutes, the impression tray is carefully removed and inspected. After rinsing and drying, the margins around the prepared tooth (teeth) are carefully examined. Any faults in this area may require repetition of the procedure.

Two–step Putty Wash Impression Technique

This technique is more time consuming but slightly easier for the beginner. The "putty–like" material is mixed and placed in the tray. An impression is then taken with this material only. After curing and removal from the mouth, the impression is rinsed and dried. The light–bodied silicone is then mixed and placed over the crown preparation as previously mentioned. The tray is then carefully replaced into the mouth in exactly the same place. After curing and removal, the resulting impression is carefully inspected.

This method is more advantageous if the preparation level is subgingival. This is because the hard set "putty–like" impression material acts as a plunger, pressing the light–bodied silicone into the sulcus, resulting in an exact reproduction of the bevelled area.

The next procedure is to take an impression of the opposite jaw, in order to provide the dental laboratory with a full occlusion. Although this impression can be made with the "putty–like" silicone, using a one–step technique, this is costly. Alginate impression material is more economical, but requires the equipment and ability to pour dental stone models immediately in the practice (see impressions and stone models, 12.16). However, if a veterinary dentist is capable of performing endodontics, crown preparation and impression taking, he/she should be able to make a stone model. Generally alginate is used for the opposing jaw, unless maxillary and mandibular crown preparations are being performed at the same time. Until the technique is mastered, slow–setting alginate should be used. Once experience has been gained, fast–setting alginate can be used.

Premeasured amounts of alginate powder are added to premeasured amounts of water in a rubber mixing bowl. This is rapidly spatulated to produce a bubble–free smooth mixture. The correct impression tray is then filled and placed in the opposing jaw. It is best to have the tray facing up, and the teeth facing down, so that the alginate does not run out of the tray. When set, the tray and alginate are carefully removed and inspected. Since alginate will distort after a few hours (see impressions and stone models, 12.16), the stone model must be poured as soon as possible, or at least within an hour or two. In order to reduce the chance of bubbles in the stone, a DEBUBBLER SOLUTION should be lightly spread on the alginate impression. The stone is then poured into the alginate impression.

Since air bubbles can easily be trapped in the stone in the canine teeth area, a VIBRATOR should be used. The tray should be held on the vibrator and the stone poured into the anterior teeth first. Any bubbles will come to the surface. The rest of the alginate impression is then filled with stone while still on the vibrator. When the tray is full of stone, it is placed, teeth up, on a further "pad" or "base" of dental stone, which can be placed on a wet paper towel on a counter top. A model BASE FORMER TRAY can also be used if available. The stone is left to set for at least one hour, or preferably overnight. The tray is then gently pried loose from the alginate, followed by careful removal of the alginate. Due to the divergence of most canine teeth, the alginate either should be cut away around these teeth or broken off with an instrument such as an old scaler. The dental stone should be inspected for any irregularities and the base trimmed.

An alternative to making a full arcade impression of the prepared site with silicone, is to make just a small silicone impression of the involved tooth and one or two neighboring teeth. A small tray or a custom–made tray can be used. Following this, both maxillary and mandibular alginate impressions are made of the full mouth. The dental laboratory will be able to fit an accurate stone model of the prepared tooth from the silicone impression, into the full mouth stone impression. This method will save some costs on the expensive silicone material, which can be important when working with large dogs.

The final procedure is to make a bite registration (see preparation of orthodontic appliances, 9.26). The impressions, stone models, bite registration and instructions are then sent to the dental laboratory.

For those veterinarians and technicians who have never had any experience taking impressions and making stone models, it is strongly recommended that professional help is sought initially. Invite a veterinary dentist, human dentist, dental chairside assistant or a laboratory technician to come to your practice and guide you in your initial attempts. Alternatively, you could go to their place of business with a plastic animal dental model (e.g., Visi-Model), and your animal impression trays (e.g., Lyman, Schein) and have them demonstrate the techniques. Wet labs at veterinary dental meetings are also excellent places to obtain hands-on experience.

CHAPTER 9

ORTHODONTICS

Orthodontics is the branch of dentistry that is concerned with the diagnosis and treatment of malocclusion and related skeletal disorders.

It is important to clarify whether the malocclusion is either skeletal or dento–alveolar in origin, or a combination of both.

While different breeds of *cats* show hardly any deviation in their occlusion, the different breeds of *dogs* show marked variations in occlusion based on the skeletal morphology of the breed.

ANGLE'S CLASSIFICATION of malocclusions in the human, which was based on the position of the maxillary first molar, has been modified for use in veterinary dentistry. The four groups, NORMAL OCCLUSION, CLASS I, CLASS II and CLASS III MALOCCLUSIONS are based on certain maxillary and mandibular relationships, and tooth positioning or abnormalities.

9.1 NORMAL OCCLUSION

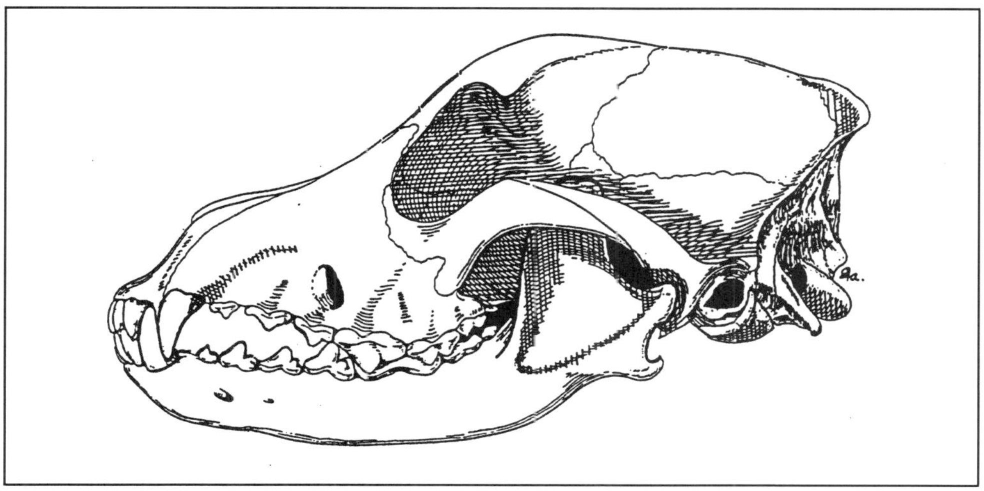

Figure 112. Normal occlusion.

Normal occlusion relates to what should be the correct skeletal and dental arrangement. However, due to selective breeding, and inbreeding, about 20 percent of dogs (e.g., Bulldog) and some cat breeds (e.g., Persians), will not meet these requirements. Although their occlusions are genetic malocclusions, they can be considered a normal standard for the breed.

NORMAL JAW RELATIONSHIP (ORTHOGNATHISM)

The most anterior point of the maxilla is slightly in front of the most anterior point of the mandible. The maxilla is straight and not bowed. The angle between the TEMPOROMANDIBULAR JOINT (TMJ), the CORONOID PROCESS and the BODY OF THE MANDIBLE should form approximately a right angle.

NORMAL DENTO–ALVEOLAR RELATIONSHIP

Incisors:

The INCISAL (or cutting) EDGE of the mandibular incisor teeth occludes with the lingual surface of the maxillary incisors (SCISSOR BITE).

Canine teeth:

The tips of the canine teeth diverge in a buccal direction. The mandibular canine teeth fit into the space between I3 and C in the maxilla. There should be no contact of these teeth.

Premolars:

P1, P2 and P3 have no occlusal contact, and mandibular P2, P3 and P4 should interdigitate between maxillary P1, P2, P3 and P4. The maxillary carnassials, P4, occlude buccally to mandibular carnassials, M1. The mesio–palatal surface of maxillary P4 also contacts the mesio–buccal surface of the mandibular M1.

Molars:

The disto–buccal cusp of the mandibular M1 occludes with the central fossa of the maxillary M1.

9.2 ACQUIRED VERSUS GENETIC MALOCCLUSIONS

As a general rule, if there is a normal skeletal arrangement of the jaws, malocclusions caused by malposition of teeth are considered *acquired*, although some malocclusions can be considered either *acquired* or *genetic,* based on the cause. These aberrations are ACQUIRED if they have been caused by outside forces either during tooth development or after the tooth has erupted. Examples and causes of *acquired* malocclusions are:

Retained deciduous teeth (some cases may be genetic), *anterior crossbite* (some genetic), *posterior crossbite* (some genetic), *lingually displaced canine teeth* (some genetic), *missing teeth* (some genetic), *impacted teeth* (some genetic), *supernumerary teeth, ectopic teeth, malformed teeth, tooth migration, temporomandibular joint trauma* and *jaw fracture.*

Anterior crossbite is considered acquired if the premolar interdigitation is normal. This is an important consideration when examining breeding and show pets. Most show judges only look at the incisor relationship, although they should be looking at the premolar and molar relationship also. It is estimated that about 50 percent of anterior crossbite cases are acquired and 50 percent are genetic. If the premolar interdigitation is *abnormal,* the anterior crossbite should be considered genetic.

Most GENETIC malocclusions tend to involve an abnormal skeletal arrangement of the jaws, with the teeth being out of alignment because of incorrect jaw growth. The most common *genetic* malocclusions are *brachygnathism* and *prognathism.* Other genetic malocclusions include *anterior crossbite* where the *jaw length* is *abnormal, level bite* (a slight degree of prognathism), *wry bite, tooth rotation, crowded teeth, missing teeth, rostral deviation of the mandibular canine tooth* in Persian cats and the *tight lip syndrome* in Shar Peis.

9.3 MALOCCLUSIONS WHICH REQUIRE TREATMENT

It is difficult to discover the reason for either decreased or increased forward growth in the jawbones, although an autosomal gene affecting cartilage growth has been incriminated. Any malocclusion that is considered genetic, or is suspected of being genetic, should not be treated orthodontically, unless the malocclusion is causing, or may cause, an oral problem.

If breeding and show pets have a *genetic* malocclusion, orthodontic corrective procedures are considered unethical and should only be performed if the pet is neutered, or if you are convinced that the owner does not plan on breeding or showing.

Any malocclusion that is considered *acquired* can be corrected orthodontically, in order to relieve the problem that it is causing, or may cause in the future. Treating acquired malocclusions in known breeding and show pets, is controversial since the AMERICAN KENNEL CLUB (AKC) and other kennel clubs do not allow the altering of any tooth structure or position. In reality, what kennel clubs, breeders and judges are saying is that they do not want a malocclusion or a dental problem covered up or corrected, which will show up in future generations. If an acquired malocclusion or a dental condition is causing, or may cause, an oral problem, then use your judgment as to what is in the best medical interest of the pet.

Oral problems caused by *malocclusions* and *dental conditions* include soft tissue trauma (sometimes leading to an oronasal fistula), tooth attrition, loosening of the periodontal apparatus, periodontal disease, alveolar bone destruction, incorrect jaw growth, incorrect tooth positioning, bowing or ventral curvature of the mandible, misalignment of the temporomandibular joint with consequential arthrosis, additional stress on the muscles of mastication, myofacial pain syndrome and sometimes difficulty in eating.

Corrective procedures for malocclusions, including orthodontic procedures, should only be performed in order to help correct the problems associated with the malocclusion, and not for cosmetic purposes.

Repairing broken teeth with restorative materials or with cast crowns in breeding and show dogs and cats is controversial. Current regulations by kennel clubs do not permit the altering or the correction of any tooth structure. However, if the broken tooth is going to cause pain, infection or an oral problem, then repairing it should not be considered unethical, as long as the procedure is not covering up a genetic defect. A broken tooth may create oral problems such as periodontal disease, periapical abscesses and tooth drifting of the occluding teeth, the neighboring teeth and even the broken tooth itself. Therefore it is in the best interest of the pet to repair the broken tooth in order to prevent such problems from developing. This requires your best judgment and consideration of the ethics involved.

9.4 CLASS I MALOCCLUSION

There is a normal relationship of all the maxillary teeth to all the mandibular teeth, but the line of occlusion is incorrect due to one or more teeth being out of alignment, rotated or changed in different ways. The skeletal relationship is the same as that of a normal occlusion. Although most Class I malocclusions are considered acquired, some can be genetic.

The following sections (9.5 – 9.18) describe the Class I malocclusions.

9.5 RETAINED DECIDUOUS TEETH

Retained deciduous teeth are one of the most common problems in cats and dogs causing Class I malocclusions. Usually the retained deciduous teeth are located buccal to the permanent teeth, except the deciduous maxillary canine teeth, which are located distal to the permanent canine teeth. Deciduous teeth should be lost as the permanent teeth begin to erupt and before the permanent teeth are in their final position. If more than half the crown length of the permanent tooth has erupted, and the deciduous tooth is still firmly in place, retention should be suspected. A retained tooth usually will prevent the permanent tooth from erupting in its correct position. Although retained deciduous teeth are considered acquired, this condition should probably be considered potentially genetic. This is still controversial. Retained deciduous teeth are seen more commonly in some breeds, especially small dogs such as Yorkshire Terriers. Removing the retained deciduous tooth before malocclusion occurs, may produce a normal occlusion. This procedure is known as INTERCEPTIVE ORTHODONTICS (see interceptive orthodontics, 9.24).

9.6 ANTERIOR CROSSBITE (ACQUIRED)

Anterior crossbite is characterized by some of the mandibular incisors being rostrally inclined, occluding in front of the maxillary incisors (Photo 80). In most cases it is only one or two teeth on one side of the mouth. This is usually considered an ACQUIRED MALOCCLUSION problem (Class I), but in some cases can be a GENETIC MALOCCLUSION (Class III).

In order to determine whether it is acquired, there may be a history of retained deciduous incisors or the puppy tugging on ropes. However be wary of this if you have not actually seen it, because naturally the owners (especially breeders) do not want to believe that it is genetic. If the condition is a genetic problem, this can usually be determined by looking at the premolar interdigitation (see anterior crossbite — genetic, 9.22).

9.7 POSTERIOR CROSSBITE

Posterior crossbite is a relatively rare condition, usually unilateral, where there is a crossbite relationship of the carnassial teeth. The mandibular first molar occludes buccal instead of lingual to the maxillary fourth premolar (Photo 81). Usually by the time it is discovered there is little that can be done. The common sequel that occurs is that heavy calculus deposits will be formed on the mandibular first molar, rather than on the maxillary fourth premolar. Although posterior crossbite is generally considered a Class I acquired malocclusion, from trauma, sucking habits or excessive mouth breathing, it can have a genetic origin, being commonly found in collies and shelties. An abnormal curvature of the hard palate often causes the maxillary carnassial teeth to occlude lingual to the mandibular carnassial teeth.

9.8 LINGUALLY DISPLACED AND BASE NARROW MANDIBULAR CANINE TEETH

This is a common malocclusion where the mandibular canine teeth are tipped lingually. The pointed crowns of the canine teeth strike the hard palate, causing necrosis of the mucosa and the underlying bone. In extreme cases, a fistula is opened into the nasal cavity allowing food particles to be impacted into the nasal cavity, causing severe nasal complications. The problem is usually bilateral, but can be unilateral. The cause is generally considered acquired, because buccally retained deciduous mandibular canine teeth force the erupting permanent mandibular canine teeth lingually. The cause can be genetic, arising from misplaced tooth germinal tissue or due to an abnormally narrow anterior mandible (base narrow mandible).

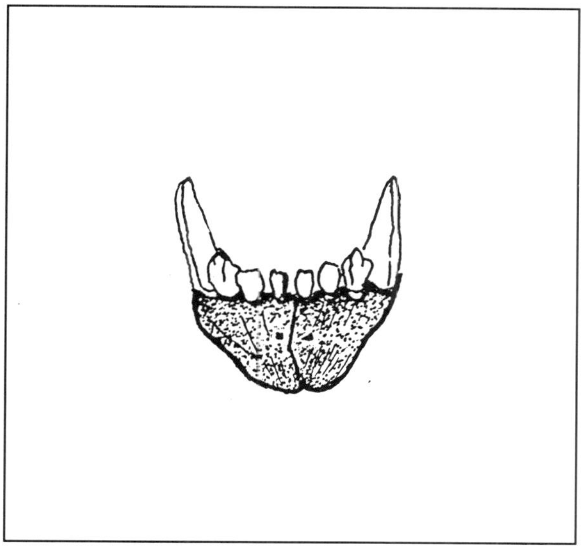

Figure 113 A. Normal canine teeth relationship.

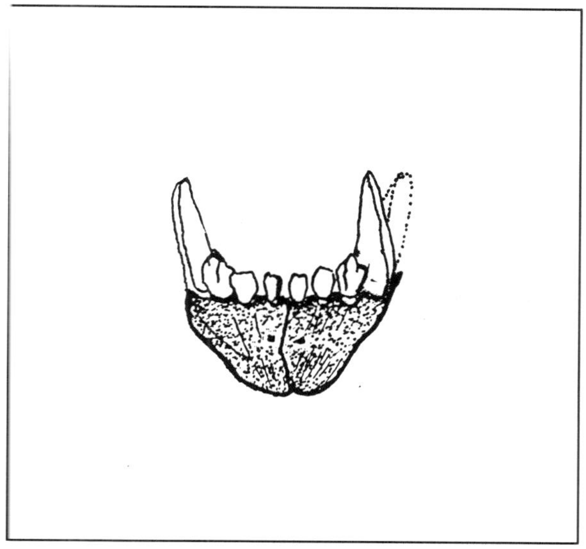

Figure 113 B. Unilateral (base narrow) (lingual) canine tooth.

The condition can be corrected by means of an inclined plane (see inclined plane appliance, 9.31), by fixing an expansion screw between the canine teeth (see expansion screws for movement of lingually displaced canine teeth, 9.33) and with a W–wire (see W–wire for the movement of lingually displaced canine teeth, 9.34).

The correction of this malocclusion is rapid, often occurring in five to ten days, if done early. Also, because of the natural dental interlock of the canine teeth, drifting back is almost impossible.

Early extraction of the retained deciduous canine teeth is the best preventive treatment if they are the cause. After extraction, the owner should be instructed to try to apply digital pressure buccally to the mandibular canine teeth as frequently as possible, if the pet will permit, in order to help them realign. If this does not work, orthodontic procedures mentioned above should be performed.

It must be remembered that this condition should be treated early (six to nine months of age) for the best results. Occasionally the cause is a malpositioned maxillary I3, which directs the tip of the mandibular canine tooth lingually. If this is the case, then the maxillary I3 should either be orthodontically treated first or extracted.

In some cases, such as older dogs or severe base narrow conditions, orthodontic movement may not be feasible. Treatment in these cases will require cutting down the crowns of the displaced canine teeth (see crown reduction, 7.16).

9.9 MISSING PERMANENT TEETH

Missing teeth are generally considered genetic in origin, unless they have been deliberately extracted. Missing teeth may also be the result of forces such as trauma to the jaws. Although more commonly found in brachycephalic breeds, missing teeth can occur in all breeds.

Several terms are given to missing teeth, depending on the numbers and types of teeth missing.

Hypodontia.

Absence of a few teeth. This is a common condition characterized by the absence of one or more teeth, and is seldom associated with other anomalies. Examples would be all P1 missing, or P1 and P2 missing, or a mandibular M3 and maxillary P1 and P2 missing.

Oligodontia.

Absence of many teeth. These teeth are usually from different groups (i.e., incisors, canine teeth, premolars and molars). Generally this condition is associated with a small size of the existing teeth and ectodermal anomalies (e.g., Mexican hairless dog).

Anodontia.

Absence of all teeth. This is a rare condition frequently associated with generalized deformities, such as hereditary ectodermal dysplasia.

Most commonly the teeth that are missing are the premolars, although incisors and molars can be involved also. Congenitally missing teeth do not require treatment, and should definitely not be replaced in breeding and show pets with implants and artificial crowns or with a bridge.

In order to confirm the absence of a missing tooth, dental radiographs should be taken. Occasionally, what was thought to be a missing tooth may prove to be an impacted or a retained tooth (see impacted and retained teeth — exposure, 10.13), or a subgingivally fractured tooth overgrown with gingival tissue.

9.10 IMPACTED TEETH

An impacted tooth results from the failure of the tooth to erupt into its normal position. The tooth may be either partially erupted or unerupted. A completely impacted tooth will be absent in the dental arcade, but visible on a dental radiograph (Photos 4, 5).

The failure to erupt can be caused by growth in the wrong direction, due to either misalignment or damage of the tooth bud, a lack of space to erupt, and inability of the tooth to penetrate the gingiva. Generally this is an acquired condition, but can be genetic. Treatment involves either removing the tooth or surgical removal of soft tissue and bone to assist in its eruption (see impacted and retained teeth — exposure, 10.13). If the tooth is not causing any problem, it can also be left where it is. Periodic radiographs should be taken since impacted tooth roots tend to form cysts.

9.11 SUPERNUMERARY TEETH

Extra or supernumerary teeth are not uncommon, usually involving the premolars but sometimes the incisors. Although supernumerary teeth are thought to be caused by a disturbance of the tooth bud development, there may be a genetic cause. A large percentage of Bulldogs and Bull Terriers are found with eight incisors.

Supernumerary teeth may cause crowding or incomplete eruption of neighboring teeth, leading to malocclusion. If a supernumerary tooth is causing malocclusion or a periodontal problem, the tooth causing the most problem should be extracted. Try to keep the teeth with normal root structure and crown shape, especially those with an anatomical position as close to normal as possible.

9.12 ROTATED AND CROWDED TEETH

Due to decades of misguided selective breeding and in some cases natural selection, skull size and jaw length and width have become dramatically changed in certain breeds. Since tooth size does not necessarily change with skeletal changes, some teeth end up with insufficient space to develop, and thus become crowded and rotated.

The tooth found most commonly rotated is the maxillary third premolar, especially in brachycephalic breeds. A tooth can be found rotated at any angle on its vertical axis, up to 90 degrees to the line of occlusion.

In breeds that have developed long narrow heads, such as dolichocephalic breeds, crowding and rotation of the incisors can occur. Since the maxillary and mandibular incisor teeth normally make occlusal contact with each other, crowding in one jaw can adversely affect the tooth alignment in the opposing jaw.

Narrow anterior jaws account for the base narrow canine tooth syndrome, which leads to lingually displaced canine teeth (see lingually displaced and base narrow mandibular canine teeth, 9.8).

Abnormal subgingival pockets often result between the rotated tooth and its neighbors. This allows food and debris to become trapped, which eventually leads to periodontal disease. Occasionally crowded teeth prevent the eruption of a tooth (see impacted teeth, 9.10), or cause the non–erupted tooth to be misplaced (see ectopic teeth, 9.13).

Many cases of rotated teeth or of crowded teeth do not need to be corrected, unless they are causing an oral problem. Treatment varies depending on the problem that is created. For slightly crowded teeth, simple odontoplasty (see odontoplasty, 9.36) of their contact points will allow for self–correction or permit enough space in order to perform orthodontic movement. In cases where orthodontic movement is not feasible, extraction or sometimes hemisection and extraction of the offending teeth or tooth part should be performed.

Since the cause of rotated and crowded teeth is of skeletal origin, except with supernumerary and malformed teeth, the condition is considered genetic. This is due to the creation and propagation of abnormal skull and jaw shapes.

9.13 ECTOPIC TEETH

These are teeth that erupt at an abnormal position, often buccal to the line of occlusion. This problem is caused by a malpositioned tooth bud and is considered acquired. Generally treatment is not necessary unless the tooth is causing a problem.

Although some cases can be treated orthodontically, extraction is often the treatment of choice if there is a periodontal or an occlusal problem.

9.14 MALFORMED TEETH

Teeth that have either an abnormal shape or abnormal size are infrequent findings but can occur in any breed. They are generally a result of disturbances of the tooth bud during initial development and are not considered heritable.

Dens in Dente (or "tooth within a tooth") is when the enamel from the crown invaginates into the dentin, in an apical direction.

Gemination of a tooth is when a single tooth bud divides, causing a single rooted tooth with two crowns. This condition is sometimes called a GEMINI or a TWIN tooth.

Dilaceration is an abnormal curvature of the apical part of the root, often in a sharp bend, making it difficult to perform endodontic therapy or extract the tooth.

Supernumerary roots are rare and usually involve triple–rooted teeth. The extra root(s) are generally abnormal in shape.

Fusion of a tooth is when two tooth buds are joined together. The result may be one tooth with two roots or two teeth fused together by their crowns and roots. A dental radiograph will be required to evaluate this condition.

Microdontia. Permanent teeth that are *smaller* than normal.

Macrodontia. Permanent teeth that are *larger* than normal.

Most malformed teeth do not cause any malocclusion, but many variations are possible that could interfere with the occlusion. If the malformed tooth is not causing a problem, either from visual or from radiographic evidence, it should be left alone.

9.15 TOOTH MIGRATION

A tooth can migrate or move abnormally in any direction. This can be due to forces on the tooth, or lack of forces on the tooth. Teeth can move or be moved in several different ways:

Extrude — outwards (coronal) movement of a tooth from the alveolar socket.
Intrude — inwards (apical) movement of a tooth into the alveolar socket.
Protrude — rostral (forwards) tipping of a tooth. This applies to the anterior teeth.
Retrude — caudal (backwards) tipping of a tooth. This applies to the anterior teeth.
Drift — movement of a tooth, usually in a mesial or distal direction.
Rotate — rotational movement of a tooth on its vertical axis.

A tooth can EXTRUDE due to the absence or the fracture of an OPPOSING or ANTAGONISTIC tooth in the opposite jaw.

This is mostly seen with the incisor teeth, especially in young dogs who have lost an opposing incisor early in life. It can also occur in cases of open bite of the incisor (see Class III malocclusion, 9.20).

A tooth can INTRUDE due to CONTACTING FORCES from an opposing tooth in the opposite jaw. An example of this is a level bite (see level bite, 9.21).

PROTRUDED and RETRUDED teeth are found in cases of abnormal contact from the opposing incisor teeth, either from a dento–alveolar malocclusion or from a skeletal malocclusion. They can also be caused by trauma and external orthodontic forces. This condition is sometimes referred to as LABIAL or LINGUAL VERSION.

Teeth can migrate or DRIFT either mesially or distally when a neighboring or a contacting tooth is missing or is misplaced. This is often seen with the incisor teeth.

ROTATED teeth are usually a result of crowding (see rotated and crowded teeth, 9.12).

There are several normal forces acting on the teeth. Forces from the tongue, lips and buccal mucosa are generally in a balance and do not change the tooth position. Changes in these forces, such as abnormal sucking habits, tongue thrusting and excessive mouth breathing can cause migration of teeth.

Orthodontic devices also cause teeth to migrate, but this is a deliberate and controlled movement.

9.16 TEMPOROMANDIBULAR JOINT (TMJ) AND JAW INJURIES

Fractures and dislocations of the temporomandibular joint and fractures of the maxilla and mandible, often result from automobile and falling accidents. There are many possibilities that can occur, and must be diagnosed by visual observation, digital palpation and radiography. TMJ dislocations are usually unilateral and displace rostrodorsally.

The injury usually involves some degree of malocclusion or misalignment of the teeth. The primary consideration when repairing these injuries is to reestablish a good occlusion of the teeth. In some cases this may require extracting teeth, sectioning part of a tooth and altering the shape of a tooth.

9.17 CAUDALLY INCLINED TEETH (RETRUSION) (DENTO–ALVEOLAR DISTAL OCCLUSION)

Usually this is a condition in which the canine teeth relationship is normal, but the mandibular incisor teeth lie so far caudally that they no longer have occlusal contact with the maxillary incisor teeth.

The condition is usually genetic in origin and is often seen in dolichocephalic breeds. Another example of this problem is the TIGHT LIP SYNDROME of the SHAR PEI. The lower lip does not develop normally and fits tightly over the mandibular incisors, tipping them caudally. Here the genetic problem of the lip causes an acquired movement of the incisors. The tension on the lip must be corrected before orthodontic movement of the teeth can be performed. Tension on the lip is relieved by cutting the rostral alveolar mucosa from canine tooth to canine tooth, and freeing the submucosa with a periosteal elevator. The mucosa is left to heal by granulation, without sutures.

Treatment of caudally inclined teeth involves tipping the mandibular incisors rostrally. This can be accomplished by means of a labial bar or a labial arch wire attached to the mandibular canine teeth with either elastics or brackets attached to each incisor tooth (Photo 86), a lingual bar and spring attached to the mandibular canine teeth or an expansion screw in an acrylic plate attached to the canine teeth and anterior premolars (see treatment of malpositioned anterior teeth, 9.28).

9.18 ROSTRALLY INCLINED TEETH (PROTRUSION) (DENTO–ALVEOLAR MESIAL OCCLUSION)

This is a condition in which the skeletal structure is normal but the incisors lie so far rostrally that normal occlusal contact is lost. The canine teeth are sometimes involved.

The condition is usually acquired by the young dog tugging on rope or other objects, pulling the incisors rostrally. It may involve only the maxillary incisors or only the mandibular incisors, or both. Also, only some of the incisors in either arch may be involved, such as is seen in anterior crossbite. Rostral deviation of the mandibular canine tooth is seen most commonly in the Persian cat. This is usually considered a genetic problem.

Treatment involves moving the involved teeth caudally. When the condition involves the incisor teeth, the aim is to return the teeth to a normal scissor bite if possible. When only the mandibular incisors are involved, it is generally considered easier to move the mandibular incisors caudally, than to move the maxillary incisors rostrally.

Rostrally deviated mandibular and maxillary incisors can be moved caudally by means of a lingual bar, with built–in hooks, which is attached to the canine teeth. Elastics are then attached from the bar to each incisor tooth by means of hooks, buttons or composite (see treatment of malpositioned anterior teeth, 9.28). These teeth can also be moved caudally by placing elastic power chain around the rostral surface of the incisors. The power chain is attached from all of the incisors and canine teeth by means of brackets bonded on these teeth (Fig. 127). If the rostral deviation of the mandibular incisors is only slight and there is near occlusal contact with the maxillary incisors, a BITE WING can be bonded on to the maxillary incisors in order to move the mandibular incisors (see bite wing appliance, 9.32). Slight odontoplasty can be performed on the rostral incisal edge of the mandibular incisors to help guide them under the inclined plane (see inclined plane appliance, 9.31).

Rostrally displaced canine teeth are generally moved caudally by means of elastic power chain, which is attached to the canine tooth and to the carnassial tooth (see brackets, buttons, hooks and elastics, 9.35).

9.19 CLASS II MALOCCLUSION — BRACHYGNATHISM

Brachygnathism is also known as MANDIBULAR BRACHYGNATHISM, SKELETAL DISTAL OCCLUSION, RETRUSIVE MANDIBLE, DISTAL MANDIBULAR EXCURSION, PARROT MOUTH, OVERSHOT JAW and UNDERBITE. This condition is commonly seen in long–skulled (dolichocephalic) breeds such as Collies, Shelties, Dachshunds and Russian Wolfhounds.

The mandible is shorter than the maxilla. In severe cases this difference in length is obvious, and in mild cases it is evidenced by the relationship of the maxillary teeth to the mandibular teeth.

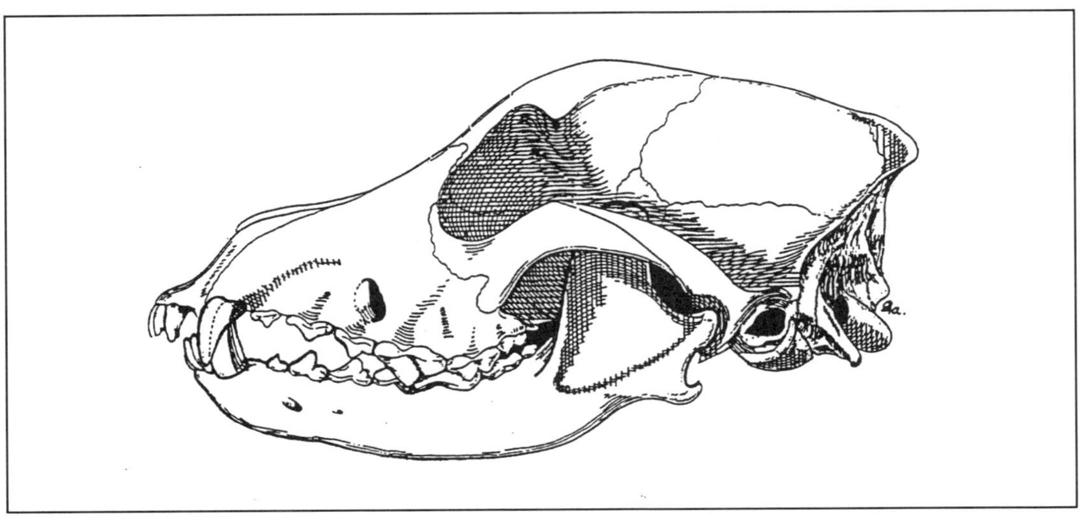

Figure 114. Brachygnathism.

With brachygnathism all the *maxillary* teeth occlude more rostrally to their *mandibular* counterparts than normal. The maxillary *incisors* are more rostral to the mandibular incisors and do not have occlusal contact with each other. The maxillary *canine teeth* either touch the mandibular canine teeth or are rostral to them. The maxillary *premolars* are displaced rostrally to the mandibular premolars and do not interdigitate normally.

In some breeds the ANGLE OF THE MANDIBLE relative to the *temporomandibular joint* may be *more* than in the normal animal.

When the maxilla has a sudden growth spurt, but not the mandible, the rostral dental interlock will often tend to drag the mandible forwards. This increases the angle of the mandible relative to the temporomandibular joint.

Although some veterinary dentists use the angle of the mandible to help determine the degree of malocclusion, it should be considered at present as an unreliable guide in many breeds. This is because there are so many variations in skull size and shape and the reference points are not always accurate.

In the human, measurements can be fairly accurate due to a reasonably constant shape and size of the maxilla and mandible, and the sophistication of CEPHALOMETRIC MEASUREMENTS. Cephalometry is the measurement of the dimensions of the head to determine the nature of abnormalities and the need for correction.

Measurements of the angle of the mandible should be based on a vertical line through the center of the ramus, parallel to the anterior and posterior edges, and a horizontal line parallel to the gingival margin starting at approximately the level of the mental foramen.

If vertical measurements are based on the palpable points of the angular process, the TMJ and the coronoid process, and the horizontal measurements are based on the ventral border of the body of the mandible, errors will be encountered. In many cases, the length of the maxilla will have a direct bearing on the vertical reference line, and the ventral bowing of the mandible will influence the horizontal reference line.

Before reference points can be reliably used to help determine the degree of malocclusion, more research is required. Accurate guidelines for cephalometric measurements based on key reference points on the skull and radiographic measurements are required.

Brachygnathic malocclusions will be evident in all degrees from mild to severe. They are considered genetic unless a history of trauma or of deciduous teeth interlock has been documented. Deciduous teeth malocclusions should probably be considered genetic.

If the degree of brachygnathism is not too severe, the principal of an ACTIVATOR can be used. This appliance is used in human orthodontics to encourage and direct the growth of the mandible. An acrylic appliance is constructed which fits both jaws, but holds the mandible in a protruded position. The condyles are held out of the fossa, which encourages more growth than would otherwise occur. This appliance is unsuitable for dogs, but the natural occlusion can be utilized. If the rostral surface of the maxillary canine teeth or the caudal surface of the mandibular canine teeth, is thickened by adding a cast crown the same effect can be attained. Alternatively the appropriate surface can be thickened by bonding acid–etch composite to the canine teeth.

The only other treatment for this condition, if possible at all, is surgery. In human medicine several operations have been described, involving segmental ostectomy or sectioning of the ascending ramus of the mandible, in order to move the mandible rostrally. In the dog and cat, surgery of the ascending ramus is not practical. The caudal teeth are usually found in a normal occlusal relationship and cannot be moved forward or backward due to the position in which the cusps occlude. Almost all procedures designed to alter the length or the position of the mandible are accomplished in the area of the second or third premolars. These procedures are high risk, complex and not usually warranted in animals (see surgical procedures in orthodontics, 9.38). In selected cases, orthodontic movement, crown reduction or extraction of teeth can be performed on those teeth that are causing oral problems.

9.20 CLASS III MALOCCLUSION — PROGNATHISM

Prognathism is also known as MANDIBULAR PROGNATHISM, SKELETAL MESIAL OCCLUSION, PROTRUSIVE MANDIBLE, MESIAL MANDIBULAR EXCURSION, UNDERSHOT JAW and OVERBITE.

This condition is commonly seen in short skulled (brachycephalic) breeds such as Bulldogs, Pugs, Boxers and Pekingese as well as some cat breeds such as Persians. Although it is a genetic malocclusion, it is considered normal for these breeds.

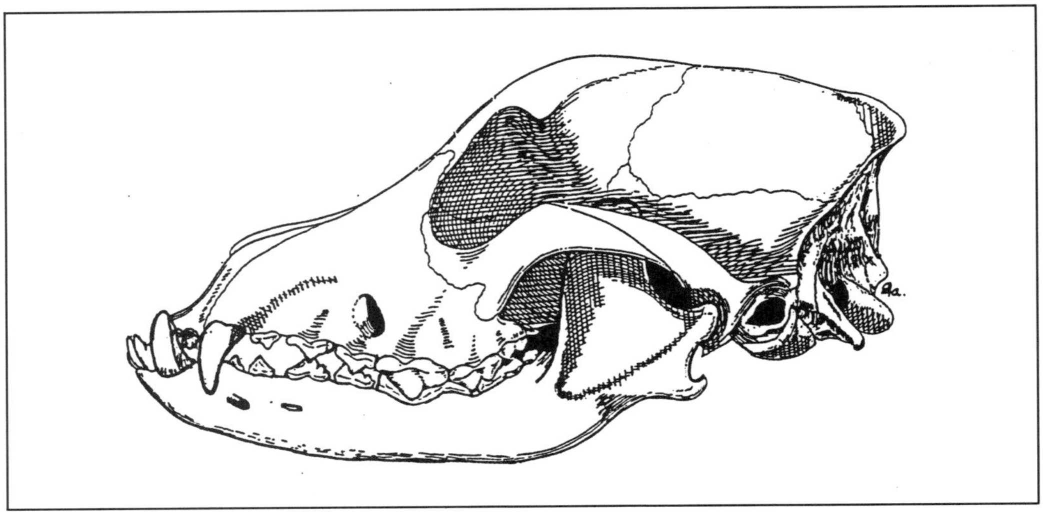

Figure 115. Prognathism.

Prognathism is caused either by an excessive growth of the mandible, a reduced growth of the maxilla or a combination of both. In severe cases, this difference in length is obvious, and in mild cases it is evidenced by the relationship of the mandibular teeth to the maxillary teeth. With prognathism all the *mandibular* teeth occlude more rostrally than normal to their *maxillary* counterparts. The mandibular *incisors* are usually more rostral to the maxillary incisors and do not have occlusal contact with each other. The mandibular *canine teeth* are usually some distance rostral to the maxillary canine teeth and are either touching the maxillary incisors or are rostral to them. The mandibular *premolars* are usually displaced rostrally to the maxillary premolars and do not interdigitate normally.

In some breeds the ANGLE OF THE MANDIBLE relative to the *temporomandibular joint* may be *less* than in the normal animal.

When the mandible has a sudden growth spurt, but not the maxilla, the mandible will grow in all directions including caudally. Often the rostral growth is restricted by the anterior dental interlock, forcing the caudal mandible more caudally.

As with brachygnathism, measurements of the angle of the mandible based on the palpable points of the angular process, the TMJ and the coronoid process are prone to errors in many breeds. More research is needed to successfully use this angle as a reliable guide to the degree of malocclusion.

In some cases of prognathic occlusion, the mandibular premolars and canine teeth are rostrally displaced, but the incisor relationship is normal. The interlocking occlusion of the incisors and canine teeth maintains the incisor relationship and often causes the mandible to curve ventrally or bow as it grows. The imaginary horizontal line between the tips of the cusps of the maxillary and mandibular premolars becomes deviated, leaving a space. In rare instances the rostral displacement of the mandible can cause an open bite between the incisor teeth. An OPEN BITE refers to a space between the maxillary and mandibular incisal edges, when the mouth is in resting occlusion.This may be due to the interlocking of the mandibular canine teeth and the maxillary lateral incisor teeth forcing the anterior part of the mandible ventrally. An open bite can also be caused by an abnormally long tongue in the puppy. The tongue tends to be carried between the incisors, which permits the canine teeth and molars to erupt into an abnormal contact. Once this is established and growth is complete, the open bite becomes permanent. If the tip of the tongue is noticed protruding out of the mouth 70 to 80 percent of the time, particularly at rest, surgical removal of the tip of the tongue can be performed.

These malocclusions will be evident in all degrees from mild to severe. They are considered genetic unless a history of trauma or of deciduous teeth interlock has been seen. Deciduous teeth malocclusions should be considered as genetic, although this is controversial at present. Although in very severe cases treatment can be surgical, consisting of partial ostectomy of the body of the mandible, such a procedure is high risk, complex and usually not warranted (see surgical procedures in orthodontics, 9.38). As with brachygnathism, in selected cases, orthodontic movement, crown reduction or the extraction of teeth can be performed on those teeth that are causing oral problems.

9.21 LEVEL (EVEN) BITE

In this Class III malocclusion the mandible has a slight degree of prognathism as evidenced by the mandibular teeth occluding slightly anterior to their normal relationship or occlusion with the maxillary teeth. This causes the maxillary and mandibular incisors to occlude tip to tip (Photo 79). The sharp INCISAL EDGES are in occlusal contact, causing the main cusps to be rapidly worn down to the level of the lobes or even further, giving the teeth an unusually wide appearance. This abrasion is worsened by biting on hard objects such as wood, leather and metal. It is important for the prognosis to know whether the incisors are so worn down that they no longer contact each other. If there is still contact, the condition can be alleviated through judicious beveling of these teeth (see odontoplasty, 9.36).

9.22 ANTERIOR CROSSBITE (GENETIC)

As previously discussed (see anterior crossbite — acquired, 9.6) this condition can be genetic in origin. This is actually a mild degree of prognathism, as evidenced by a slight rostral displacement of the mandibular teeth. The mandibular premolars will not have a correct interdigitation with the maxillary premolars, especially P1 and P2, and the mandibular canine teeth will probably be touching the maxillary lateral incisors.

9.23 WRY BITE (MOUTH)

Wry bite is an unclassified malocclusion, since it can be partly Class II or partly Class III or partly both. This is a condition where one side of the maxilla or the mandible grows forward more than the other side, developing a unilateral prognathism or a unilateral brachygnathism, often with a normal shaped skull. In most cases involving the maxilla there will be a deviation of the midline of the head, visible from the nose to the occipital crest. Most soft tissue structures will appear abnormal on the deviated side. There will be an asymmetry between the teeth of each side, as well as the hard palate. There may be a sloping OPEN BITE of the incisors from one side to the other. It is considered a genetic deformity. If the genetic defect lies in the maxilla, then often the mandible will be influenced secondarily due to the mechanical interlock of the teeth, and often the occlusion of the incisors and canine teeth will be normal, but with all teeth deviated rostrally on one side.

If the mandible is the primary source of the genetic defect, there is usually a malocclusion of the maxillary and mandibular rostral teeth.

Occasionally trauma to the skull may give the appearance of a wry bite and should be carefully evaluated with radiographs.

9.24 INTERCEPTIVE ORTHODONTICS

Each quadrant of the mandible and maxilla grows independently of each other. Sudden growth spurts of one jaw and not the other at a very young age, can cause an abnormal dental interlock between the maxillary and mandibular deciduous incisors and canine teeth. This interlocking of the teeth can block the forward growth of the jaw, which did not have the growth spurt, causing an eventual skeletal malocclusion. In order to permit the jaws to grow to their full genetic potential, the deciduous incisors and canine teeth should be removed as soon as the problem is noticed. This procedure is usually referred to as INTERCEPTIVE ORTHODONTICS. Extracting the deciduous incisors and canine teeth will relieve the mechanical obstruction to jaw growth that they are causing. Although all the deciduous incisors and canine teeth can be extracted, it is only necessary to remove those teeth from the shorter jaw, which are preventing the forward growth of that jaw. Try to leave those deciduous teeth that would either inhibit additional abnormal jaw growth or would stop the jaw growth when the correct relationships are obtained.

Firmly retained deciduous teeth that remain after the permanent teeth have erupted, should be removed to allow the permanent teeth to grow into their natural occlusion. This is also considered *interceptive orthodontics.* The rule of thumb as to whether to extract firmly retained deciduous teeth is that *there should never be two teeth of the same type in the same place at the same time.*

9.25 ORTHODONTIC TREATMENT

The principles and techniques of orthodontic treatment are similar to those in human orthodontics, although usually less complicated, precise and sophisticated. Before orthodontic treatment is undertaken a veterinary dentist has to evaluate the overall picture of the teeth and jaw bones, the reasons why an orthodontic procedure should be performed, what is best for the pet and any ethical considerations involved.

The most reliable reference points are the canine teeth and the premolars. The angle of the mandible relative to the temporomandibular joint may be important, but more research and classification of breed types is necessary.

Orthodontic treatment in veterinary medicine largely involves fixed appliances, although in some cases removable appliances have their advantages. Many devices can be made by the veterinary dentist, providing the materials such as wires, elastics, brackets, buttons, hooks, expansion screws, acrylics, cements and impression materials are available (see dental materials, Chapter 12). More sophisticated devices, such as cast bilateral or cast unilateral telescoping inclined plane appliances, have to be made by a dental laboratory (see inclined plane appliance, 9.31).

The RETENTION PERIOD of the tooth, which is the period that a tooth is held in position after it has been orthodontically moved, is usually as long as the MOVEMENT PERIOD (often 2–3 months). Retention is generally done with wire (or wire and acrylic). In some cases (e.g., lingual canine teeth) retention can be obtained by the natural dental interlock of the surrounding teeth.

9.26 PREPARATION OF ORTHODONTIC APPLIANCES

If possible, it is wise for the veterinarian to make an orthodontic appliance "in situ." This lowers the costs and eliminates the necessity of making impressions and stone models, as well as additional anesthetic procedures. If it is necessary to have the appliance made by a dental laboratory, the first procedure under anesthesia will be to make impressions and stone models of the mandibular and maxillary anterior teeth, and to make a bite registration. Impression trays for dogs and cats (Fig. 153) are now available, although as a compromise disposable trays made for humans can be used. The region distal to the second premolars is generally of no importance, thus human impression trays of suitable size can be used in many cases. The most important part of the impression is at the CINGULUM of the tooth, where the free gingival margin contacts the tooth. When the tray has been tried for size, it is filled with impression material and placed over the maxillary teeth. It is pressed into place and held until the impression material has set. The tray should then be carefully removed. Pulling on the handle may remove the tray, leaving the impression material in the mouth. To prevent this from occurring the tray and impression material should be loosened first, at the sides, to break the suction. The procedure is repeated for the mandibular teeth.

A further mix of silicone impression material is then made. This is rolled into a "sausage" and placed on the occlusal surface of the mandibular teeth. The jaw is then closed, being careful not to trap the tongue or the lips between the teeth. This is generally made when all procedures are completed and as soon as the endotracheal tube has been removed. This process is called BITE REGISTRATION. A sheet of BITE REGISTRATION WAX can also be used. The two impressions and the bite registration are sent to the dental laboratory for pouring and articulation of the stone model. If the impressions are to be sent to a dental laboratory an elastomeric material must be used. If the stone models are to be poured by the veterinarian, alginate can be used (see impression and stone model technique, 8.15).

For an accurate representation of the bite, the models should be returned on an ARTICULATOR. This is a device that holds the maxillary and mandibular models in the correct relationship to each other, with a hinge that mimics more or less the movements of the temporomandibular joint. This allows not only for construction of suitable appliances, but also allows examination of the occlusal relationship itself. The veterinarian should design the appliance, and draw an outline of the various parts in pencil on the stone model. It is advisable to discuss the design with the laboratory technician, describing which tooth movements are required, and especially the method of fixation, since most human dental laboratories are not familiar with veterinary procedures. Although an articulated model is ideal, it is more difficult and expensive to make. Most veterinary orthodontic appliances can be made satisfactorily without articulating the model.

9.27 FIXATION OF ORTHODONTIC APPLIANCES

FIXED ORTHODONTIC APPLIANCES

Most orthodontic appliances are attached in the region of the anterior teeth (i.e., incisors and canine teeth). There is a simple and effective method of retaining orthodontic appliances in dogs, which makes use of the large surface area and divergence of the canine teeth. Secure attachment to these teeth is obtained by acid–etching the enamel and bonding the appliances or the brackets to the canine teeth. In some cases orthodontic wire can be twisted around these teeth and incorporated into an acrylic appliance.

If additional retention anchorage is required, the first or the second premolars can be included in the appliance.

Direct bonding of brackets, hooks or buttons to the incisor teeth enables these teeth to be moved via the orthodontic appliance. There are numerous brands of luting cements to bond these devices to the teeth (see luting cements, 12.10). Wires can be twisted around the incisor teeth and secured with composite or incorporated into acrylic.

REMOVABLE ORTHODONTIC APPLIANCES

If orthodontic movement of the teeth is going to take several weeks to perform, some appliances can be designed to be removable. These can be easier for the clients to adjust and keep clean, and allow variation in the time intervals that pressure will be applied.

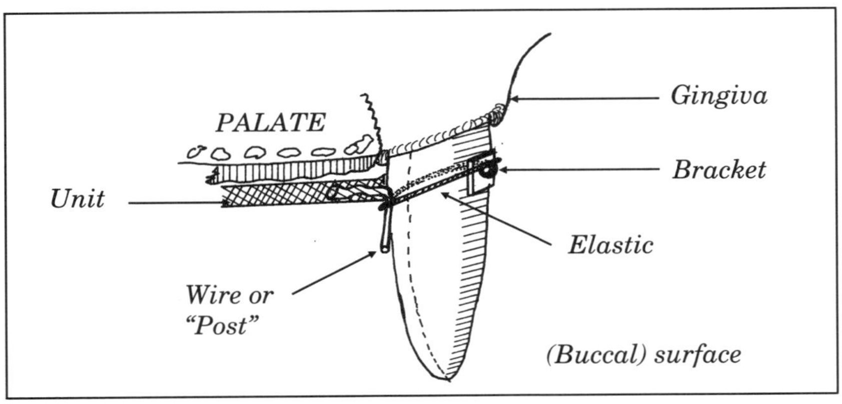

Figure 116. Removable orthodontic appliance.

The basic design of the removable appliance is similar to a fixed appliance, except where it is fixed to the teeth. A FIXATION WIRE (or "post") is built into the appliance, extending coronally on the lingual surface of the canine teeth (and incisor teeth if necessary). The length of these wires (or "posts") should be about half the length of the crown. Brackets are bonded on to the buccal surfaces of the teeth involved, as close to the gingival margin as possible. Small elastic bands hook over the bracket and encircle the tooth and the fixation wire (or "post"). Usually elastics on the canine teeth and the lateral incisors are adequate for retention of most appliances.

In order to allow the dog to get accustomed to the device and to prevent its removal with the front paws, an Elizabethan collar should be used for the first few hours. Wiring the device in place for the first 48 hours can also be done, then substituting the wires for the elastics.

The owner should remove the unit daily, clean it with a toothbrush and soapy water, and leave it out of the mouth during meals and for one to two hours afterwards.

9.28 TREATMENT OF MALPOSITIONED ANTERIOR TEETH

There are many positions in which the incisor teeth and canine teeth can be malpositioned:

1. Rostrally inclined mandibular incisors.
2. Rostrally inclined maxillary incisors.
3. Caudally inclined mandibular incisors.
4. Caudally inclined maxillary incisors.
5. Rostrally inclined mandibular canine teeth.
6. Rostrally inclined maxillary canine teeth.
7. Caudally inclined mandibular canine teeth.
8. Caudally inclined maxillary canine teeth.
9. Lingually displaced mandibular canine teeth.
10. Lingually displaced maxillary canine teeth.
11. Buccally displaced mandibular canine teeth.
12. Buccally displaced maxillary canine teeth.
13. Buccally displaced incisors.
14. Rotated and crowded incisors.
15. Intruded incisors.
16. Extruded incisors.

ORTHODONTIC PROCEDURES should only be performed on those teeth that are causing either mechanical or periodontal problems, or may lead to future oral problems. In some cases more than one type of treatment may be required to correct the position of a single tooth (e.g., rotation and tipping). Several treatments are possible depending on the situation:

1. Rostrally inclined mandibular incisors.
Lingual bar or lingual arch wire with elastics.
Labial bar with a spring activator.
Elastic power chain.
Bite wing and odontoplasty.

2. Rostrally inclined maxillary incisors.
Palatal bar or palatal arch wire with elastics.
Elastic power chain and buttons.

3. Caudally inclined mandibular incisors.
Labial bar or labial arch wire with elastics.
Lingual bar with a spring activator.
Expansion screw in an acrylic plate.
Arch wires attached to bands.

4. ***Caudally inclined maxillary incisors.***
   Labial bar with elastics.
   Palatal bar with a spring activator.
   Expansion screw in an acrylic plate.
   Bite wing and odontoplasty.
   Arch wires attached to bands.

5. ***Rostrally inclined mandibular canine teeth.***
   Elastic power chain and buttons, hooks or composite.
   Crown reduction.
   Extraction of interfering maxillary lateral incisor.

6. ***Rostrally inclined maxillary canine teeth.***
   Elastic power chain and buttons, hooks or composite.
   Crown reduction.

7. ***Caudally inclined mandibular canine teeth.***
   Inclined plane appliance.
   Crown reduction.
   Expansion screw in an acrylic plate.

8. ***Caudally inclined maxillary canine teeth.***
   Crown reduction.
   Expansion screw in an acrylic plate.

9. ***Lingually displaced mandibular canine teeth.***
   Inclined plane appliance.
   Expansion screw with wire and composite.
   W–wire spring appliance.
   Bite wings.
   Crown reduction.

10. ***Lingually displaced maxillary canine teeth.***
    Expansion screw with wire and composite.
    Inclined plane appliance.
    W–wire spring appliance.
    Crown reduction.

11. ***Buccally displaced mandibular canine teeth.***
    Elastic power chain with either brackets or composite.
    Expansion screw (in reverse) with wire and acrylic.
    Crown reduction.

12. ***Buccally displaced maxillary canine teeth.***
    Elastic power chain with either brackets or composite.
    Expansion screw (in reverse) with wire and composite.
    Crown reduction.

13. ***Buccally displaced incisors.***
    Elastic power chain and buttons.
    Odontoplasty.
    Extraction.

14. Rotated and crowded incisors.
Arch wire and slotted brackets.
Odontoplasty.
Expansion screw with wire and composite.
Extraction.

15. Intruded incisors.
Elastic power chain and buttons.
Arch wire and slotted brackets.
Gingivectomy and fibrotomy.

16. Extruded incisors.
Elastic power chain and buttons.
Arch wire and slotted brackets.
Crown reduction.

9.29 LINGUAL, PALATAL AND LABIAL BARS

The LINGUAL BAR and the PALATAL BAR are metal bars which are fabricated by the dental laboratory. It is a curved bar that fits across the mouth just caudal to the incisors, with bands soldered to each end that slip over the canine teeth. These bands are bonded to the canine teeth.

If this device is used to move the incisor teeth caudally, it may have either hooks or buttons soldered along its length in line with each incisor tooth that requires movement. Small elastic rings are attached from the hooks or the buttons to each incisor tooth. The method of attachment to the incisor tooth can vary. A hook with a mesh base can be bonded to the caudal surface of the incisor tooth. A button with a mesh base can be bonded to the rostral surface of the incisor tooth. A small amount of composite can be bonded to the rostral surface of the incisor tooth, with a small groove cut in the composite to retain the elastic.

If a lingual bar or a palatal bar is used to move teeth rostrally, activating springs are soldered to its rostral surface that will make contact with the lingual surfaces of the incisors. This gentle pressure gradually moves the teeth rostrally. The tension may have to be adjusted periodically to obtain the desired effect.

A LABIAL BAR is basically the same as a lingual bar, except that it is designed to lie rostral to the incisors, from canine tooth to canine tooth. The principles of attachment of elastics and springs are similar to the lingual bar, except they are reversed.

These are complicated devices to make, and impressions and stone models must be made and sent to the dental laboratory. A second anesthetic procedure must be performed to cement the device.

In cases where the incisors are to be moved caudally, a LINGUAL or a PALATAL ARCH WIRE can be used instead of a lingual or a palatal bar. This is a heavy gauge wire that can be hand crafted by the veterinary orthodontist, eliminating the need for dental impressions and models, as well as additional anesthesia or sedation. Small hook–like bends can be built into the wire for attachment of the elastics. Although not as strong as the lingual or the palatal bar, it can be useful for minor orthodontic movement.

Some appliances may not be suitable or may have to be modified because the opposing teeth hit the appliance on occlusion.

9.30 EXPANSION SCREW IN AN ACRYLIC PLATE

In order to move the maxillary or the mandibular incisors rostrally, an expansion screw incorporated into an acrylic plate can be used (Photo 84).

Since the fabrication of an acrylic appliance involves an exothermic reaction (producing heat), it is best to make the appliance on a stone model and then cement it to the teeth. Although the appliance can be made in the mouth, using plenty of vaseline to cover the oral soft tissues, it would mean a prolonged anesthetic time to fabricate and fit the appliance.

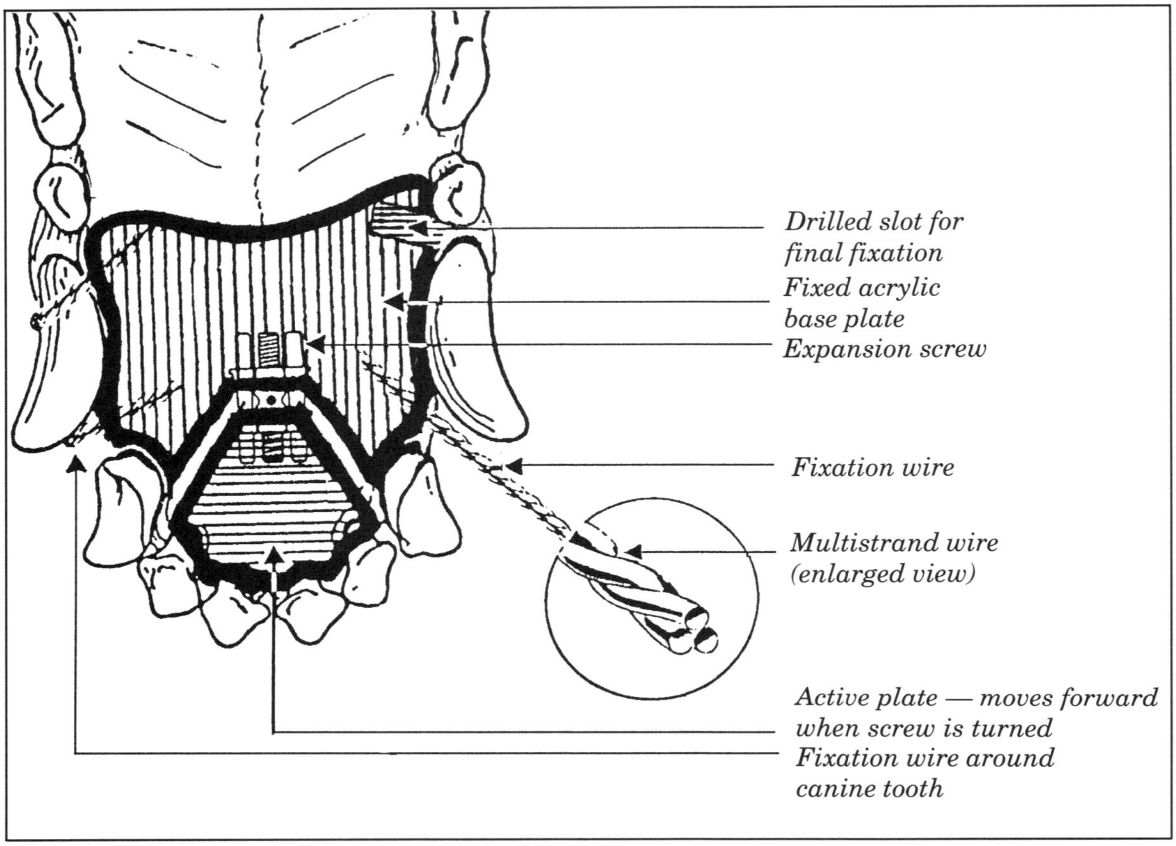

Figure 117. Fixation of acrylic appliance with the aid of wire loops on the canine teeth.

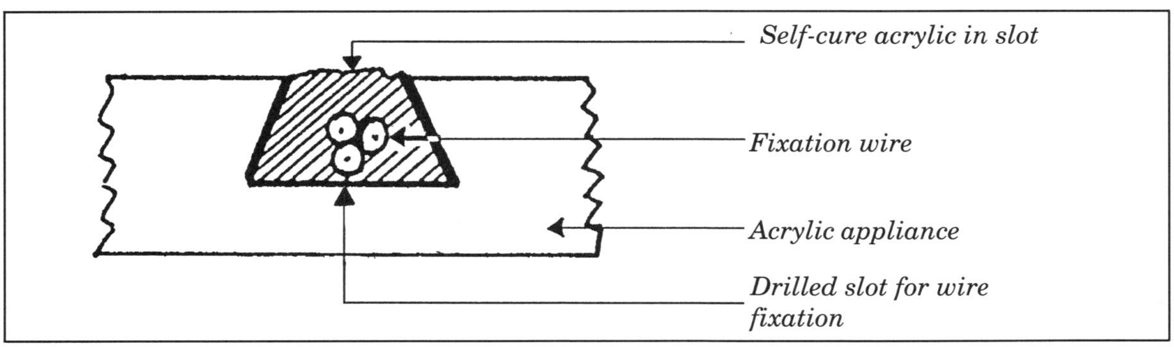

Figure 118. Cross–section of acrylic appliance at fixation area.

The acrylic appliance is made in the laboratory with two short pieces of braided wire exiting buccally just rostral to the canine teeth. Braided wire with three or more strands is commonly used in human orthodontics because of its flexibility. A retention groove is cut in the acrylic device just caudal to the canine teeth. The finished appliance is tried in place, and any necessary adjustments are made. The canine teeth are then acid–etched as previously described, and the braided wires passed around these teeth and twisted together in the midline. The part of the wires passing around the teeth is bonded to the teeth with composite. Once bonded to the teeth, the ends of the wires are untwisted and cut off so that the wires fit into the retention grooves. These ends are secured in the retention grooves with self–cure acrylic. Any excess acrylic is trimmed with a bur.

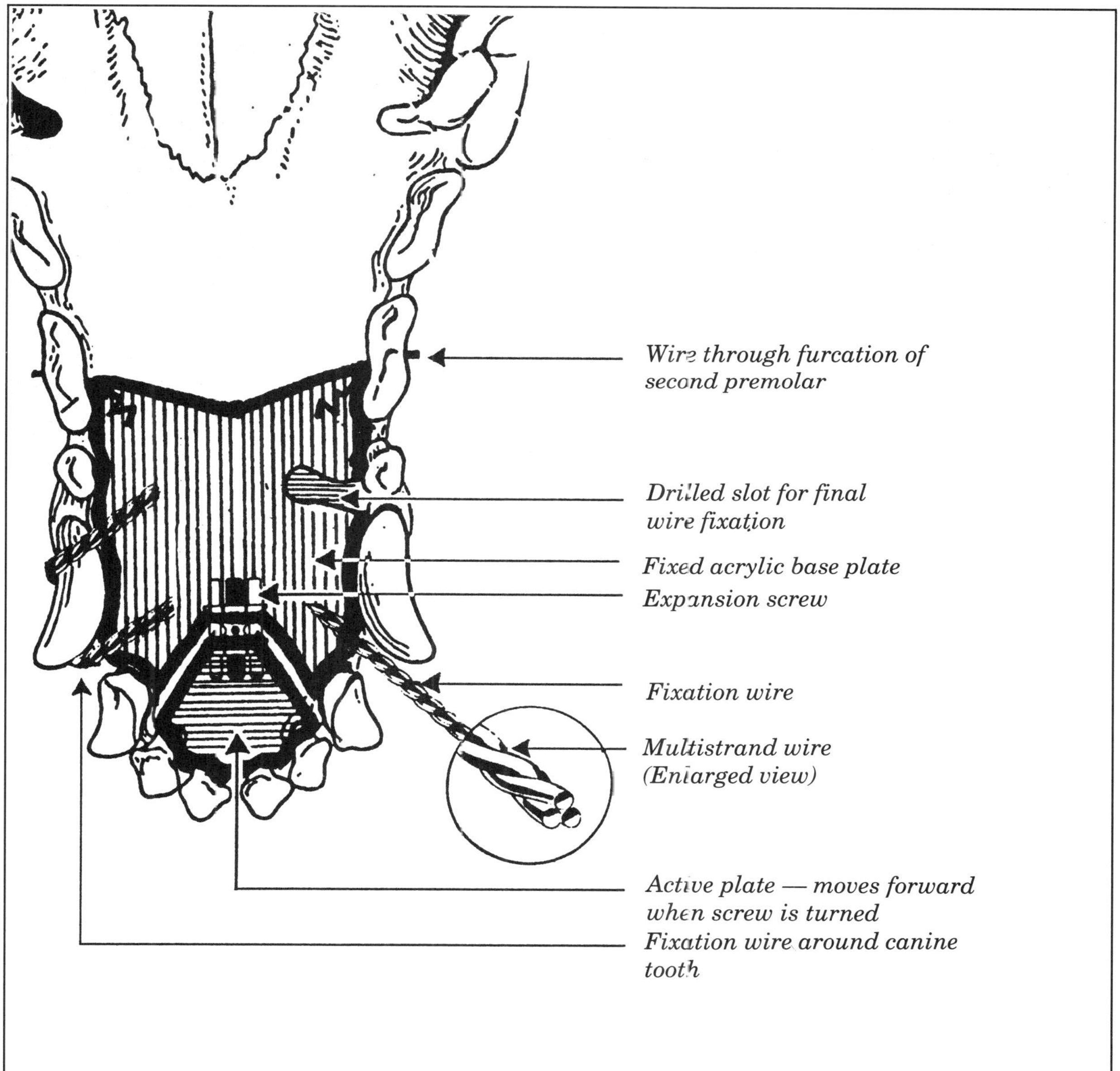

Figure 119. Elongated acrylic appliance with additional wire support through furcation of second premolars.

If the retention from the canine teeth is inadequate, such as when the canine teeth do not diverge enough, the appliance can be extended distally. Two extra stainless steel wires are embedded in the base of the appliance, and pushed under the bifurcation of the second premolars to hold the distal end of the appliance in place. If necessary, the bifurcation can be opened slightly with a round bur. This type of secondary attachment can irritate the gingiva but, for the generally short period of orthodontic treatment, this is acceptable. If a single incisor tooth needs to be moved, the acrylic plate can be made as described, with a PISTON SCREW built into the acrylic instead of the expansion screw. The piston screw is placed in the acrylic lingual to the tooth that is to be moved. The tip of the screw is positioned in contact with the tooth. Both types of screws should be turned one quarter of a complete rotation every four days.

9.31 INCLINED PLANE APPLIANCE (DEVICE)

A type of inclined plane appliance used to move lingually displaced canine teeth consists of an acrylic or a metal appliance that fits over the canine teeth of the jaw opposite the lingually displaced canine tooth. When the mouth closes, the displaced canine tooth (or teeth) contacts the inclined plane part of the device, which forces the tooth buccally into its correct position (Photos 88, 89, 90). These devices can have a unilateral or a bilateral inclined plane groove, depending on whether one or both of the mandibular canine teeth have to be moved. Metal appliances are the most efficient and reduce the time taken to perform the procedure. The latest appliances for young dogs, six to ten months of age, have a telescoping bar with cast bands on each end, which slip over the two maxillary canine teeth. They are called CAST BILATERAL (and UNILATERAL) TELESCOPING INCLINED PLANE APPLIANCES. The telescoping bar allows for the growth of the teeth and maxilla while the device is in place, and makes positioning on divergent canine teeth easier. A solid bar, rather than a telescoping bar, is adequate for adult dogs whose teeth and jaw growth is completed.

Lingually displaced canine teeth are usually found and treated in young dogs six to 10 months old, while the skull is still growing. The procedure using a metal appliance is usually a three–stage process. The first step, under sedation, is to take impressions of the canine teeth. A stone model is then poured. A wax or a silicone bite registration is also made (see preparation of orthodontic appliances, 9.26). These are then sent to the dental laboratory for casting of the device. Be sure to use a laboratory that is familiar with its construction, making sure that the wing(s) of the inclined part are wide enough so that the teeth make definite occlusal contact in the groove. There is some of lateral movement in the mandible of dogs and it is possible that, if the tip of the mandibular canine tooth catches the medial edge of the inclined plane, the tooth could be forced lingually and not buccally.

The second step is to bond the appliance on the maxillary canine teeth. Try to get the appliance returned from the laboratory within five days, since the mouth and teeth are still growing in most young dogs. Before bonding the device, try it in place with the dog awake to make sure that it fits and works properly. Then sedate the dog and bond it on, using acid–etch technique and a suitable metal–to–enamel bonding agent (e.g., Ketac–Cem).

Tooth movement is usually rapid in young dogs, six to ten months old, often being completed in five to ten days. In older animals, movement will take up to three to five weeks.

The third step is the removal of the device, which may or may not require sedation. A special orthodontic bracket removing instrument can be used to crack it off or it may have to be drilled off. The natural dental interlock of the mandibular canine teeth between the maxillary canine teeth and lateral incisor will retain the orthodontically repositioned teeth in place.

An alternative to a telescoping metal inclined plane device is to make your own ACRYLIC INCLINED PLANE APPLIANCE "in situ," across the maxillary canine teeth. With the dog under anesthesia, a slotted bracket is bonded on to the buccal surface of each maxillary canine tooth, just coronal to the gingiva. Orthodontic wire, 22– or 24–gauge, is passed around these teeth, through the slots in the brackets and twisted together in midline. This will reinforce the acrylic splint and prevent it from coming off. A trough or a dam of play dough, plasticine, silicone putty or similar material is made across the mouth to include the canine teeth and the wire. Vaseline, plastic or wax paper should be placed on the hard palate to prevent direct contact with the acrylic (because of the exothermic reaction). Powdered acrylic (polymer) is then placed in this trough and the liquid part (monomer) added. The mixture is built up until it forms a bridge across the teeth, building up more layers where the inclined plane groove is required. When the acrylic is hard, in about five minutes, the correct angulation of the groove is made with an acrylic trimming bur in a low–speed handpiece. The appliance should be tested by closing the mouth, and trimmed as necessary, to create the correct incline. Testing usually requires either removing the endotracheal tube or pushing the end carefully into the mouth, enough to permit occlusion of the teeth. Some dogs will allow the bite registration to be taken when fully awake.

Additional acrylic may have to be added to the appliance in order to get the correct angle of the inclined plane.

The second stage of this procedure is the removal of the appliance. Sedation or anesthesia will usually be required, since it may be necessary to cut the appliance off with a tapered bur in a high or a low–speed handpiece.

Both methods work well, and the choice depends on the skill of the operator, the costs involved, the age of the dog and the number of visits anticipated.

9.32 BITE WING APPLIANCE (DEVICE)

If the mandibular canine tooth is only slightly inclined lingually, an alternative to making a full inclined plane appliance is to make a BITE WING APPLIANCE, which is a type of inclined plane. This fits only from the maxillary canine tooth to the maxillary lateral incisor. These bite wings may be either unilateral or bilateral.

A figure–of–eight wire loop, 22– or 24–gauge wire, is made around the maxillary canine tooth and the maxillary lateral incisor. A bracket bonded to the buccal surface of each tooth provides additional retention for the wire. Self–cure acrylic is then molded around these two teeth, incorporating the wire, and an inclined plane groove is cut with an acrylic trimming bur.

Sedation or anesthesia is not generally required for removal of the appliance.

Bite wings made of wire incorporated in either composite or acrylic can also be used to move other teeth, especially mandibular incisors that are in a slight rostral deviation. In these cases, an inclined plane is placed on the incisal edge of the maxillary incisors (Photo 87). The inclined plane can either be made of acrylic that is formed around the teeth, or made of composite that is bonded on the incisors using an acid–etch technique. In order to strengthen and attach the acrylic or the composite, orthodontic wire is first attached to the teeth. The acrylic or the composite is then placed over the wire and shaped to leave an inclined plane at the incisal edge of the maxillary incisors. The incisal edge of the mandibular incisors can be bevelled slightly (odontoplasty) to help guide these teeth into the inclined plane.

9.33 EXPANSION SCREW FOR MOVEMENT OF LINGUALLY DISPLACED MANDIBULAR CANINE TEETH

This treatment for lingually displaced mandibular canine teeth is performed with the use of an EXPANSION SCREW held in place with wire and composite (Photo 85). A normal expansion screw, designed for use in human removable appliances, is supplied by several manufacturers in a variety of sizes. It consists of two metal plates each with three parallel holes. The outer holes hold rods that stabilize the structure and the inner hole is cut with a thread for the actual screw. A key is provided to turn the screw. Expansion screws with removable rods are more practical for fixation with wire.

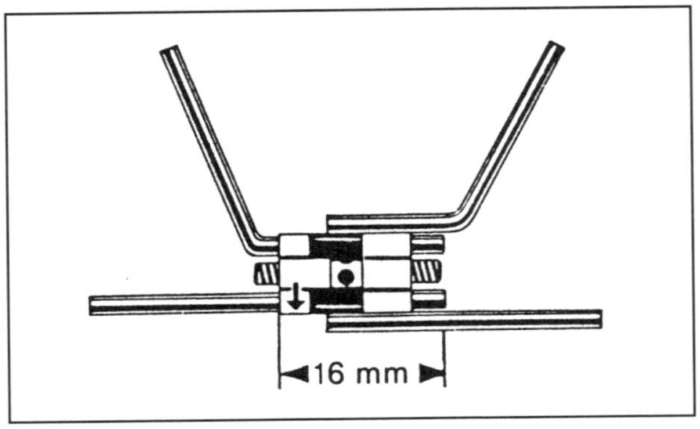

Figure 120. Hydrax–Biederman expansion screw.

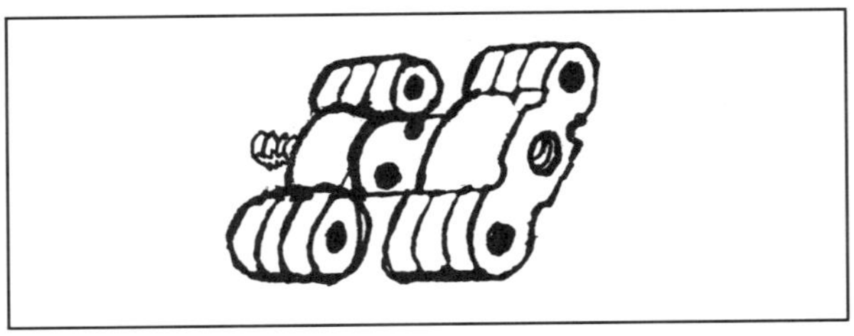

Figure 121. Unitek expansion screw.

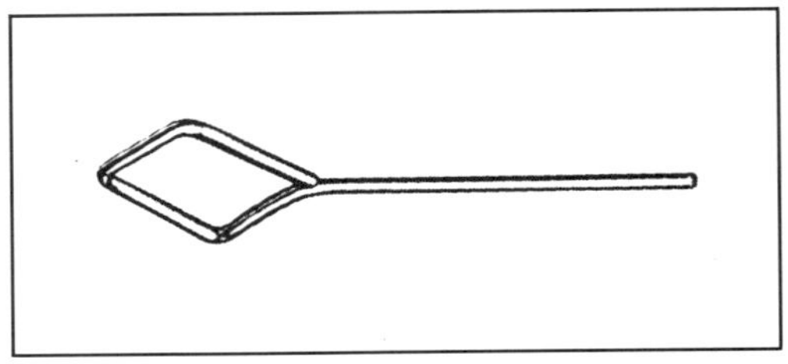

Figure 122. Adjustment key.

Fixation of the Expansion Screw

A screw is chosen that fits as close as possible between the two canine teeth in its original (closed) position. A wire is threaded through both holes left in one of the plates after the rods have been removed, and left with the ends sticking out. The other plate is similarly prepared. The two canine teeth are first etched, followed by a layer of composite resin. The wire will cut into the relatively soft resin, reducing the tendency of the wire to slip off the conical–shaped canine tooth. Composite is then placed over these wires to secure them to the teeth and cover any exposed ends of the wires. Although the device may prevent complete closure of the mouth, this is advantageous since it will permit the misaligned teeth to move laterally. Every four days, the screw should be turned one quarter of a complete rotation with the key (make sure the owner knows which direction!). This can be left to the owner, although it is recommended that a string be tied to the key to prevent its loss and/or swallowing should the dog try to pull away. Depending on the seriousness of the malocclusion, a treatment time between two weeks and two months can be expected. The appliance should be checked every 10 days or so to ensure that it sits tightly and the desired end point has not been passed.

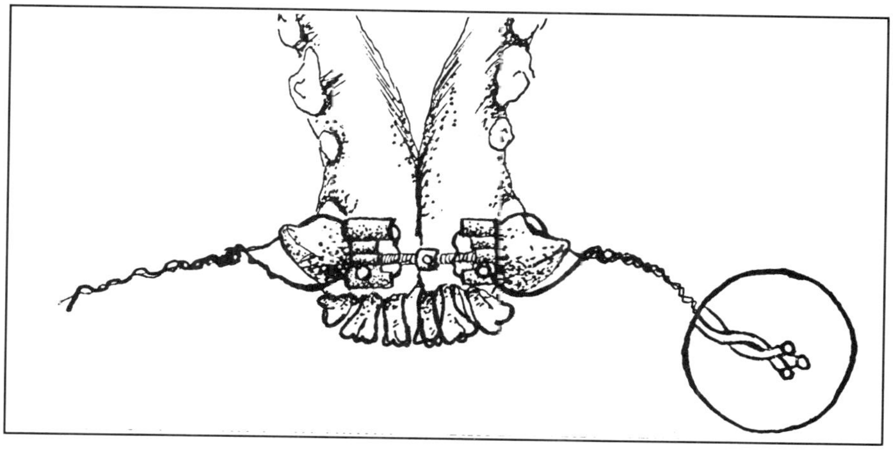

Figure 123 A. Expansion screw being wired around canine teeth.

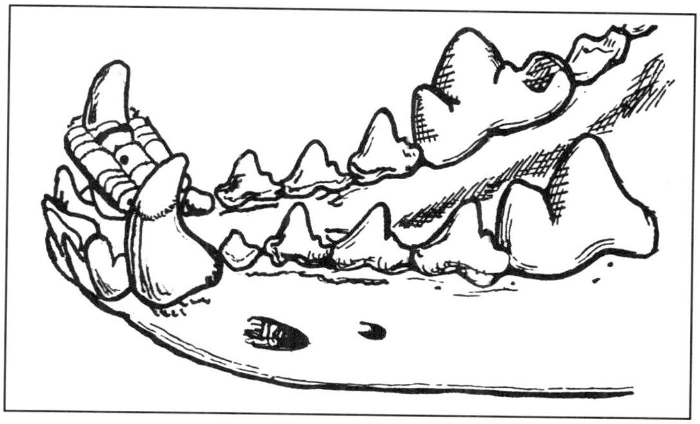

Figure 123 B. Expansion screw wired and bonded around canine teeth.

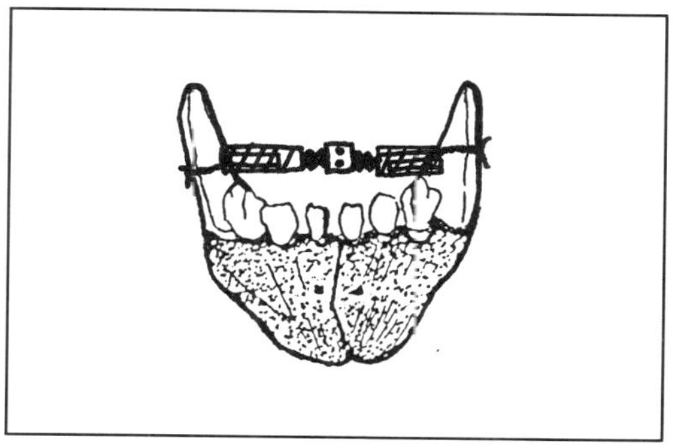

Figure 123 C. Horizontal positioning of expansion screw delivers equal forces to both canine teeth.

UNILATERAL LINGUALLY DISPLACED MANDIBULAR CANINE TOOTH

Often only one mandibular canine tooth is displaced. In this case the screw should be set at a slant, with the screw attached as coronally as possible on the tooth to be moved, and as gingivally as possible on the other tooth. The tooth with the more coronal leverage point will move the most. The other canine tooth will still tend to move but more slowly, although after the screw has been removed it should move back into its original position.

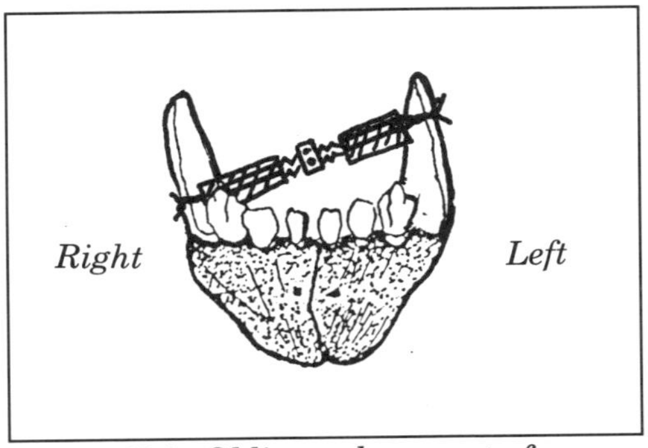

Figure 124. Oblique placement of expansion screw delivers more force and leverage to left canine tooth.

WIDE INTERCANINE DISTANCE IN LARGE DOGS

In some wide–skulled breeds of dogs, the distance between the canine teeth is too large for the biggest expansion screw available. A suitable expansion device can be custom made in the laboratory. Alternatively, the human expansion screw device can be fitted with one side attached as described above, while the other end is left free. Long wires are then attached to this end and, after crossing, twisted around the other tooth. The crossed wires are then embedded in self–cure acrylic. The floor of the mouth should either be smeared with vaseline or protected by a plastic strip while the acrylic cures to prevent thermal damage. Excess acrylic should be removed during or after polymerization.

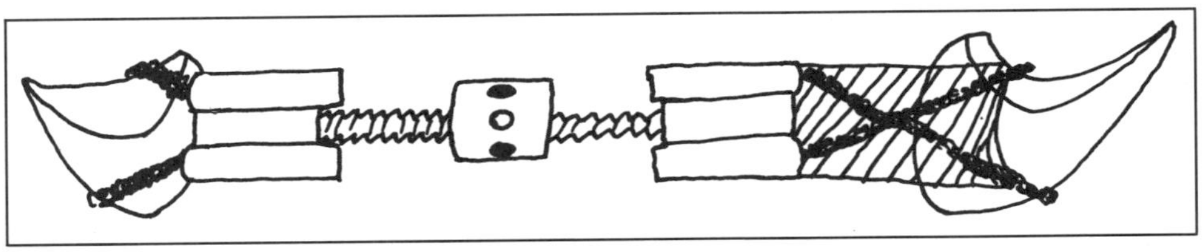

Figure 125. Method for large breeds Additional wire and acrylic used to bridge excess space.

A special screw device for larger dogs is being designed but is not yet available.

Warning: Too rapid or too much movement can cause opening of the mandibular symphysis. However, this will close again after removal of the expansion device. A four–day period between each turning of the screw has proven to be the most effective and physiologically sound interim time.

9.34 W–WIRE FOR THE MOVEMENT OF LINGUALLY DISPLACED MANDIBULAR CANINE TEETH

A spring–loaded expansion wire, called an OMEGA or "W–wire," can also be used to move lingually displaced canine teeth. The expansion wire is formed in a W–shape, with the vertical sides of the "W" being attached to the lingual side of each canine tooth, and the center of the "W" lying on the floor of the mouth. Although this method appears to work, it may not give as controlled or as rapid a movement of the teeth as the inclined plane appliance or the expansion screw.

9.35 BRACKETS, BUTTONS, HOOKS, WIRES AND ELASTICS

BRACKETS are used as attachments in human orthodontics. They have a slot into which specially prepared RECTANGULAR or SQUARE WIRES fit. The metal brackets are either attached to BANDS, which fit around the tooth, or to special METAL BASES (preferably with a mesh or a grooved backing). The base of the bracket is cemented on the tooth (LUTING) with luting cement, after acid–etching the tooth. Special ARCH WIRE is then bent to form SPRINGS, which apply the desired force to the teeth. The wire is slotted into the brackets, which hold it in place. These devices are known as BRACES (Photo 86). The whole procedure is complicated and expensive, and the opportunity for error is great. It is best left to those skilled in veterinary orthodontics, or to obtain the help of a human orthodontist.

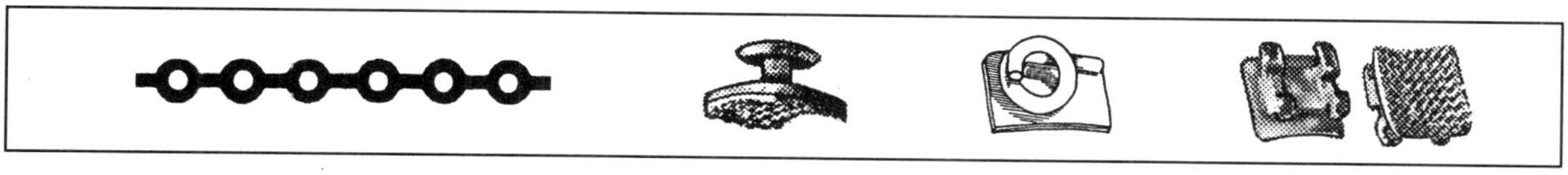

Figure 126. Elastic power chain. Button. Hook. Bracket.

The use of buttons, hooks and elastics is easier than slotted brackets. BUTTONS are supplied with a mesh or a grooved base for additional retention. HOOKS are either supplied similar to buttons (there is a hook instead of a button) or can be hand made by twisting wire around the tooth and making a hook from the twisted ends (Photo 83). A *composite* button or slotted bracket can also be custom made on the tooth. The composite is bonded on to the tooth surface and shaped with a bur to retain an elastic chain. ELASTIC POWER CHAINS or ENERGY CHAINS are elastic chains supplied in different sizes by orthodontic and dental suppliers. If the buttons are placed at different heights on different teeth, and then joined with an elastic chain, the force of the elastic will pull the teeth to the same height (Fig. 127). The chain fits exactly over the button, so placement is relatively easy.

Remember that an outward force (EXTRUSION) on one tooth will produce an inward force (INTRUSION) on the neighboring teeth, and the elastic will tend to pull all the teeth together and ROTATE the end teeth. If this is a potential problem, the teeth that are not required to be moved can be bonded together with composite or secured with an acrylic splint. Be sure that the surface area of the root(s) of the anchor tooth (teeth) is greater than that of the tooth (teeth) to be moved, otherwise the anchor tooth (teeth) may be moved too.

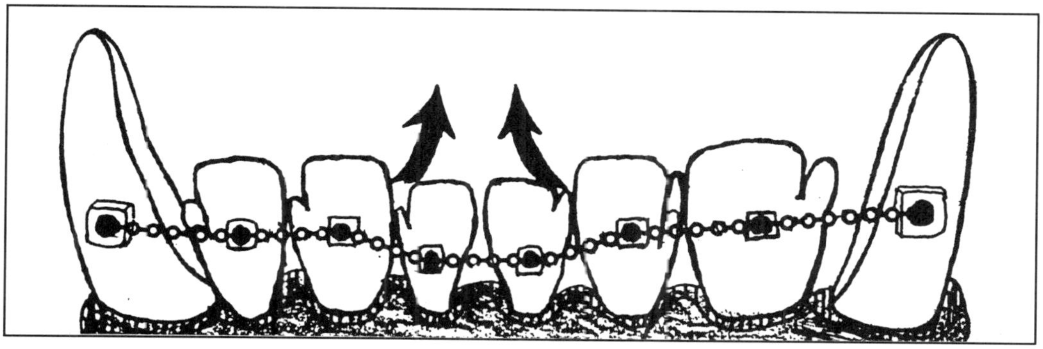

Figure 127. Retrusion of intermediate and lateral incisors.
Brackets are bonded to labial surfaces of incisors and canine teeth.
Extrusion of central incisors is caused by more apical placement of brackets.

The carnassial tooth is generally used as an anchor tooth in order to move a canine tooth with elastic power chain (Photo 82). To increase the surface area of the anchor tooth, the neighboring molar tooth can be wired and bonded with composite to the carnassial tooth. The force required to move teeth with elastic power chain should be between one and three ounces. In order to achieve this pressure, the elastic chain should be measured from button to button and then stretched about one third of its length before being attached.

ELASTIC RINGS or ELASTIC BANDS, which are used with lingual or with labial bars, are available in a wide selection of sizes and force values. This assures a precise degree of required control with continuous gentle force. ELASTIC LIGATURE THREAD is also available for certain orthodontic procedures.

The most common movement of teeth that is performed in veterinary dentistry involves TIPPING. When a force is applied to the tip of a crown, it moves the tip of the tooth and not the root apex. The FULCRUM, or axis of movement, is about one third of the way up the root from the apex forcing this point against the alveolus, which slowly resorbs, allowing movement.

Some orthodontic movements may require more than one type of appliance or procedure in order to achieve the desired effect. Care must be taken that one orthodontic procedure does not create another orthodontic problem. Careful monitoring of the progress with frequent examinations is recommended. The client should be thoroughly informed about what is to be expected and any problems that may occur.

9.36 ODONTOPLASTY (REMOVAL OF PART OF THE TOOTH STRUCTURE)

Odontoplasty (grinding of a portion of the enamel and sometimes the dentin of a tooth) is often necessary before, during or after an orthodontic treatment, but it can occasionally be used alone as a corrective measure.

In cases of CROWDING of the mandibular incisors, expansion of the canine teeth cannot always provide enough space, or the canine tooth position is such that expansion is not desirable. Careful odontoplasty of the mesial and distal surfaces of the incisor teeth can provide the additional space required. After this, muscle force from the tongue and lips is sometimes adequate to align the teeth, although in more severe cases orthodontic devices may be necessary to move the teeth. When moved, the teeth should stay in place by their natural dental interlock.

Depending upon the tightness of the interdental spaces, a thin diamond disc, either single– or double–sided depending on the teeth involved, or a thin pointed diamond bur or tapered fissure bur should be used. Following odontoplasty, the cut surface of the tooth should be smoothed with finishing diamonds, sanding discs or sanding strips. A new air-driven sanding attachment for a low-speed handpiece (e.g., Profin Directional system, Weissman Technology International, Inc.) is extremely effective for smoothing enamel and dentin, as well as even performing odontoplasty in some cases. The instrument uses reciprocating diamond-coated metal sanding tips.

Occasionally food and debris become impacted in periodontal pockets below the cingulum of slightly misaligned and tightly contacting teeth. Removal of the contact points aids in preventing this impaction, by allowing it to be licked or flushed away (Photo 58). After odontoplasty, the teeth should be pressed together to confirm that no

After odontoplasty, the teeth should be pressed together to confirm that no CONTACT POINT (EDGE) (SURFACE) between the teeth has been missed below the gingiva. No tooth should be reduced more than the others, or too much on one side. A certain amount of lateral movement can be expected, if space is available. Often the ground teeth will move a little, and then lock again in a slightly different configuration. Repeated grinding is indicated here. Be sure to use water cooling, or to allow time for cooling, especially in juvenile teeth that have thinner dentin and are more liable to damage through overheating.

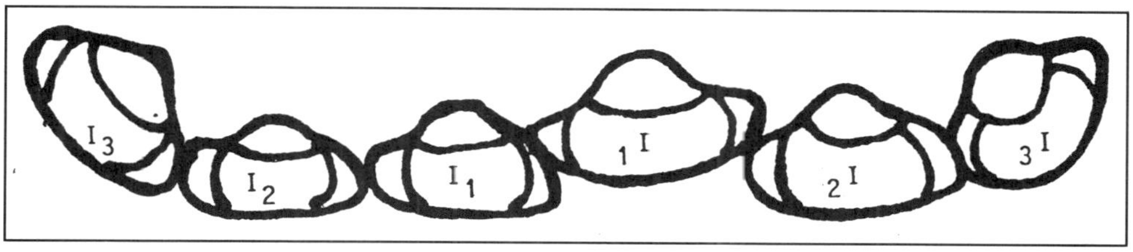

Figure 128 A. Crowded mandibular incisors. Lingual positioning of lower incisors.

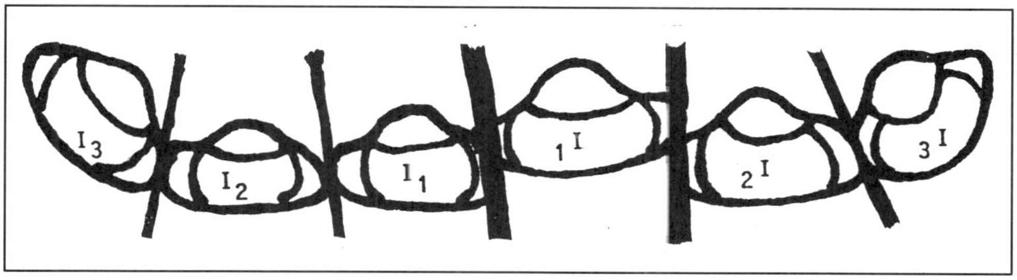

Figure 128 B. Odontoplasty of contact surfaces allows teeth to be moved. Tongue pressure alone will sometimes cause rostral movement of tooth in minor cases. In more severe cases use orthodontic devices.

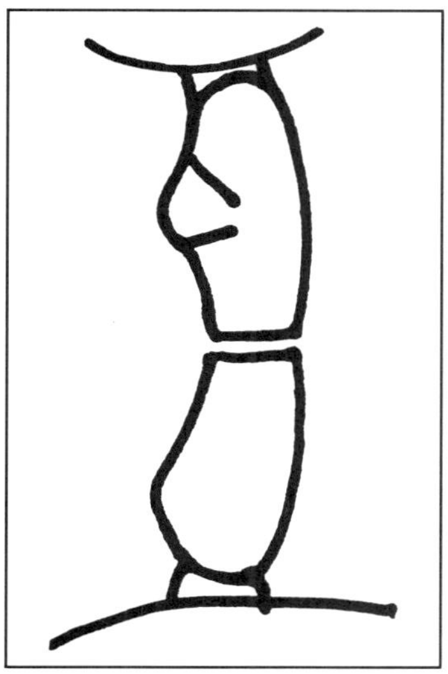

Figure 129 A.

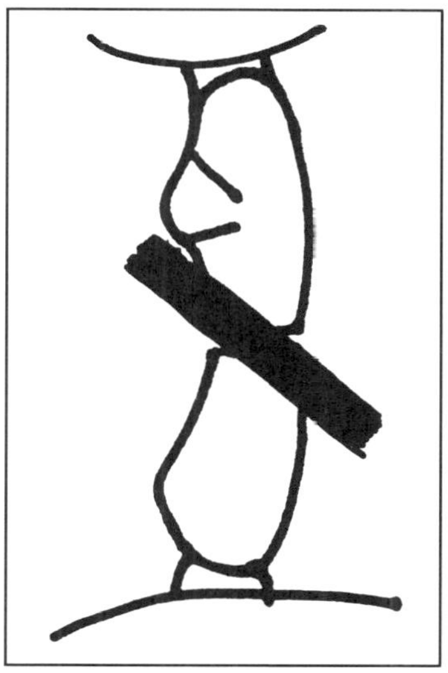

Figure 129 B.

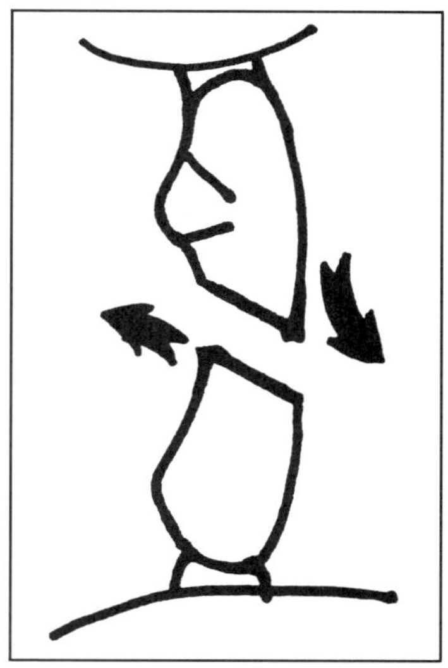

Figure 129 C.

129 A. Level (even) bite of incisors. Causes traumatic intrusion and horizontal attrition of teeth.
129 B. Creating a chisel edge shape to incisors.
129 C. Scissor bite is now established and causes protrusion of upper tooth and retrusion of lower tooth as well as slight extrusion of both teeth.

In cases of *level bite* of the incisal edge, angular grinding (odontoplasty) can alleviate the problem. The contact point on the incisal edge has normally been ground flat through constant attrition. The odontoplasty should be performed at an angle of 45 degrees (Fig. 129 B) and polished. Normally the constant force of the occlusion has INTRUDED (pushed inwards) these teeth or prevented normal eruption. Once they are not in traumatic contact, the intruded teeth should EXTRUDE (push outwards) by themselves, re–establishing a normal tooth length. The inclined plane created by the odontoplasty will PROTRUDE (push forwards) the maxillary teeth and RETRUDE (push backwards) the mandibular teeth, reestablishing the correct relationship.

9.38 SURGICAL PROCEDURES IN ORTHODONTICS

Open reduction of the length of the mandible in cases of severe prognathism has been published. A section of the mandible on each side is removed and the fragments joined with plates. Methods for *open extension of the length of the mandible* in cases of severe brachygnathism also exist.

These BLOCK or SEGMENTAL OSSEOUS RESECTION procedures are performed in the body of the mandible at the level of the second to fourth premolars. Extraction of one or two premolars is usually necessary. The mandibular bone is cut either in a "stair–step" or a "vertical sagittal" cut. The angles and length of the cuts must be adequate in order to leave good bone to bone contact in the final position.

The greatest problem with changing the length of the mandible is that the maxillary and mandibular arch widths are fixed at the level of the canine teeth. In most cases, either rostral or caudal repositioning of the mandible will put the canine teeth in traumatic occlusion. It is very difficult to reestablish the correct occlusion, and in most cases several teeth have to be removed, because the screws for the plates would destroy their roots. If a dental handpiece and bur are used to make the bone cuts, the contents of the mandibular canal can be saved if great care is used. These nerves and blood vessels will usually stretch or compress adequately to compensate for the change in bone length and will remain functional. Be careful that the stabilization pressures do not injure these tissues, during and after the fracture fixation. If the mandibular nerve is damaged or is destroyed, there is a loss of sensation in the lip, which leads to drooling and difficulty in eating and drinking.

Elongation and reduction of the length of the mandible are complex procedures, and are usually not warranted. Since it is not ethical to perform such a procedure on show dogs, it would only benefit dogs with either such a severe malocclusion that the tips of the teeth were traumatizing the opposing oral soft tissues, or the malocclusion was making eating difficult. In such cases these problems can be better treated by extracting, reducing or orthodontically moving the offending teeth.

Another form of *block resection* is to cut the bone around an *individual tooth* or *group of teeth* (i.e., incisors) and reposition the bone. Although this technique does not damage the periodontal structures, there is a risk of losing the blood supply to the osseous block being moved. Because the roots of the incisors lie very close to each other and converge apically, the procedure is very difficult and prone to failure. Retention splints are required for four to six weeks, which can cause periodontal damage.

Surgical repositioning of individual misaligned teeth can be performed in selected cases. The technique is to partially sever the periodontal ligament and gently lever the tooth into the new position. This method can be used to reposition a permanent canine tooth that is displaced by a retained deciduous canine tooth. After the deciduous tooth has been removed, the periodontal ligament of the permanent canine tooth is carefully severed in the coronal half of the alveolus, using an elevator. The tooth is then gently levered into the space left by the deciduous tooth. If there is not enough space in the alveolus, it must be created surgically with a bur. The repositioned tooth is retained in place with gingival sutures. This procedure is only practical in young dogs, four to six months old, or before the apex of the root closes. Care must be taken not to disrupt the apical blood supply of the tooth. If total blood loss occurs, the tooth will become non–vital and the tooth will require endodontic therapy. If all the periodontal fibers are broken, the tooth may not reattach. The disadvantages occur infrequently and can usually be avoided if reasonable care is used in the movement. The advantages are that subsequent orthodontic treatment, anesthesia and expense can be avoided. The procedure can be the answer to minor occlusal problems in the young four to six months old puppy and kitten.

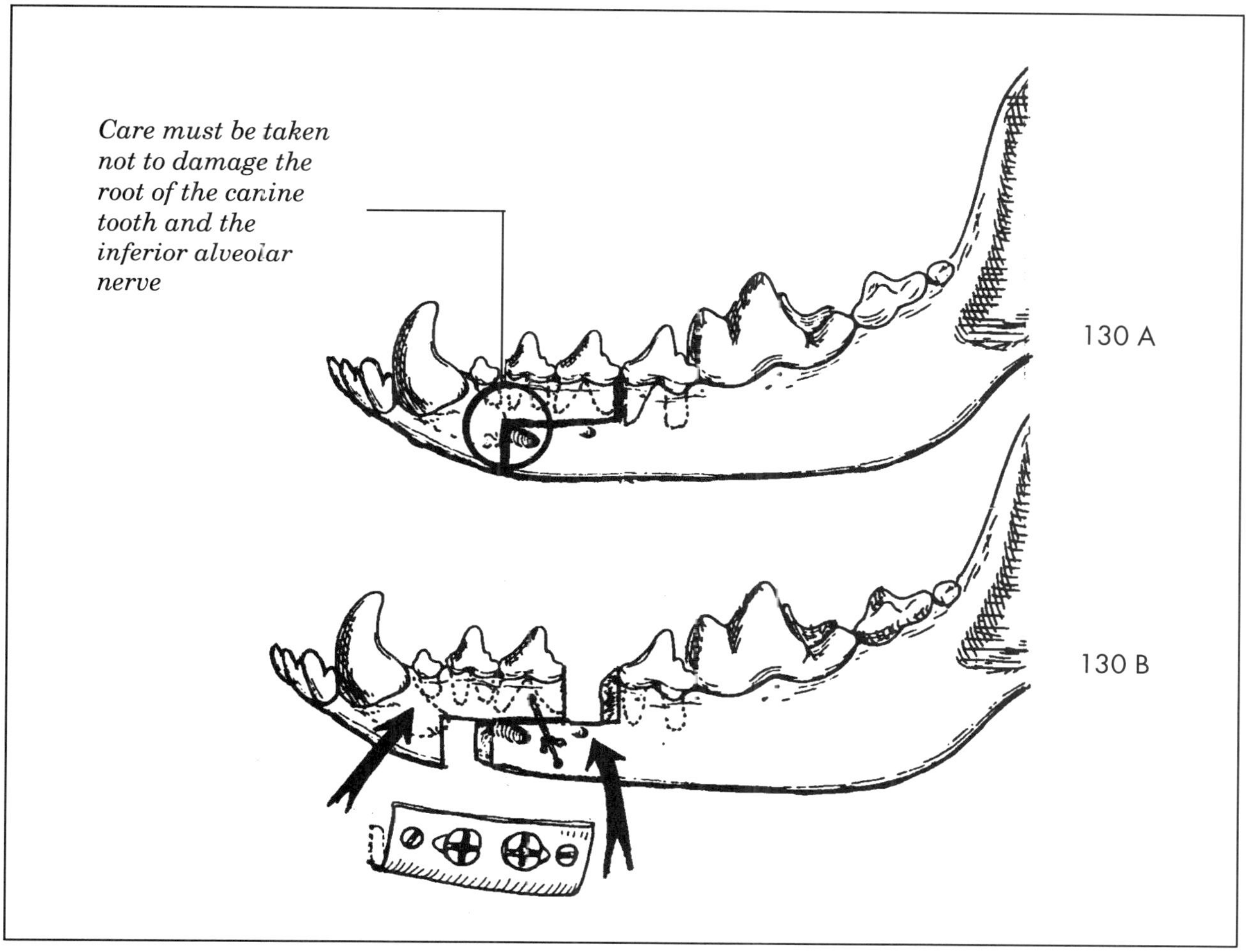

Figures 130 A–B. "Stair–step" segmental osseous resection of the mandible.

130 A. The anterior segment is cut in the shape of a step. Care should be taken not to damage the apices of the teeth.

130 B. The two segments are wired together in the desired position. Additional support is necessary with an intraoral acrylic splint.

CHAPTER 10

ORAL SURGERY

10.1 FRACTURES OF THE JAWS

Fractures of the jaw occur commonly as a result of falls or from automobile accidents. Often these fractures are not noticed by the owner, and therefore a thorough examination of the jaws is recommended after any accident for medical and legal reasons.

Symptoms of a jaw fracture include abnormal position of the jaws, inability to close the mouth properly, abnormal movement of the jaws when palpated, swelling, crepitation, pain, poor eating ability, tooth loss, bleeding, lacerations of the lips and gums.

Radiographs should always be taken in two views if you are suspicious of the jaw fractures.

10.2 FRACTURES OF THE MANDIBLE (LOWER JAW)

Therapy is dependent upon the site of the fracture (or fractures). The most difficult fractures to diagnose and treat involve the condyles. These fractures, fortunately, heal well if left alone since a pseudoarthrosis can develop. Fractures of the body of the mandible can be treated by plating the fracture (Fig. 132), or for other options consult an orthopedic surgery text. Fractures or separation of the MANDIBULAR SYMPHYSIS can be stabilized with wire. If the canine teeth diverge, 24– or 26–gauge wire is twisted in a FIGURE–OF–EIGHT pattern around the canine teeth and covered with self–cure acrylic. The floor of the mouth should be coated with vaseline to protect the sensitive mucosa from the exothermic reaction of the curing acrylic and from the irritation of the acrylic monomer. Alternatively this "figure–of–eight" wire can be secured to the canine teeth with composite following acid–etching of the teeth (Photo 91). If the canine teeth do not diverge buccally in their correct position, CIRCUM–MANDIBULAR WIRING should be performed. The wire is attached to a large curved needle and passed into the gums rostral to one canine tooth, under the mandible and out through the gums caudal to the other canine tooth, around the canine tooth itself, and then back the other way from rostral to caudal. The ends are then twisted together. Additionally a wire can be led around the front of the incisors from one canine tooth to the other. The ends of the wires are then covered with acrylic to prevent irritation of the soft oral tissues and lips (see acrylic splints, 10.6).

10.3 BIOMECHANICS OF MANDIBULAR FRACTURES

The pull and forces of the mandibular muscles tend to dislocate the fragments of bone at the fracture site.

The masseter, temporalis and medial pterygoid muscles are attached to the mandible and are used to close the mouth. The digastric muscle is attached to the symphysis and is used to open the mouth. The forces of both sets of muscles tend to separate the fragments. The method of fixation must be chosen to prevent these forces from being able to separate the jaw fragments. Radiographs should be used to determine the exact position and angle of the fracture so that the operation can be planned properly.

Teeth in the fracture site present a problem. In the past these teeth used to be extracted as a matter of course but, with the introduction of modern techniques, many of these teeth can be saved.

Teeth in the fracture site that are luxated, fractured or infected usually are removed. Teeth that are involved in the fracture site, but do not hinder fracture closure, and where the periodontium is not damaged (or only slightly), can be retained, at least temporarily if needed, for support of wire and acrylic splints. Antibiotics are necessary as the periodontium can provide a direct route into the fracture site for infection from the oral cavity. The affected root of a multirooted tooth can be sectioned and extracted, as long as a vital pulpotomy or endodontic therapy is performed to protect the other root(s).

As a simple rule of thumb, if in doubt, any mobile tooth in the fracture site should be extracted immediately, unless it contributes to fracture stability.

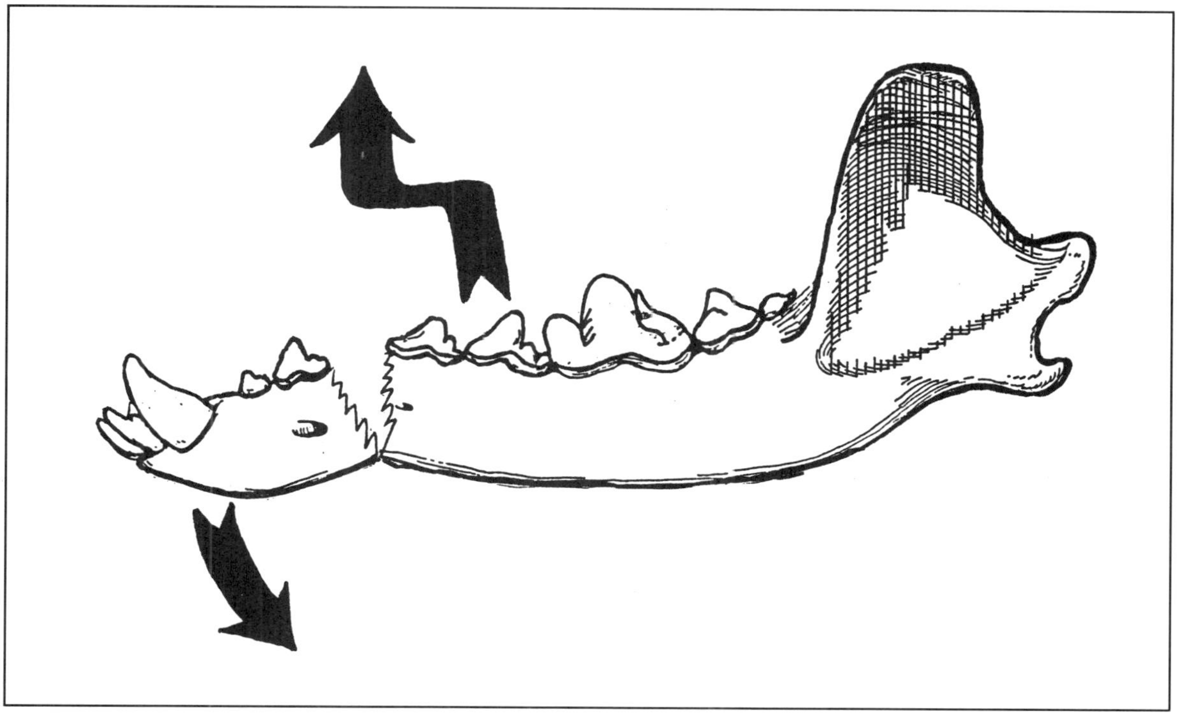

Figure 131. Biomechanics of fractured mandible.

Muscle forces tend to pull the rostral segment ventro–caudally, and the caudal segment rostro–dorsally. Depending on the angle of the fracture this can be either favorable or unfavorable.

10.4 PLATING AND PINNING

COMPRESSION PLATES, REGULAR BONE PLATES, LAG SCREWS and INTERMEDULLARY (I.M.) PINS can be used in some cases of fractured jaws, but only in selected places. The jaw bones *do not* lend themselves well to this type of INTRAORAL FIXATION because of their shape and size. The roots of the teeth occupy much of the jaw and can easily be damaged by the plate screws and the I.M. pins. Intramedullary pins placed along the length of the mandible will usually destroy the blood vessels and nerves in the mandibular canal. When repairing a fractured mandible, *maintaining the dental occlusion is more important than the fracture alignment.*

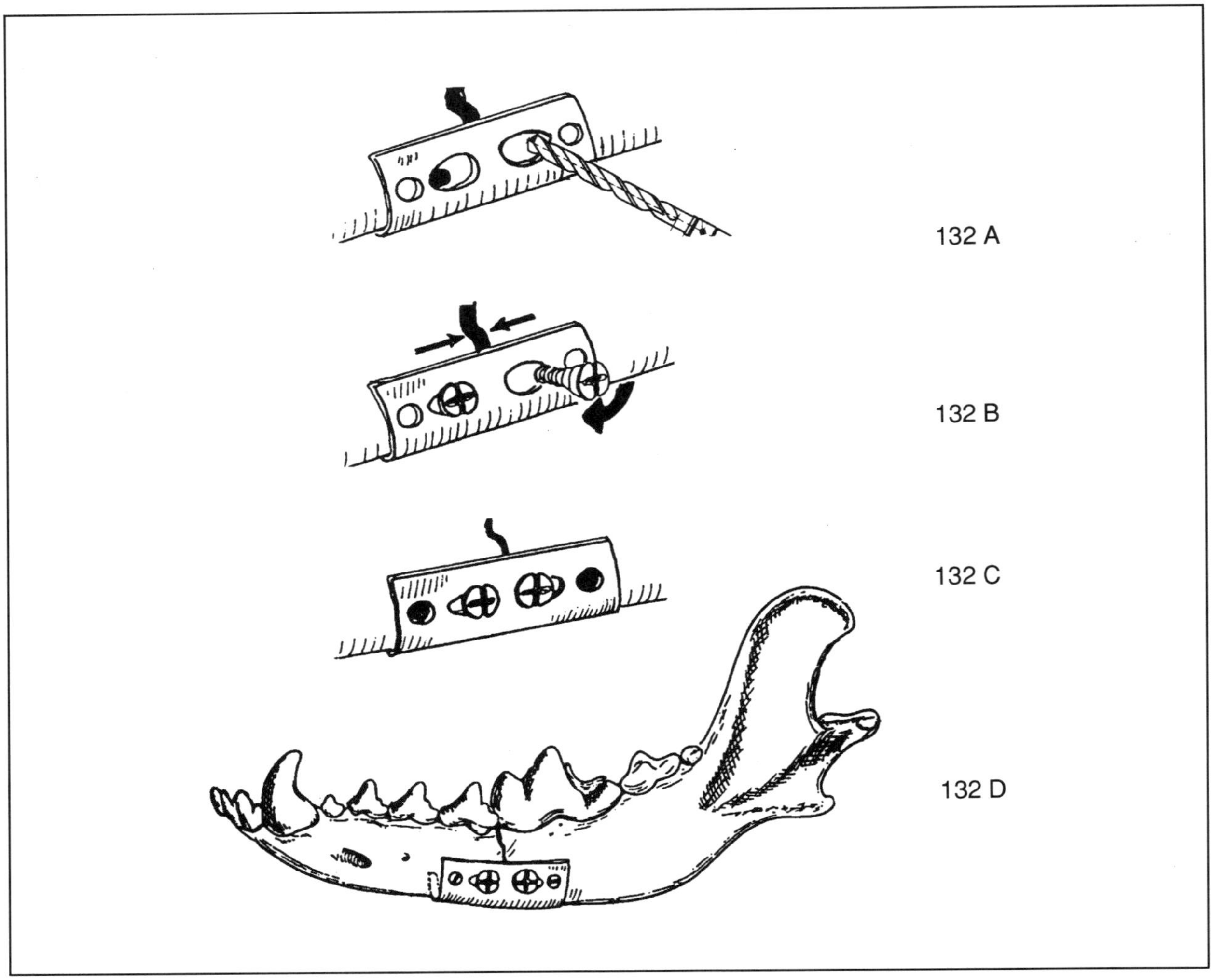

Figure 132 A–D. Stabilization of vertical fracture sites.

Compression plate alignment. Due to elongated plate slots, the two segments are brought together when the screws are tightened.

132 A. Drilling holes at ends of elongated slots.
132 B. Placing tapered screws in holes, causes compression of segments.
132 C. Screws tightened. Two more holes are drilled for further fixation.
132 D. Segments compressed and held by four screws.

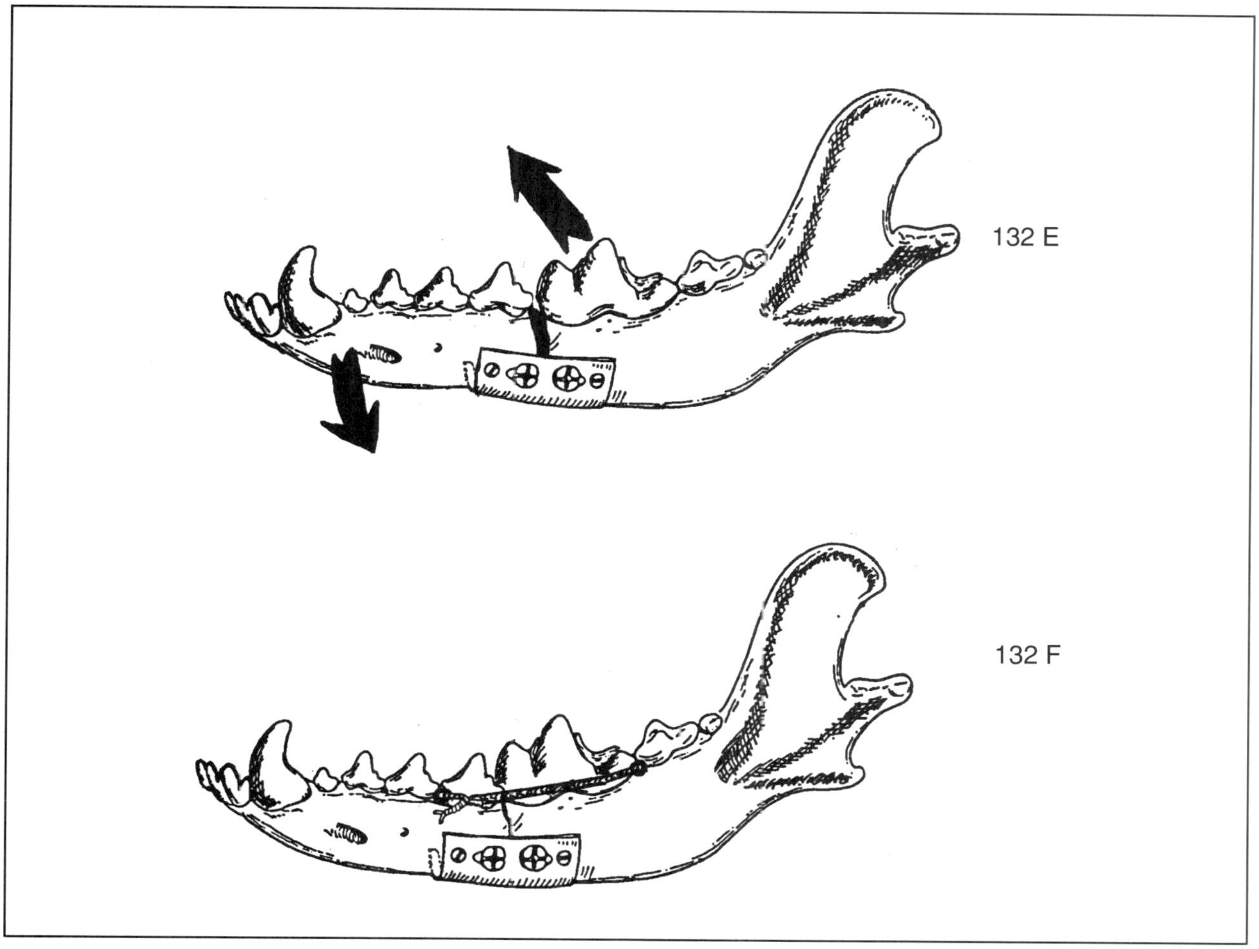

Figure 132 E–F. Stabilization of vertical fracture sites.

132 E. Muscle forces tend to open dorsal fracture site. Additional support may be necessary.
132 F. Additional interdental or interosseous wiring will stabilize the fracture site.

EXTRAORAL SPLINTING with a KIRSCHNER–TYPE APPARATUS can be used in selected cases, but is not necessary if alternative methods can be used. They are awkward for the pet and difficult to apply successfully.

Intramedullary pins are placed percutaneously into the bone each side of the fracture site and fixed together with self–cure acrylic.

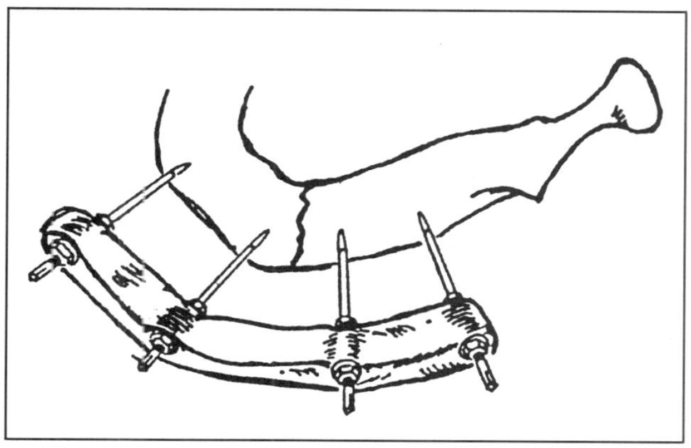

Figure 133. Percutaneous extraoral splint (Kirschner–type apparatus).

Wiring and acrylic splinting is now considered the method of choice in most cases of jaw fractures (see wiring, 10.4 and acrylic splinting, 10.6).

Occasionally lag screws alone can be used to stabilize fractures (Fig. 134). If plates, lag screws and I.M. pins are used, it is often wise to provide additional fixation with wire, since the masticatory forces will tend to open the fracture site around the plate or the pin.

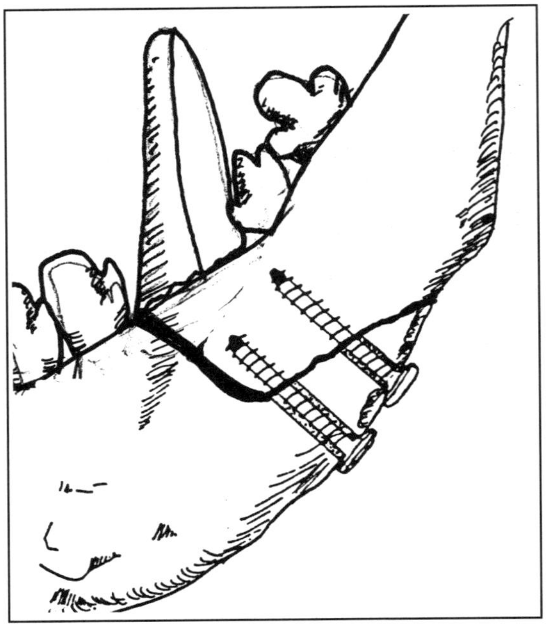

Figure 134. Lag screw fixation.

The external holes are larger than the screws; the internal holes match the screw size. When tightened the bones are compressed.

10.5 WIRING

Wiring of oral fractures is easier than plating and pinning and can be less traumatic. For simple stable fractures, wiring is the treatment of choice. For more complex fractures, additional support and stability can be obtained with acrylic splints incorporated around the wire (Photo 19). Correct wiring techniques and acrylic splinting can be used satisfactorily for most jaw fractures and are less prone to complications. The commonly used wiring techniques include INTEROSSEOUS WIRING (through two pieces of bone), CIRCUMFERENTIAL WIRING (around the bone), INTERARCADE WIRING (between the jaws), INTERDENTAL WIRING (between the teeth) and FIGURE–OF–EIGHT (around the teeth).

The GAUGE OF WIRE used for most BONE WIRING should be either 20– or 22– gauge. For INTERDENTAL WIRING and STABILIZING ACRYLIC SPLINTS, either 24– or 26–gauge wire may be used.

A loop of wire can be used to assist pulling the fixation wire through the holes drilled in the bone (Fig. 136).

Several different wiring methods have been used for interdental wiring including IVY LOOP, STOUT, ESSIG and RISDON methods (see *BOJRAB* and *THOLEN*, Small Animal Oral Medicine and Surgery).

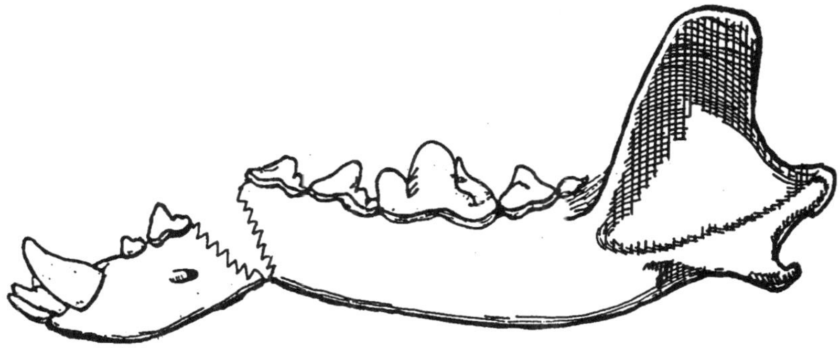

135 A Dorso-ventral oblique fracture (unfavorable)

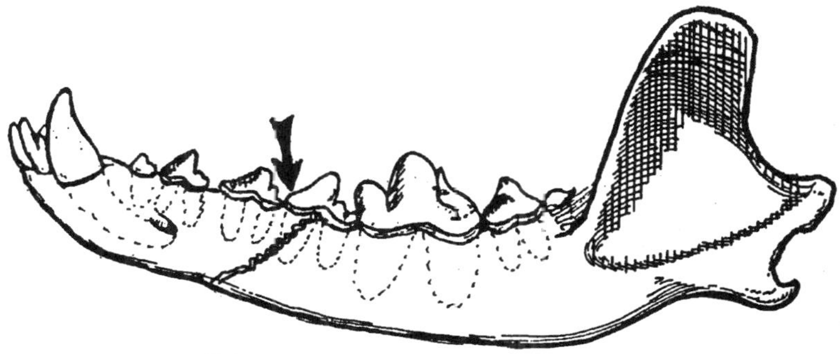

135 B Ventro-dorsal oblique fracture (favorable)

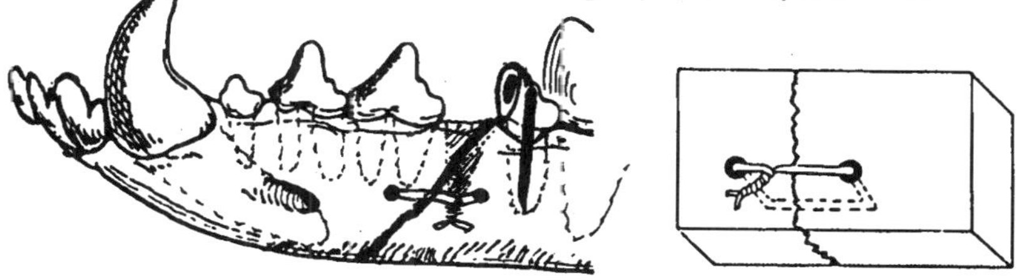

135 C

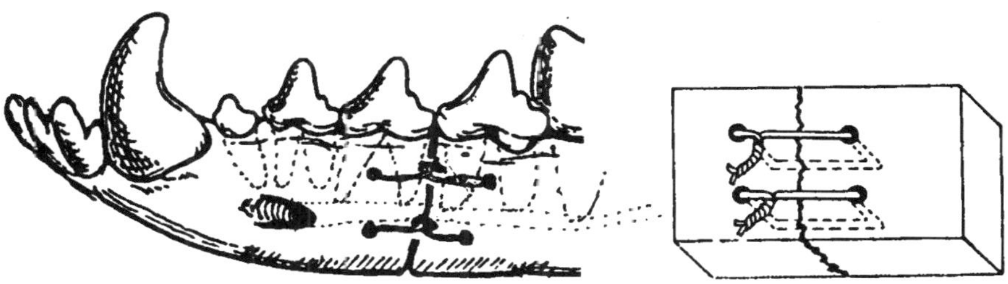

135 D

Figure 135 A–D. Wiring of mandible.

135 A. Fracture site opens up considerably, due to muscle pull.
135 B. Muscle pull helps to self stabilize the fracture. Note the fourth premolar in fracture site (arrow).
135 C. Single interosseous wiring is sufficient to stabilize some fractures. Fourth premolar should be removed or hemisectioned.
135 D. Double interosseous method wiring. Meticulous positioning of holes is necessary to avoid roots and mandibular canal.

A wire loop can facilitate returning the wire from the lingual side.

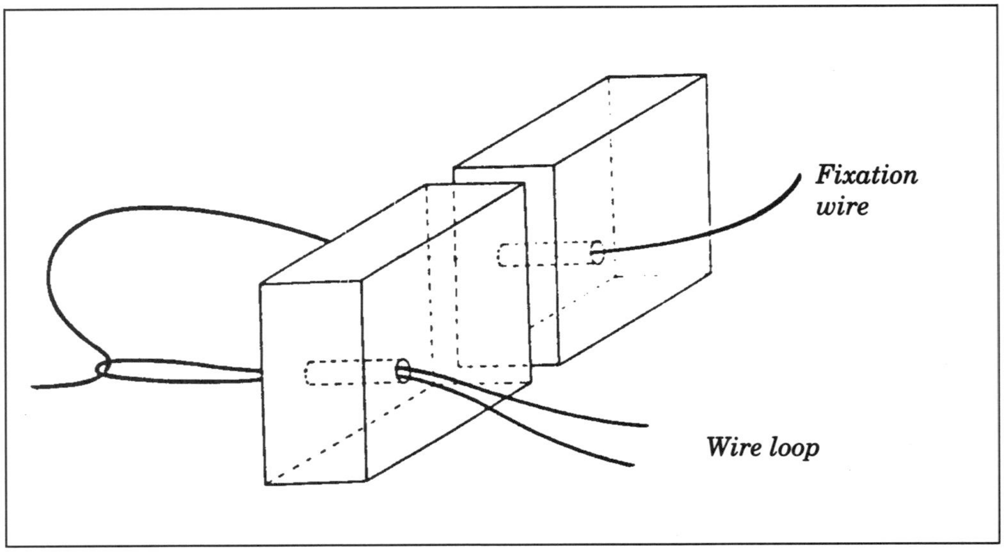

Figure 136. Wire loop to pull fixation wire through bone.

10.6 ACRYLIC SPLINTS – INTRAORAL

Acrylic splints can be used for several intraoral procedures, including stabilizing bone fractures, splinting loose teeth and reimplanting avulsed teeth (Photos 16-19). These splints are extremely practical for jaw fractures rostral to the first molars (Photo 19).

When the mandible has been fractured, especially rostral to the first molar, acrylic splints with wire are often the treatment of choice. Before an acrylic splint is made, the fracture site has to be either stabilized or reduced. This can be done either manually or with wire. The most important consideration is to reestablish a proper occlusion. No matter how good the fracture reduction is, all will be in vain if an adequate occlusion is not attained. The interdigitation of the teeth is very precise and there is little room for error.

The acrylic is built up in layers incorporating the wire supports, using putty or Playdough to form a trough (dam) (Photo 18). The acrylic should be 1.5–2 mm thick, placed coronal to the gingival margins, and *mostly* on the *lingual* surface of the *mandibular teeth* and on the *buccal* surface of the *maxillary teeth.*

Since the reaction by which self–curing acrylics harden is an EXOTHERMIC REACTION (heat is produced), and since the acrylic monomer is irritating, care must be taken not to damage the soft tissues of the mouth. In order to avoid this, the splints can be made on a stone model. This is often not practical because of the extra time, anesthesia and costs involved. To minimize heat damage when an acrylic splint is made in the mouth of the animal, the soft tissues can either be smeared with a thin layer of vaseline, or covered with wax paper, aluminum foil and plastic. Vaseline is used most commonly.

Before satisfactory wiring can be accomplished, sheets of a pliable LIGHT–CURED ACRYLIC SPLINTING MATERIAL (Densply's "Triad") can be placed over some jaw fractures for temporarily holding the reduced bone and teeth in place. The soft sheet of acrylic is cut and molded over the site, then light–cured. Additional self–curing acrylic and wire can then be added to secure the splint.

When cured, all acrylic splints are trimmed with either carbide burs or acrylic trimming burs, carefully removing any flash and making sure that no pockets and crevices are left for food and debris to collect.

10.7 INTERARCADE FIXATION

ZETNER'S INTERARCADE FIXATION method can be used to hold jaw fragments together. This technique is good for cats and small dogs. TMS PINS are placed in the buccal surfaces of all four canine teeth. The jaws are then brought together, so that the teeth are in their proper occlusion, and the pins joined with wire and/or self–cure acrylic. The animal is fed by squirting liquid food into the cheek pouches. It is possible with this method to fix the jaws slightly apart. Although this allows the animal to feed itself, it is difficult to position the fragments accurately. Small discrepancies in occlusion can be corrected by grinding the early occlusal contact points, but larger discrepancies will necessitate the extraction of one or more canine teeth, or refracturing the jaw later to get the correct occlusion.

The composite around the teeth should be carefully removed after the fracture has healed. The pins can be either cut off and polished flat, or removed by unscrewing or by drilling out, and the resulting holes filled with composite.

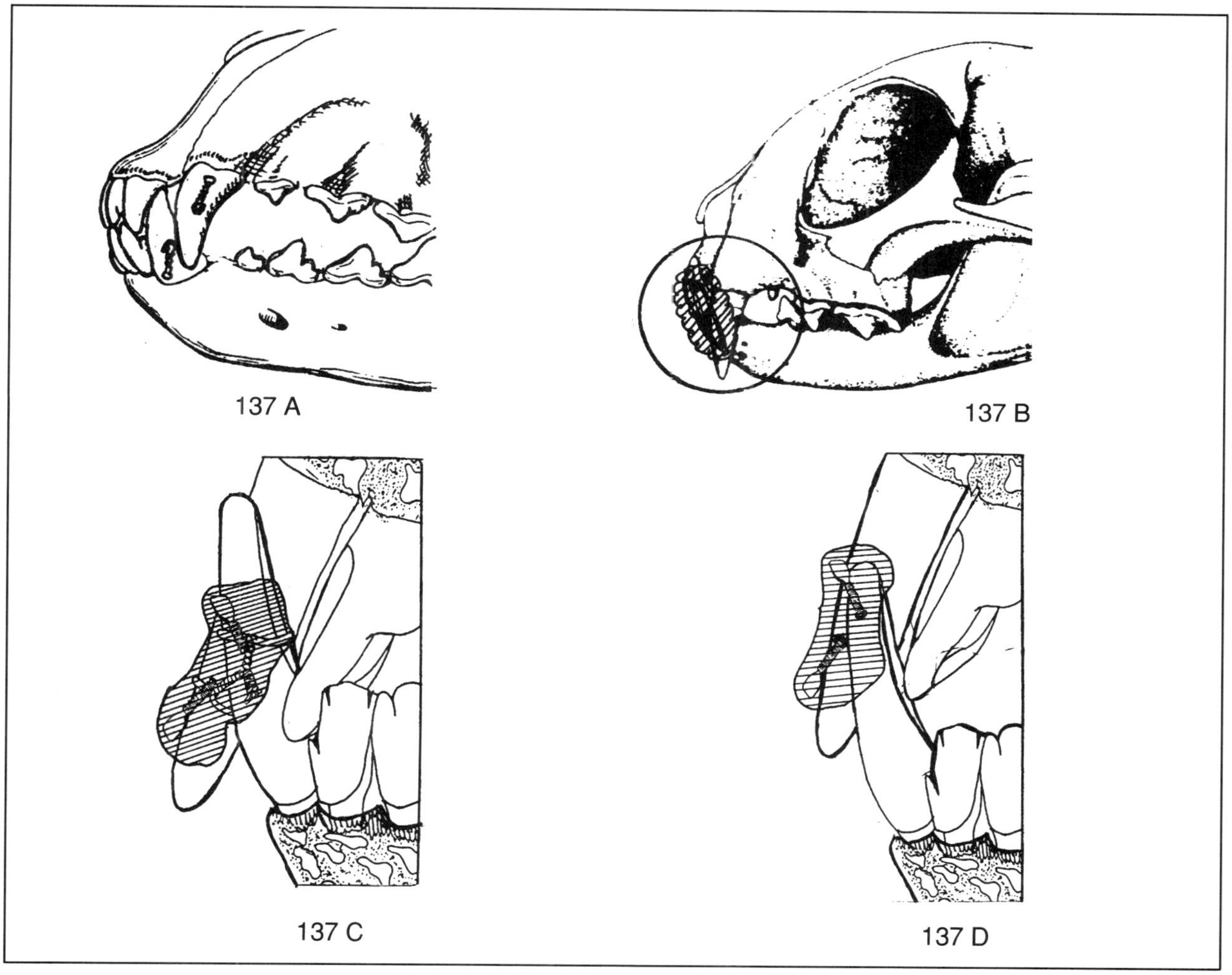

Figure 137 A–D. Interarcade fixation (Zetner).

137 A. Parapulpal pins in canine teeth.
137 B. Pins are linked by either composite or by wire, or both together, locking the jaws together.
137 C. Mouth in full occlusion. Pins and additional wire embedded in composite.
137 D. Mouth in partial occlusion. Pins alone embedded in composite.

Care should be taken to avoid damaging the pulp, especially in juvenile teeth.

This procedure should not be performed on animals that tend to vomit, such as longhaired cats that get hairballs. The risk of inhalation pneumonia would be considerable, and could cause the death of the pet.

10.8 JAW FRACTURES OF PUPPIES

Metal plates are definitely contraindicated in puppies because the tooth germinal tissue in the jaw bone would be irreparably damaged, the growth of the mandible would be retarded. Because of the delicate nature of the bone itself, the operation is technically very difficult. Although wires, acrylic splints or interjaw fixation can be used, in many cases a simple TAPE MUZZLE is just as effective. To facilitate easy removal of a tape muzzle, the tape should be wrapped or placed once around the muzzle with the sticky side out, and then folded back on itself and wound around again so that a non–sticky side is also on the outside. This type of sling can be removed and replaced as necessary. Generally four to eight weeks will be required for healing.

10.9 AVULSED TEETH – REIMPLANTATION

AVULSED TEETH are teeth that have come completely out of the socket or alveolus, usually as a result of trauma. The teeth most commonly involved are the incisors and the canine teeth.

The successful reimplantation of a tooth is greatly influenced by the length of time that the tooth is out of the socket. Ideally a completely avulsed tooth should be put back into the socket immediately and held there until treatment can be performed. If this is not possible, it should be placed in milk to protect the remains of the periodontal ligament and keep it moist. Reimplantation should be performed within a few hours to be successful, and preferably within one hour.

Providing that the avulsed tooth is intact, it should be washed with water, as well as the socket, and reseated. The remains of the periodontal ligament should not be scraped off. It is wise to closely examine and radiograph the socket area for signs of trauma. When large maxillary canine teeth are avulsed buccally by trauma, the thin bone medial to the root apex is often fractured, due to the root apex being forced into the nasal sinus.

Retention of avulsed teeth involves stabilization with wires, composites and acrylics, depending on the case. One of the best methods to hold a large canine tooth in place is to bond a slotted orthodontic bracket on to the buccal surface of each canine tooth, close to the gingival margin. Wire is then passed through the slots of the brackets and twisted together in the midline. The brackets prevent the wire from slipping off the conically shaped canine teeth. An ACRYLIC SPLINT is then poured over the wire and around each canine tooth using a dam of putty, Playdough, or similar material, to make the form (Photos 16-19). Be sure that there is a space (1–2 mm) between the acrylic and the hard palate or the sublingual tissues, and that the mouth can close properly. After a period of one to two months, the acrylic and wire splint is cut in the midline with a bur and the reimplanted tooth tested for stability. If the tooth is securely reimplanted, the acrylic device can be removed. If it is still loose (2 mm or more of lateral movement at the tip of the crown), more self–cure acrylic can be added to the midline cut to reform the bridge and the testing process repeated a few weeks later.

All completely avulsed teeth are non–vital, because the blood and nerve supply has been disrupted. Therefore, at some stage a root canal therapy has to be performed. It is best to wait until you are sure that the tooth has reseated properly. Endodontic treatment should not be performed on the avulsed tooth prior to reimplantation. Every minute the tooth is out of the socket compromises the success of the procedure, and apical root canal filling materials can jeopardize the healing process. The extra cost of a root canal procedure should also be considered, which may be unnecessary if reimplantation does not succeed, except in cases of INTERNAL ROOT RESORPTION. Although internal resorption of the root can initially be visible as a pink hue to the crown of the tooth due to pulpal hemorrhage, it can also occur without any external signs. A radiograph should be taken two to four weeks after reimplantation to check for any signs of internal resorption. If this is found, endodontic therapy should be performed as soon as possible to prevent further internal resorption.

For incisors or some small canine teeth that are avulsed, retention is obtained by wiring, splinting and bonding to the adjacent teeth, applying the same principles as previously described.

With smaller teeth, such as incisors, which are not subject to strong masticatory forces, the retaining devices can be removed earlier, even after two to four weeks, to test the degree of success.

For teeth that are only partially avulsed or subluxated, the same techniques usually apply. For TEETH that are simply MOBILE, generally only stabilization is necessary (Photo 93) and not endodontic treatment, since the blood supply to the tooth should still be intact. However, after trauma there is a high chance the pulp will become non-vital, thus close follow-up is required.

The owner should always be advised that any reimplanted tooth is a compromised tooth. Failure can occur any time for the rest of the dog's life, from external and internal resorption of the root, ankylosis and further trauma.

10.10 FRACTURES OF THE MAXILLA (UPPER JAW)

Signs of fracture of the maxilla include bleeding from the nose and abnormal mobility of the tooth carrying bone. The most common type is a separating fracture of the MAXILLARY PROCESS, normally a fracture across the maxilla at the level of the premolars, so that the frontal part of the maxilla is highly mobile. The thinness of the bone precludes plating, thus wire and acrylic splints are the treatment of choice. A length of either 24– or 26–gauge stainless steel wire is formed along the palatal surface of the maxillary teeth. The ends are bent outwards at the level of the bifurcation of the second or the third premolar, and cut off leaving about 5 mm after the bend (Fig. 138). The bifurcation of the chosen premolar can be opened with a bur if necessary, and the wire passed through the burification and bent forward to secure the distal ends. The rostral part of the wire is attached by ligating to the front teeth with thinner wire (either 26– or 28–gauge). In some cases wire alone may be sufficient to support the fracture. If more strength is needed, self–cure acrylic is mixed and placed along the palatal surface of the first three premolars and incorporated with the wire. The acrylic should not be placed on the palatal surface of the fourth premolar, due to possible problems with occlusion. In some cases where additional strength may be necessary, extra wire and acrylic can be placed across the width of the hard palate. There should be no contact between the acrylic and the hard palate, otherwise severe inflammation and necrosis may occur. Ideally the acrylic splint should only contact the teeth, and not the gums. A thick layer of vaseline should be placed over the gingival tissue before fabrication of the splint. The splint should be left in place for four to six weeks.

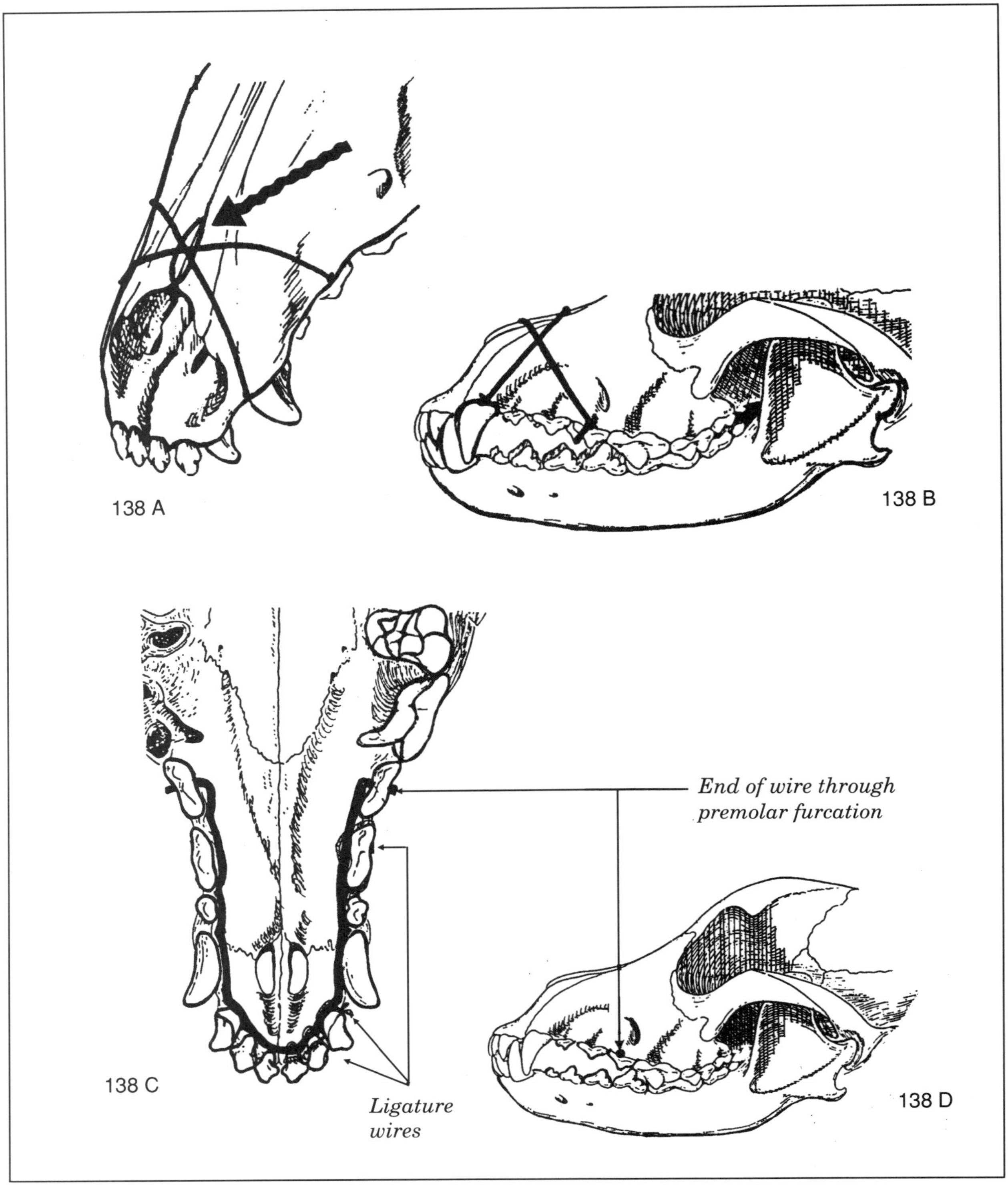

Figure 138 A–D. Fractures of the maxilla.

138 A. Cutaneous incision on nose (arrow) assists placement of wires.
138 B. Subcutaneous circumferential wiring. Wires are placed around the canine teeth and between the furcation of the premolars (3rd or 4th) or through holes in the alveolar bone.
138 C. Maxillary wire (before application of acrylic).
138 D. End of wire through premolar furcation.

Longitudinal fractures of the maxilla can be recognized by the ability to twist both canine teeth apart. Stabilization is obtained by splinting wire from one canine tooth to the other, either directly, or around the incisors or both. Additional support can be obtained by encasing the wire in acrylic (see acrylic splinting, 10.6 and inclined plane device, 9.31). Remember to protect the hard palate with vaseline, a strip of plastic or a strip of wax paper while making the acrylic splint in the mouth. An alternative method of stabilizing a rostral maxillary fracture is to pass a wire subcutaneously over the top of the nose from canine tooth to canine tooth. An incision is made in the skin on the bridge of the nose in line with the canine teeth. A long curved needle with wire attached is inserted through the incision and over the periosteum lateral to one canine tooth, and pushed down until it comes out of the attached gingiva caudal to this canine tooth. The other end of the wire is then inserted in the incision and pushed down the other side of the nose until it comes out of the attached gingiva caudal to the opposite canine tooth. This wire is passed behind the canine tooth and back into the attached gingiva rostral to the canine tooth. Then it is passed back up to the incision and down the other side, as before, to exit through the attached gingiva, rostral to the first canine tooth. The two ends are then passed around this first canine tooth and twisted together. Be sure that the twisted ends of the wire do not irritate the buccal mucosa. Covering the twisted ends of the wire with self–cure acrylic will accomplish this. Prophylactic antibiotic coverage is required in order to control any infection that may occur.

The animal should be fed liquid food or soft food only, and prevented from playing with hard objects. Acrylic splints and wiring devices should be either cleaned regularly with a mild disinfectant such as hydrogen peroxide or flushed with chlorhexidine solution.

10.11 GINGIVAL FLAP AND OSTEOTOMY

A gingival flap and osteotomy are often used to surgically remove *root remnants, retained deciduous teeth, difficult to remove teeth and ankylosed teeth.* ANKYLOSED TEETH result from the fusion of the cementum and alveolar bone, with the obliteration of the periodontal ligament.

ROOT REMNANTS (or FRAGMENTS) deep in the alveolar bone, some RETAINED DECIDUOUS TEETH, DIFFICULT TO REMOVE TEETH such as the maxillary or the mandibular canine teeth (or remains of) and ANKYLOSED TEETH are often difficult to remove. In these cases the overlying gingiva often needs to be reflected and the bone covering the root removed (Photos 2, 10). The gingiva is freed with a scalpel or a periosteal elevator along the gingival margin, and one or two releasing incisions are made beside the tooth to be extracted, slightly diverging from the horizontal incision at the sulcus (OPEN GINGIVAL FLAP). These flaps may include only the ATTACHED GINGIVA or may extend into the MUCOSA also. Both the PERIOSTEUM and the attached gingiva are raised together with a periosteal elevator, and the FULL THICKNESS FLAP retracted with a hook, or a suture. The periosteum is not raised when performing a MUCOSAL FLAP. Next, a large round bur in a low–speed handpiece is used to remove the bone covering the root (OSTEOTOMY). All the bone covering the root should be removed before the root fragment is removed with an elevator. Any sharp edges of the alveolus (socket) are shaped and smoothed with a round bur or a bone file (ALVEOLOPLASTY). With multiple extractions in a row, remodeling any rough or infected CRESTAL BONE between the alveoli (OSTEOPLASTY) is also performed using a round bur or a bone file. The flap is repositioned and sutured into place with catgut, silk or synthetic sutures. The most suitable SUTURING NEEDLES for oral surgery are 3/8–inch circle, reverse cutting, atraumatic needles with a swedged 3–0 or 4–0 SUTURE MATERIAL. Some small flaps may not require suturing. Silk and synthetic sutures should be removed after about seven to 10 days. It is important to note that the releasing incision should be made over healthy bone that will remain, and not over the bone that will be removed. The angle of the incision should diverge slightly from the gingival margin, to ensure an adequate blood supply and to aid in repositioning.

It should be noted that THERMAL NECROSIS of the BONE is always possible when drilling, unless copious amounts of water are used. For those without drilling equipment, rongeurs and chisels can be used, although less effectively than with a high–speed drill.

Incision is made caudal to root and a full thickness gingival and mucosal flap is raised using a periosteal elevator.

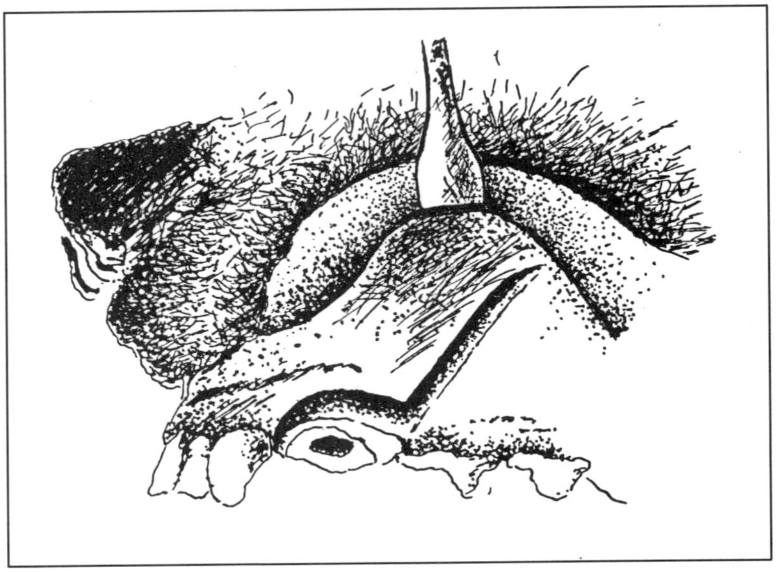

Figure 139 A. Lateral flap technique for extracting teeth.

After removal of overlying bone (osteotomy) with chisel or bur, the root can be elevated and removed.

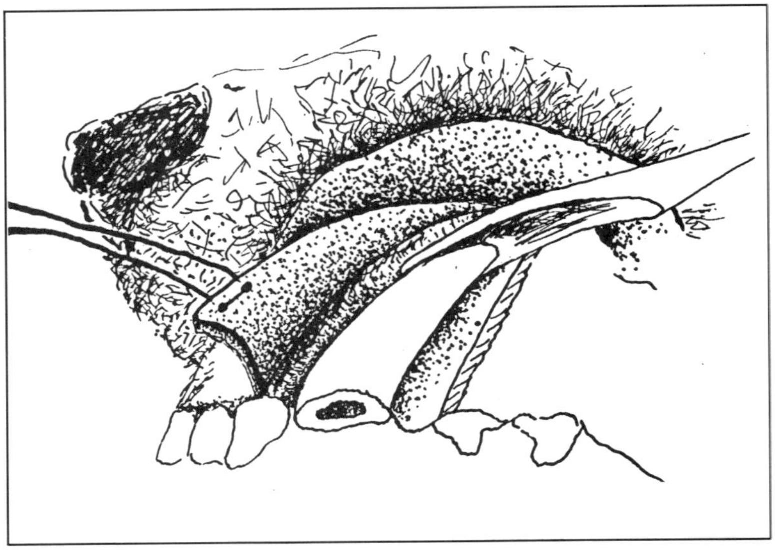

Figure 139 B. Root removal.

10.12 APICOECTOMY (APICECTOMY)

Apicoectomy is the excision of the apical portion of a tooth through an opening made in the overlying alveolar mucosa and bone. A percutaneous incision is often made to access the root apex of the mandibular canine teeth (Photo 54). It is ordinarily performed in conjunction with apical curettage and with, or as an adjunct to, root canal therapy. An apicoectomy is also termed a ROOT RESECTION, a ROOT END RESECTION and a SURGICAL ENDODONTIC PROCEDURE. The fracture of a tooth, especially the canine tooth, can lead to a massive OSTEOLYTIC PROCESS at the apex of the involved tooth. This is due to infection passing down through the exposed coronal pulp and out through the apex of the tooth into the surrounding periapical tissues. This will develop into a PERIAPICAL ABSCESS or a GRANULOMA. Sometimes during root canal therapy an endodontic instrument breaks or it perforates the apex of the tooth. During obturation of the canal, some of the filling material may accidentally pass beyond the apex into the periapical tissues. Sometimes conventional endodontic procedures fail.

140 A. Location of canine tooth root apices in maxilla and mandible (circles). Access areas. Maxilla — mucosal. Mandible — mucosal or percutaneous.

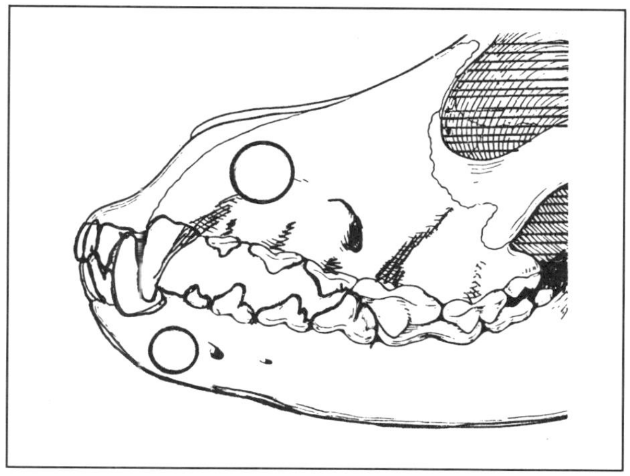

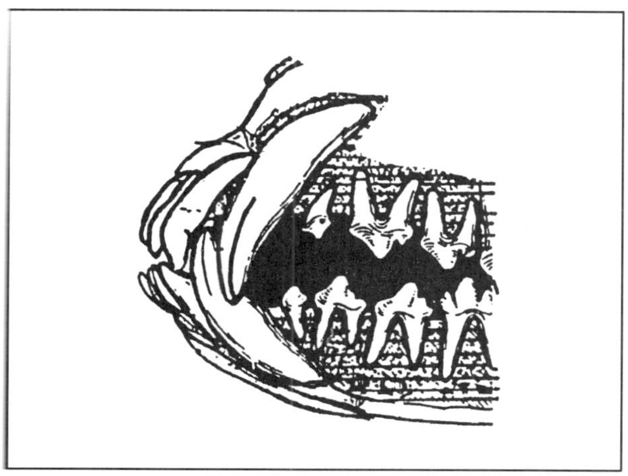

Figure 140 B. Apex relationship to premolar roots.

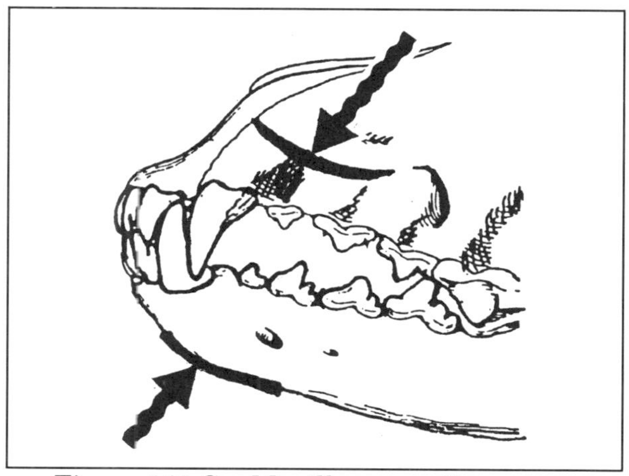

Figure 140 C. Maxilla — semilunar mucosal incision to raise flap. Mandible — percutaneous incision following contour of mandible.

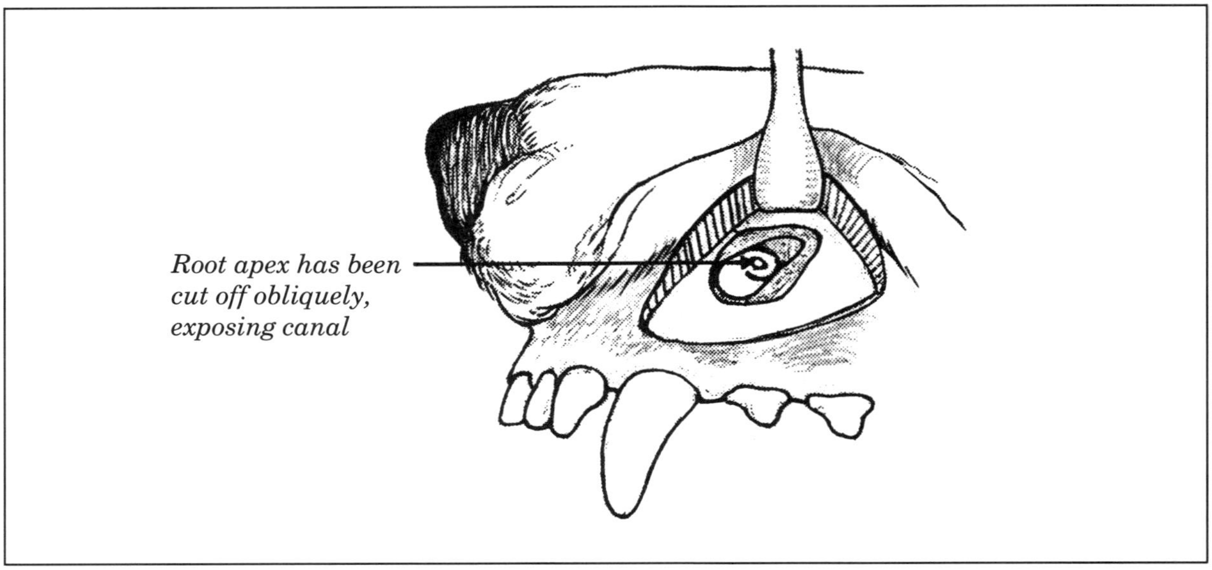

Figure 140 D. Surgical exposure of root tip, following flap procedure and alveolar bone removal.

These defects are clearly seen in radiographs of the region. When any of these situations arise, an apicoectomy should be considered. Endodontic therapy must be performed on the tooth, which is then filled and sealed coronally with a material of choice. For the maxillary canine tooth a semilunar incision is made in the mucosa at about the level of the midline of the root (Fig. 140C). A MUCOSAL FLAP is raised with a periosteal elevator, and the bone overlying the apex of the root is removed with a high speed bur to reveal the root tip.

In order to differentiate between the apical portion of the tooth and the surrounding bone or the granulation tissue, 1% METHYLENE BLUE dye or stain can be applied to the exposed area with a cotton pledget. It should be left for five seconds and then rinsed and dried. The bone and any granulation tissue of infected bone *will be stained* deeply by the dye. The root does *not stain.* Accessory canals, fractures and cracks in the root *will stain*.

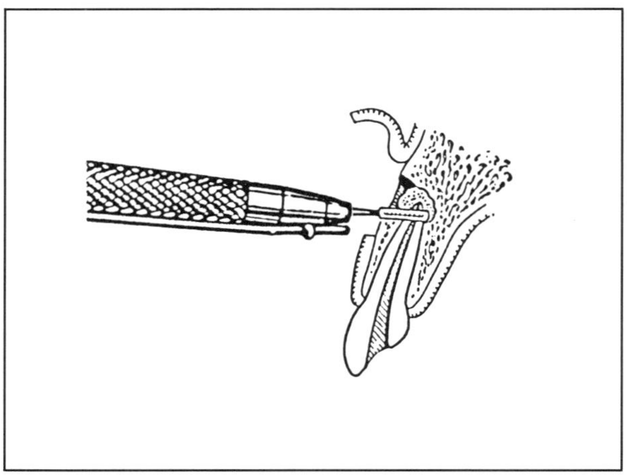

Figure 141 A. Removing 2–3 mm of root apex with a bur.

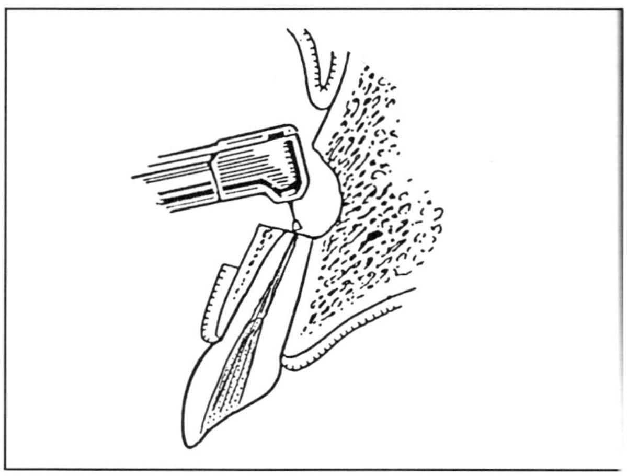

Figure 141 B. Using an inverted cone bur to open up the apical canal.

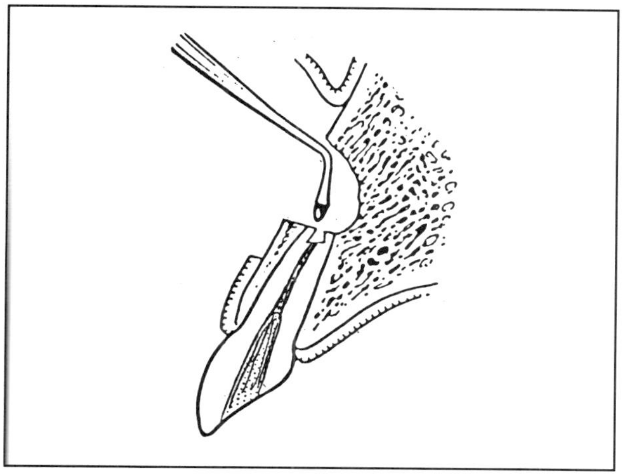

Figure 141 C. Applying an apical seal of the restorative natural.

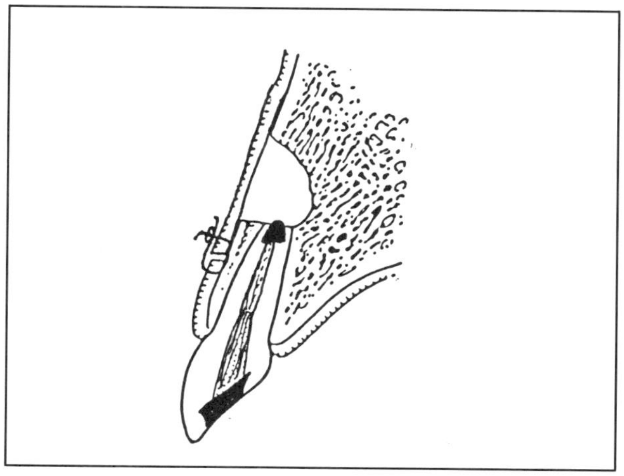

Figure 141 D. Amalgam filling in root apex and crown. Incision resutured.

The root tips of the canine teeth in the dog are usually located directly in line with the mesial roots of the second premolars. About 2–3 mm of the tip is cut off with a round or a straight fissure bur at an angle of about 45 degrees, so as to ensure a clear view of the end of the root canal. A small inverted cone bur is used to open up the root canal leaving a slight undercut, and a RETROGRADE FILLING of ZINC–FREE AMALGAM, or glass ionomer is placed to completely seal the root canal from the apical end. Zinc–free amalgam contains less than 0.01% zinc. The necrotic remains of the osteolysis and any amalgam chips are carefully removed, and the flap replaced and sutured.

10.13 IMPACTED AND RETAINED TEETH — EXPOSURE

It is not uncommon for a tooth, especially the canine tooth or the first premolar to become INPACTED in the jaw. This is either because its position in the alveolus is such that it is incapable of eruption into its normal position, or because it has been driven into the alveolar process (socket) or the surrounding tissues as a result of trauma. Traumatically impacted teeth may or may not be exposed or visible. This naturally causes problems in show dogs, since the teeth are assumed to be missing. The existence of the tooth germinal tissue can be demonstrated by means of radiographs, copies of which should be taken to the show ring to prove it, plus a letter from the veterinarian.

If the tooth is not actually impacted, but simply RETAINED in the jaw unerupted, it is possible that eruption can be encouraged by exposing the crown. A flap should be raised in the mucus membrane, directly above the crown of the tooth, to expose the alveolar bone. This bone may then be carefully removed with a round bur to expose the crown. Enough bone should be removed to create a tunnel, slightly larger than the diameter of the crown, and extending down to the neck of the tooth. A straight elevator can be carefully used to slightly loosen the coronal part of the root. This will free the tooth from any ankylosis, and will also encourage the further production of dentin at the growing root. In this way the tooth will begin to move outwards normally (extrude), and hopefully erupt into occlusion.

Figures 142 A–D. Exposing impacted tooth.

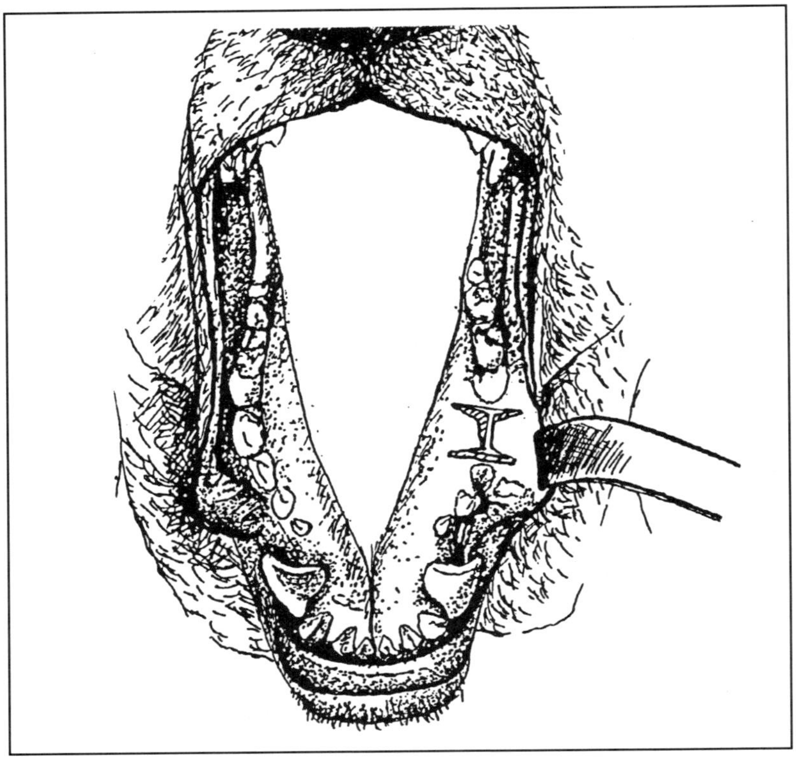

142 A. Make an "H" shape incision over the impacted tooth.

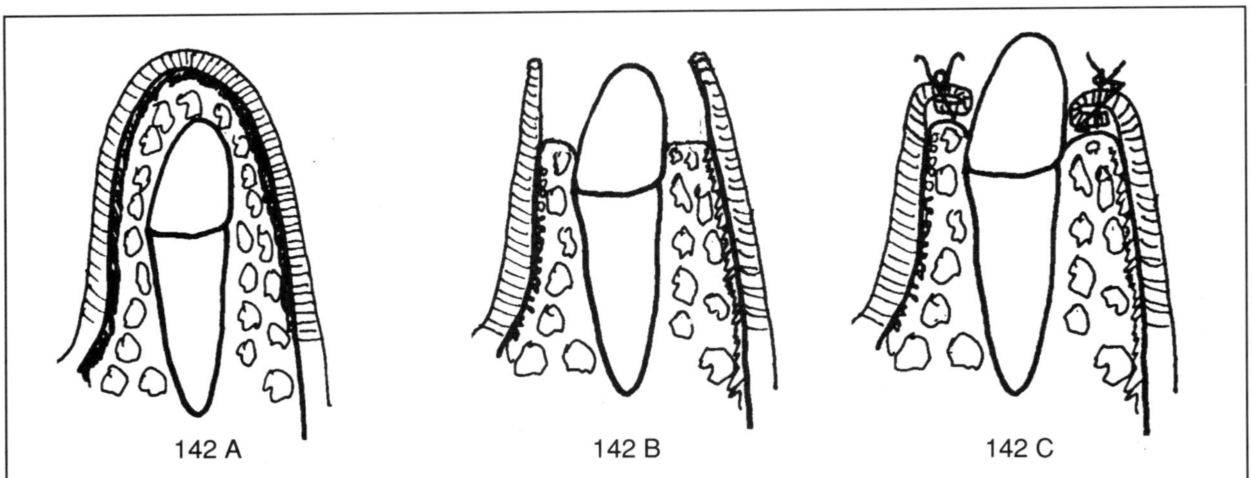

142 B. Cross section of impacted tooth.
142 C. Alveolar bone removed to expose crown, after full thickness flaps have been raised.
142 D. Epithelium is rolled and sutured (mattress) to prevent tooth being covered by rapid reepithelialization.

Operations of this type are generally only successful on the growing tooth, since after the apex has closed it is less likely that the tooth will erupt further without additional help. In this case, after the crown has been exposed, an orthodontic bracket can be bonded to the crown, using the acid–etch technique previously described. Similar brackets can be attached to the teeth rostral and caudal to the retained tooth. A short length of wire can then be attached to these two brackets, and an elastic band or a metal spring passed from the center of the bridging wire to the bracket on the retained tooth. In this way the retained tooth is brought slowly under continuous traction into occlusion. This is called EXTRUSION. The procedure is not always as easy as it sounds and can result in extraction of the tooth. It should only be undertaken by those with experience in veterinary orthodontics (or with the help of a human orthodontist). For both types of operation, the epithelium should be prevented from closing over and healing the wound. Each of the two flaps of the H–incision should be folded over and sutured to themselves (Fig. 142). This allows good healing of the transverse wound and reduces the tendency of the epithelium to grow back.

Partially erupted teeth can be encouraged to erupt further by removing some of the surrounding gingival tissue with electrosurgery. This can be followed by cutting some of the fibrous gingival tissue (FIBROTOMY) around the neck of the tooth, using a scalpel.

Traumatically impacted maxillary teeth are often driven into the nasal passage or the sinus. This results in an oronasal fistula or a direct connection between the mouth and nasal tissues. This must be corrected surgically (see oronasal fistula closure, 10.14).

10.14 ORONASAL FISTULA CLOSURE

Occasionally, after loss of a maxillary canine tooth, a fistula appears which connects the nasal passage and the mouth. This fistula develops when the canine tooth is lost from trauma and more frequently from extraction. Severe complications can arise from loss of this tooth due to the extremely thin layer of bone medial to the canine root tip (Photo 11). Such a fistula can be expected when the bone medial to the canine root tip is fractured, and also when the mucous membrane in the nasal passage is torn.

Within a few days, a large FISTULA (epithelium lined tube) forms. Through this opening large amounts of food and saliva are often trapped and impacted into the nasal cavity, causing serious infectious complications. The condition of the patient is generally one of serious illness. Pus coming through the nose, sneezing (sometimes bloody), painful and slow feeding, pawing and rubbing the nose and loss of the sense of smell can be seen in these patients.

A simple SLIDING BUCCAL FLAP (SINGLE FLAP TECHNIQUE or BUCCAL ADVANCEMENT FLAP) is used to repair a small oronasal fistula. A flap is raised from the loose mucous membrane on the inside of the lip. Care must be taken to ensure that the flap can be laid completely over the fistula without tension. The bony edge of the fistula should be smoothed with a bur or with rongeurs and then the flap is sutured into place. Since passing a suture needle through the dense palatal tissue at the cut fresh edge of the defect can be difficult, it is wise to slightly raise this tissue first with a periosteal elevator.

If the oronasal fistula causes a large defect, a DOUBLE (REVERSE) FLAP TECHNIQUE may be required. A trapezoid–shaped flap is raised from the palatal mucous membrane and folded into the defect, where it is sutured into place. A second flap is then raised from the alveolar mucosa and placed over both the palatal flap and the donor site (Photo 12). The mucosal flap is carefully sutured into place. The oral side of the palatal flap forms the new floor of the nasal cavity and the mucosal flap covers the exposed surface of the palatal flap. The operation is not easy. The palatal flap is especially difficult to prepare without impairing the blood supply and becoming necrotic. The medial edge of the flap should not be made too near to the median raphe in order to avoid damage to the palatal artery, leading to profuse bleeding. Normally a flap extending from half way between the alveolar ridge of the lost canine tooth and the middle of the palate is adequate.

After extraction of a maxillary canine tooth, it is often wise to close the defect with a flap. A sliding buccal flap is usually sufficient. Probing the apex of the alveolus should be undertaken with extreme care, and only when absolutely necessary, because of the high risk of perforation of the thin bone medial to the apical extend of the alveolus.

An OROANTRAL FISTULA is a fistulous tract, which develops into the nasal sinuses, in areas where the roots of the teeth are in close proximity with a sinus. In some cases both oronasal and oroantral fistulas can develop (Photos 13, 14, 15).

10.15 MANDIBULECTOMY AND MAXILLECTOMY

There are often conditions involving the maxilla and mandible that require radical surgical treatment. These include malignant and benign tumors, severe fractures, chronic infection and bone necrosis.

The procedures necessary to treat these conditions include a COMPLETE or a PARTIAL MANDIBULECTOMY or MAXILLECTOMY, or a COMPLETE or a PARTIAL HEMIMANDIBULECTOMY or HEMIMAXILLECTOMY. Although the surgical removal of an entire bone or a segment of bone (OSTECTOMY) may seem drastic, the animal seems to adapt well. These procedures are not as difficult as they may seem, and lend themselves to surgical bone removal using a high–speed drill. For further details see *HARVEY'S* Veterinary Dentistry.

10.16 SUBLINGUAL AND BUCCAL MUCOSA RESECTION

ABNORMAL PROLIFERATIVE SUBLINGUAL MUCOSA is occasionally found in the dog under the tongue on each side, running parallel to its surface. These thin stretched folds of mucosal tissue protrude laterally on each side of the base of the tongue, from the area of the frenulum linguae attachment to the caudal sublingual area. These mucosal folds are the result of chronic SELF–INFLICTED SUBLINGUAL TRAUMA. Constant tongue movements, such as with open mouth breathing, excessive panting and barking, stretch the sublingual tissue. This thin sublingual mucosal tissue eventually becomes caught between the opposing caudal teeth when the dog eats and is stretched further (Photos 95, 96).

ABNORMAL PROLIFERATIVE BUCCAL MUCOSA is occasionally found in the dog and rarely in the cat, in the buccal mucosa along the occlusal plane near the caudal teeth. These lesions are usually bilateral and are seen as thickened areas of cheek buccal mucosa protruding medially and parallel to the cheek teeth. The lesions start just caudal to the commissures of the lips. The buccal mucosa becomes caught between the cheek teeth and constant chewing propagates the problem, resulting in chronic SELF–INFLICTED BUCCAL TRAUMA. These problems are found more commonly in brachycephalic and small breeds or in pets with a wide skull shape in the caudal teeth area. Abnormal proliferative sublingual and buccal mucosa can be found at the same time in some pets.

The condition has been described as CHEWING GUM–LIKE SYNDROME and was first described by *HAWKINS* (1988). Due to the discomfort and pain caused by this self–inflicted trauma, the dog often exhibits chewing movements of the jaws, which resembles someone chewing gum. Unexplained barking or yelping, fearful behavior, difficulty in eating and unidentified oral pain similar to periodontal and endodontal problems are also seen. Dental examination and radiographs often reveal no reason for the symptoms. Occasionally these abnormal lesions are found in dogs that are exhibiting no symptoms of pain or discomfort.

Both conditions are probably more common than is reported, because they are generally missed on examination. Correction of the sublingual lesions involves surgical resection of the entire length of the involved mucosa. Correction of the buccal folds involves surgical resection of the involved buccal mucosa.

If both types of lesions are present they should be resected at the same time. Closure of the cut edges should be performed using a 4–0 absorbable suture material with a continuous suture pattern, to avoid the necessity of anesthetizing the patient for removal of the sutures, and to prevent irritation from the ends of simple interrupted sutures. Patients should be placed on a tranquilizer and analgesic for one or two days postoperatively. This is especially important in sublingually involved patients to prevent any excessive panting, mouth breathing and barking from irritating the surgical site.

Results of surgical resection of these lesions are rewarding and the symptoms usually resolve in a week or two. However many of these pets are predisposed to the problems recurring. This may be due to the behavior habits, the shape of the tongue and buccal mucosa or the shape of the skull. Clients should be advised that there is always a possibility that these lesions may recur in the future.

CHAPTER 11

RADIOLOGY (RADIOGRAPHY)

Radiology is probably the most important diagnostic tool in determining the status of the crown and root of the tooth, and the surrounding tissues.

11.1 USES

Dental radiographs can be used to check for:

1. The degree of periodontal disease.
2. The condition of the alveolar bone.
3. The degree of bone loss or bone regression.
4. Osteomyelitis.
5. The size and shape of the root canal and apex.
6. Periapical cysts.
7. Periapical granulomas.
8. Periapical abscesses.
9. Caries.
10. Unerupted, impacted and missing teeth.
11. Fractured crowns and roots.
12. Subgingival lesions.
13. Position of endodontic instruments in the pulp cavity.
14. Broken endodontic instruments in the pulp cavity.
15. The progress throughout endodontic treatment.
16. Dental and oral pathology and neoplasia.
17. Fractures of the maxilla and mandible.
18. The condition of the temporomandibular joint (TMJ).

Before dental radiology can be used successfully, it is important to be familiar with the normal radiographic anatomy of the various breeds and species at varying ages

(Fig. 6). As an animal ages, the *lamina dura becomes less distinct,* the *alveolar bone regresses apically,* the *trabecular pattern of the surrounding bone becomes more coarse,* the *apical foramen closes* and the *pulp canal narrows.* One must know the overlying structures that can confuse the picture, such as the middle mental foramen, the posterior mental foramen and the mandibular canal. These sometimes give the appearance of an "APICAL HALO," or a radiolucent area around the apex, which could be confused with a periapical problem.

11.2 FILM

The intraoral films used in human dentistry are well suited for small animals, and are considerably easier to use than the larger film cassette, as well as giving much better results. They are flexible, and can be adapted to fit almost any region, although excessive bending should be avoided. The following ultra–speed, non–screen HUMAN DENTAL INTRAORAL FILM sizes (Kodak) are the most useful for dogs and cats:

DF–54	Size "0"	7/8" x 1 3/8"	(22 x 35 mm)	(PEDIATRIC PERIAPICAL)
DF–58	Size "2"	1 1/4" x 1 5/8"	(31 x 41 mm)	(ADULT PERIAPICAL)
DF–50	Size "4"	2 1/4" x 3"	(57 x 76 mm)	(OCCLUSAL)

It is best to have all three sizes of film available, in order to be able to radiograph the teeth of any pet.

11.3 SETTINGS

There are many types of human dental X–ray (radiology, radiographic) machines (equipment), some with variable kVp, mA and exposure time, and some with just a variable exposure time. For veterinary purposes those with only a variable exposure time are generally sufficient. The kVp is fixed at about 70 and the mA at about 10. Although the timers usually have settings from 1/60 to 4 seconds, most veterinary dental radiographs will be taken at settings of 0.6 to 1 seconds. In order to familiarize yourself with a new machine, take a series of radiographs of the same tooth at different settings to see which exposure is the best.

If intraoral film is used with a regular veterinary X–ray machine, the mA should be set at 100, and the kVp set between 65–85, depending on the size of the animal. The exposure time should range from 1/12 to 1/10 seconds, and the film focal distance set at 12 inches. The best setting should be at 10 mAs.

When using a high–speed screened film cassette with a regular veterinary X–ray machine, the mA should be set at 100, the kVp set between 65–85, the time set at 1/20 seconds and the focal distance set at 30 inches.

11.4 FILM PROCESSING

In order to develop intraoral film, a PORTABLE (CHAIRSIDE) DARKROOM is useful (e.g., Microcopy's Insta–Veloper) with a RAPID DEVELOPER/FIXER system (e.g., Microcopy's Insta–Neg/Insta–Fix). Automatic dental film processing machines are available, but they are costly, problem oriented and take longer than manual processing. A regular veterinary processing system can also be used to process a dental film by holding the film with hemostats and dipping it in the solutions. Alternatively, a large automatic processor can be used by taping the dental film to the trailing edge of an old radiograph. There is always the risk that the film may come off as it goes through the rollers.

11.5 ERRORS

When TAKING and PROCESSING dental radiographs, many ERRORS are possible. Most of these errors can be avoided by following the points listed below:

1. Place the stippled side of dental film envelope towards the beam.
2. Place the "DOT" stamped into the film and envelope towards the beam.
3. Place the "DIMPLE" stamped into the film and envelope towards the tongue.
4. Place the film in the mouth at the correct angle.
5. Position the beam at the correct angle.
6. Do not move the dental film.
7. Do not move the X–ray machine.
8. Do not move the patient.
9. Do not bend the film excessively.
10. Hold the button down until the buzzer stops.
11. Set the correct kVp.
12. Set the correct mA.
13. Set the correct time.
14. Set the correct developing time.
15. Set the correct fixing time.
16. Set the correct developing/fixing temperature.
17. Do not double expose the film.
18. Do not use weak (or overused) developer.
19. Do not use weak (or overused) fixer.
20. Do not use old (or expired) film.
21. Do not use film that has been improperly stored.
22. Do not use an insufficient amount of developer in the container.
23. Do not use an insufficient amount of fixer in the container.
24. Do not contaminate the film with dirty fingers.
25. Do not scratch the film.
26. Do not leave fingernail artifacts.
27. Do not splash developer on the film before developing.
28. Do not splash fixer on the film before developing.
29. Make sure that the clips are clean and dry before use.
30. Make sure that there are no light leaks in the chairside developer or darkroom.
31. Make sure that the safe light is not to close to the film.
32. Make sure that the bulb in the safelight is not too strong.

11.6 TECHNIQUE (HUMAN DENTAL X–RAY MACHINE AND DENTAL FILM)

HUMAN DENTAL X–RAY MACHINES are inexpensive when compared to regular X–ray machines and will soon repay their investment. If cost is a problem, used dental X–ray machines are often for sale locally at a fraction of the new cost. However, if you are going to offer modern dentistry as a service, a human dental X-ray machine is a necessary investment.

Incisors, Canine teeth and Maxillary Premolars and Molars

In order to radiograph all the maxillary teeth and the mandibular incisors and canine teeth, the BISECTING ANGLE TECHNIQUE has to be used (Fig. 143). The dental film is placed intraorally, as parallel to the tooth as possible, and an imaginary line is calculated which bisects the angle created by the film and the long axis of the tooth. The cone of the X-ray machine is then positioned at right angles to this imaginary line. With practice this technique can soon be mastered.

Mandibular Premolars and Molars

Due to the lingual vestibule caudal to the mandibular canine teeth, dental film can be placed parallel to the mandibular premolars and molars. The center of the X-ray beam can be aimed perpendicularly through the tooth. This is called a PARALLEL BEAM TECHNIQUE (Fig. 144). This technique cannot be used for any of the teeth of the maxilla or the mandibular incisors and canine teeth, since the anatomy of palatal arch and anterior lingual vestibule does not permit perpendicular film placement and would result in an over-elongation of the tooth. If for some reason the film cannot be placed parallel to the tooth (or is more than 15 degrees to the tooth), then the bisecting angle technique should be used.

Excellent radiographs can be achieved by means of the positioning techniques recommended above for cats and dogs, and these principles can be applied to other animals.

Occasionally animals will permit some views to be taken without sedation. Generally it is wise to sedate or to anesthetize the animal to get the best views. Although a human dental X–ray machine produces only about 1/10 of the radiation of a regular machine, it is still important to wear a lead apron if you are within six feet of the patient and wear lead gloves when holding the film either with a film holder or an instrument such as a hemostat. Alternately, the dental film can be wedged in place using a crumpled paper towel or a film holder (Shipp's dental film holder), so that you may step away from the patient while the radiograph is being taken. If you are either evaluating or treating a case for a referring veterinarian, it is a good idea to use a DOUBLE FILM PACK, so that you can send a film copy to your colleague. This is not only good medicine but good public relations.

Processed dental film should be stored in either cardboard or plastic mounts, or in special envelopes, either with the patient record or in a separate filing system. To prevent the films from turning brown or discoloring with age, the film should be put back in the fixer for an additional 10 minutes, and then washed thoroughly for up to 30 minutes.

11.7 TECHNIQUE (VETERINARY X–RAY MACHINE AND FILM CASSETTE)

Regular VETERINARY X–RAY MACHINES can be used but the results will not be as accurate as a human dental X–ray machine. The film cassettes have to be placed extraorally for the premolars and molars and can be placed intraorally for the incisors and canine teeth.

Incisors and Canine Teeth

The incisor region and canine teeth can be radiographed by placing the film cassette in the mouth, as far as possible caudally. For the maxilla, a ROSTRAL MAXILLARY PROJECTION (anterior dorso-ventral) is used (Fig. 145), and for the mandible, a ROSTRAL MANDIBULAR PROJECTION (anterior ventro-dorsal) is used (Fig. 146). To obtain an accurate representation of the teeth, the bisecting angle technique should be employed.

PREMOLARS AND MOLARS

In order to radiograph the premolar and molar teeth on one side of the jaw, a LATERAL OBLIQUE TECHNIQUE is best (Figs. 147, 148). The jaw must be positioned so that the teeth from the opposite arcade do not overlap or superimpose. The angle between the teeth and the X-ray film should be between 30 and 45 degrees.

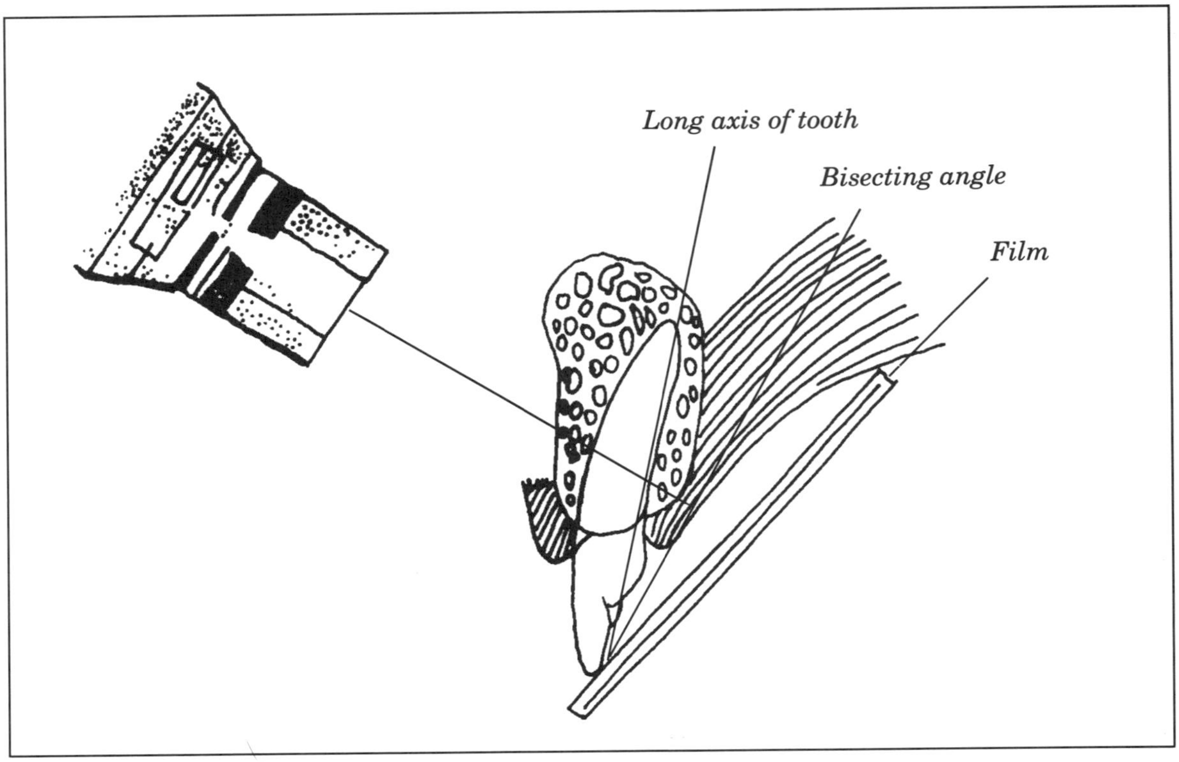

Figure 143. Bisecting angle technique.

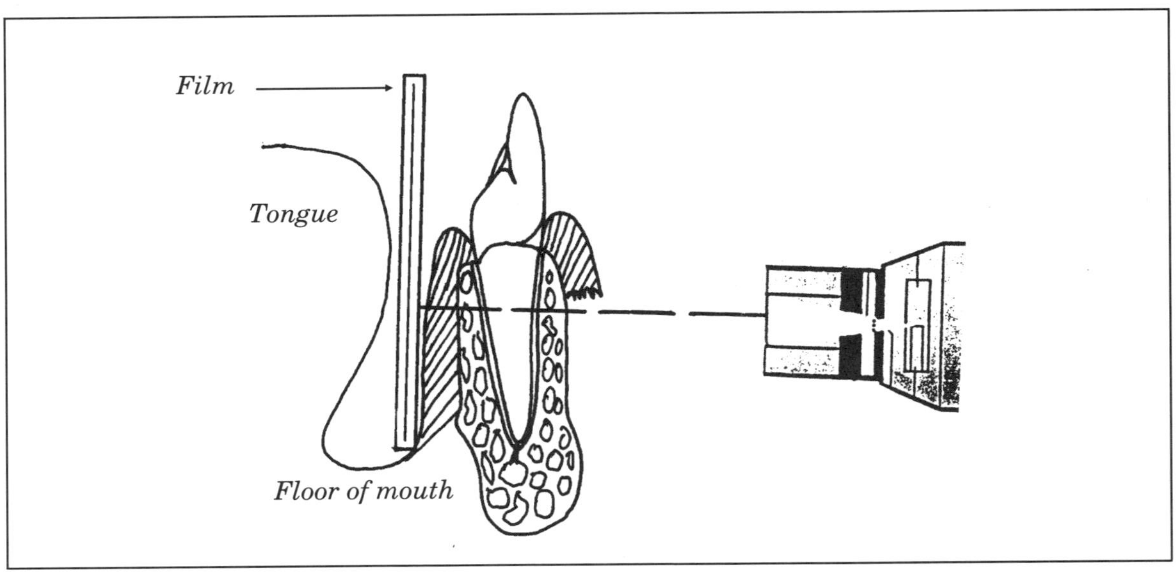

Figure 144. Parallel beam technique.

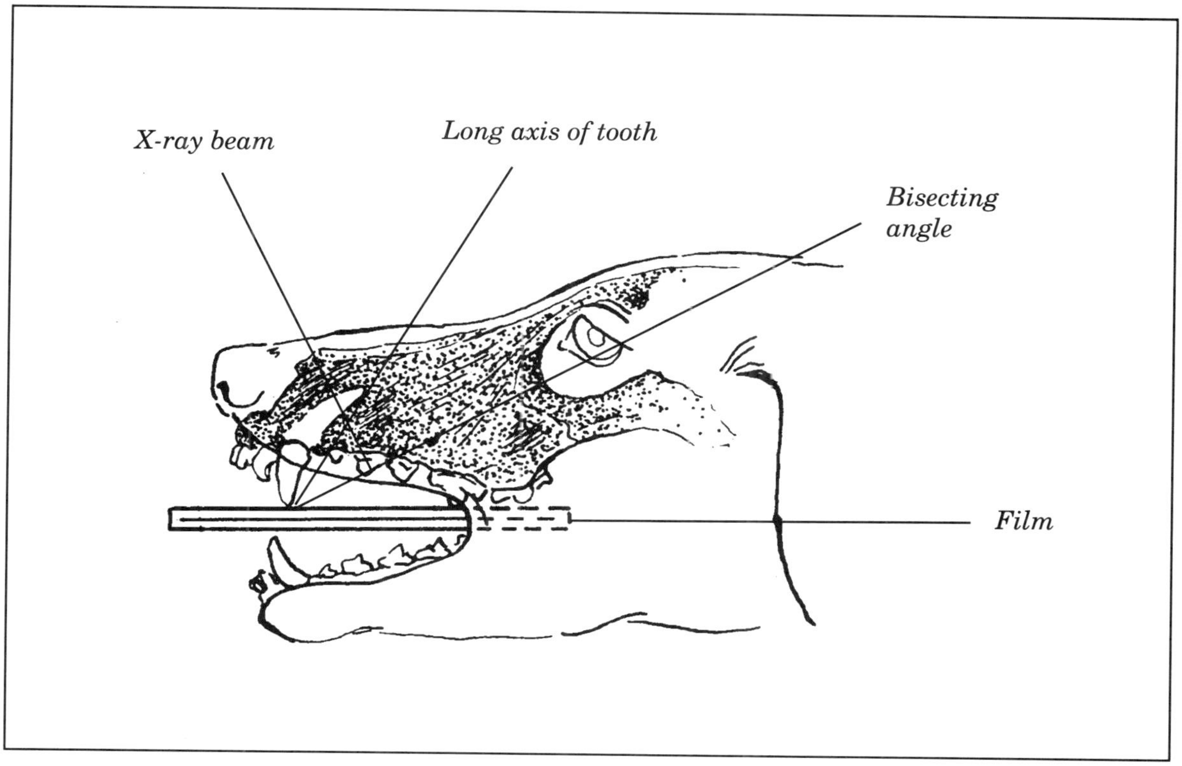

Figure 145. Rostral maxillary projection (incisors and canine teeth).

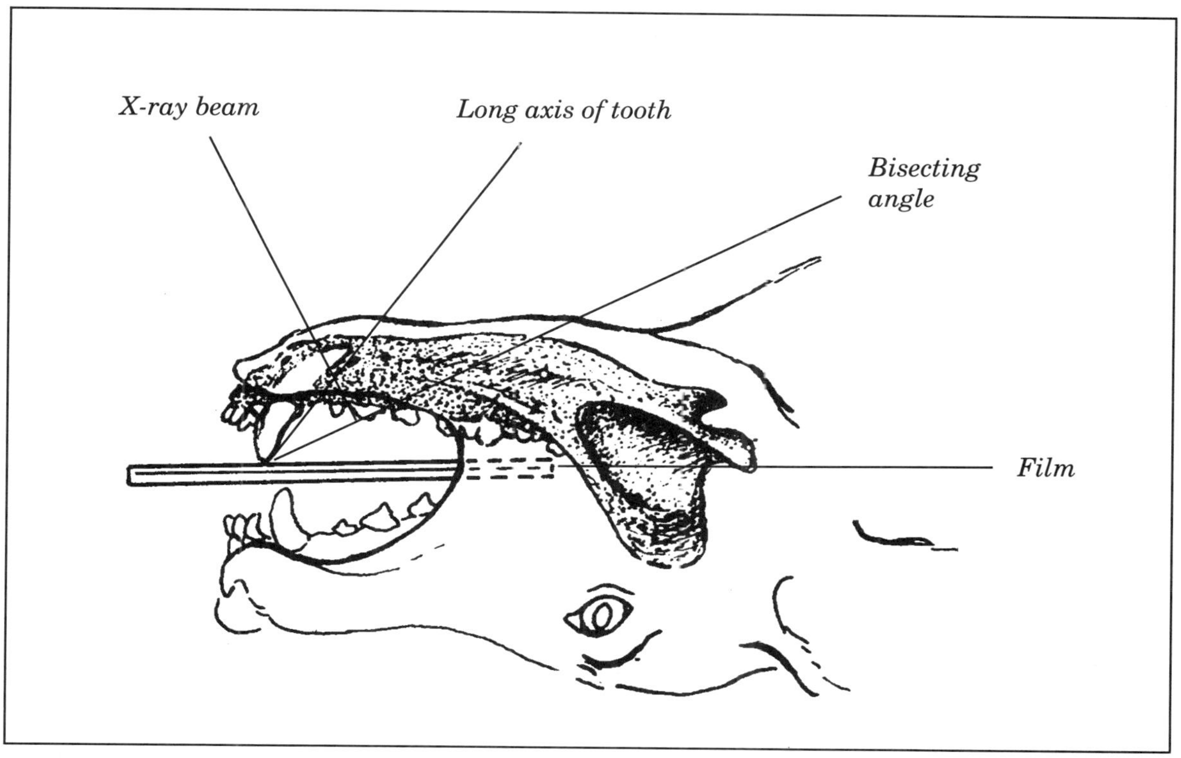

Figure 146. Rostral mandibular projection (incisors and canine teeth).

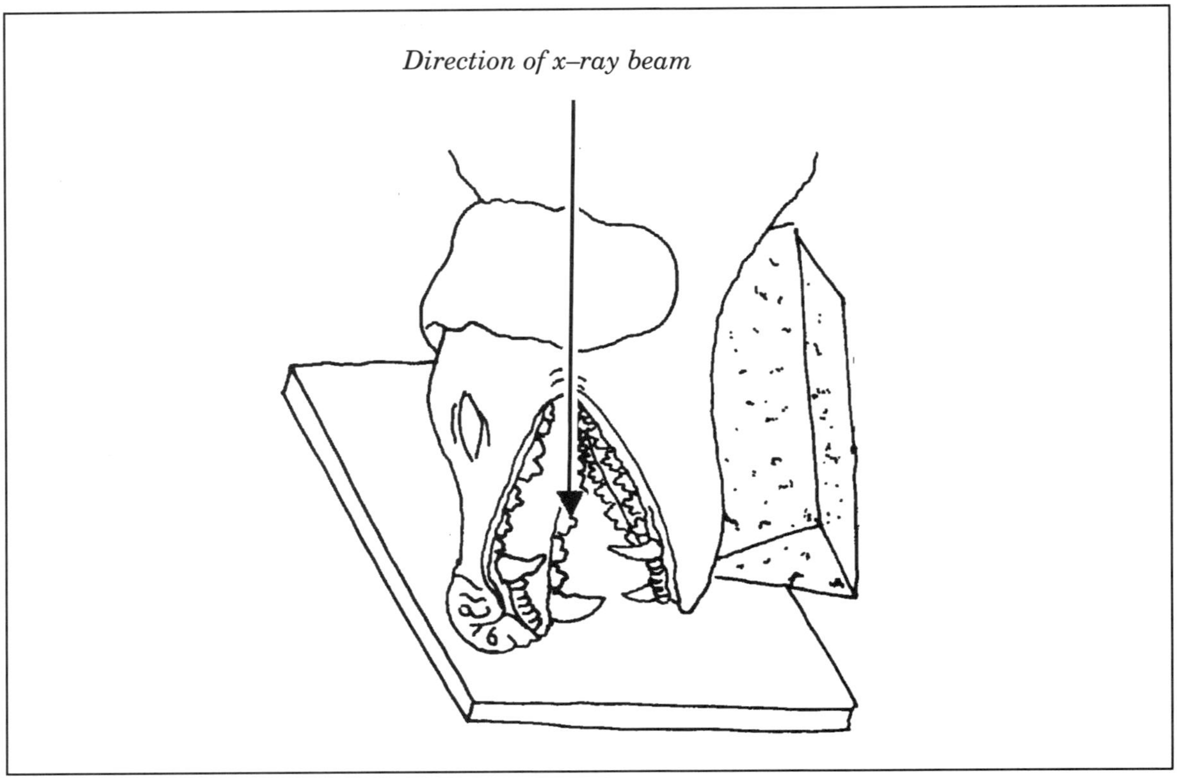

Figure 147. Lateral oblique technique (maxillary premolars and molars).

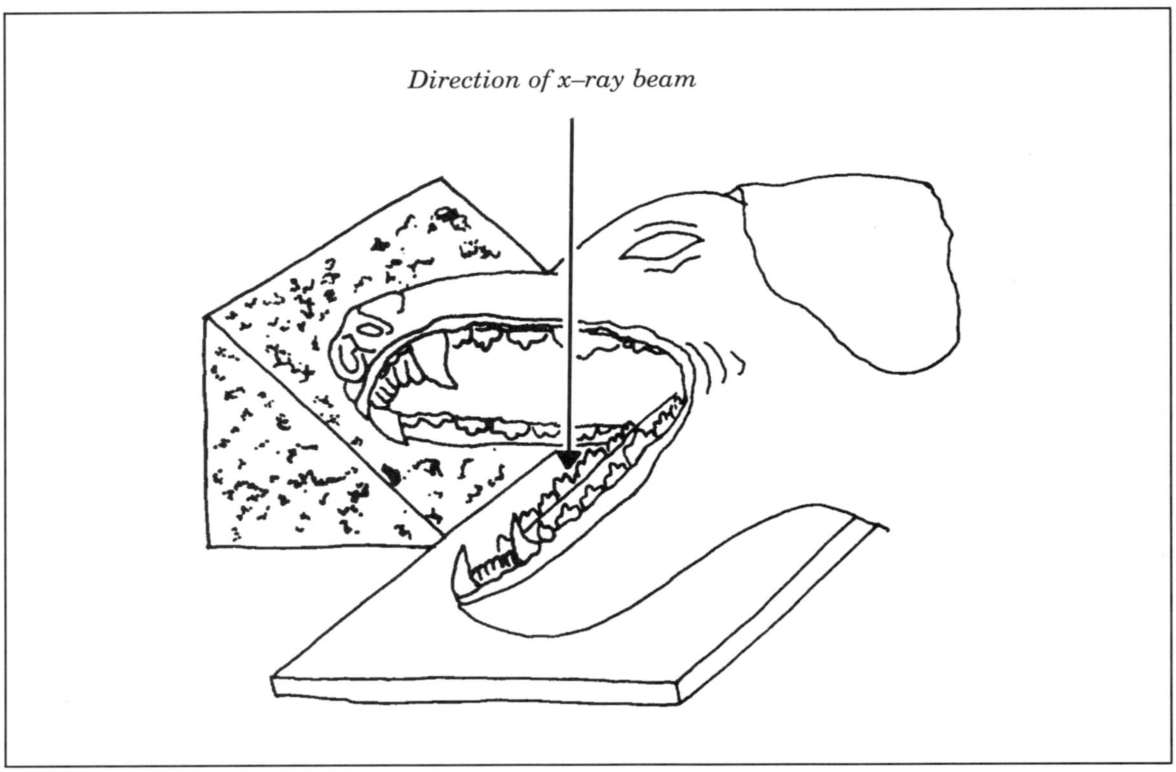

Figure 148. Lateral oblique technique (mandibular premolars and molars).

CHAPTER 12

DENTAL MATERIALS

To successfully complete advanced dental procedures, all the necessary dental materials must be available. This can be a complex task for those starting in veterinary dentistry, especially since this is one area that is constantly changing due to rapid research and development.

In order to choose which materials to purchase, it is important to know about their characteristics and applications.

The materials that we need to understand and use include: *cavity liners, varnishes* and *bases, amalgams, composites, glass ionomers, root canal filling materials, pins* and *posts, impression* and *stone materials, metals for crowns, orthodontic wires* and *elastics, orthodontic brackets, buttons* and *hooks,* and *acrylic splints.*

Since many of these materials have a short shelf life, and are only used infrequently, establish a working relationship with human dentists and purchase half full bottles or small amounts of products from them. Most dentists are very interested in veterinary dentistry and are willing to support us. They may be willing to work out a trade arrangement for veterinary services.

12.1 CAVITY LINERS, VARNISHES AND BASES

These materials are placed over the pulp and sensitive parts of the dentin prior to placement of the final restorative material. It is important to know how these materials protect the pulp and dentin in order to understand when they should be used. This can be confusing since varnishes are liners, and bases can be used as liners. Glass ionomers can also be used as bases or as liners.

12.2 CAVITY LINERS

Liners protect the pulp from irritation and reduce the sensitivity of freshly exposed dentin. Calcium hydroxide (CaOH) is a liner that should be used whenever there is less than 0.5 mm of dentin covering the pulp. It stimulates the formation of reparative dentin when placed over exposed pulp. If a thin layer of CaOH is used as a liner, it does not provide sufficient thermal insulation and strength. Thus, a cement base (or an intermediate restorative material) must be placed over the CaOH before the final restoration is placed.

"DYCAL" is a good example of a CaOH liner. It is made as two pastes that are mixed together, and may be placed with a special CaOH applicator instrument that comes with the kit. Although "Dycal" cures in one or two minutes, the newer light–cured CaOH materials can be cured in 20–30 seconds.

Low viscosity ZINC OXIDE–EUGENOL (TYPE IV) is another material that can be used as a liner, although it should not be used over exposed pulp or under a composite restoration.

LIGHT–CURED GLASS IONOMERS (TYPE III) (e.g., Vitrebond) or self–cure glass ionomers (e.g., Ketac–Cem) are excellent liners. They can be quickly applied and cured and have all the advantages of a glass ionomer (see glass ionomers, 12.8). If the pulp is close to the surface, 0.5 mm or less, CaOH should be applied first. When using *light–cured* glass ionomers as liners, conditioning of the dentin surface with polyacrylic acid is not required. Conditioning the dentin surface in order to remove the smear layer, is recommended with self–cure glass ionomers (see glass ionomers, 12.8). Light–cured glass ionomers can also be used for PIT AND FISSURE SEALING.

12.3 CAVITY VARNISHES

Technically both varnishes and liners are cavity–lining agents, since they are both used as protective coatings for freshly cut tooth material. However, varnishes not only protect the pulp from chemical irritation, but they seal the margins of an amalgam restoration and reduce microleakage. If an acid–etched composite restoration is to be used, any varnish remaining on the enamel edge of the preparation should be removed first (see liners and bases, 6.4). Varnishes are not used much today, since other materials such as glass ionomers are more effective as a liner/base material. Varnishes are not necessary if a glass ionomer is used as a liner/base. Varnishes are primarily natural gums or sometimes synthetic resins, with an organic solvent. Some varnishes contain fluoride (e.g., Copanol–F). The solvent evaporates leaving a resin film that protects the tooth structure. Varnish should not be used under either zinc oxide–eugenol or polycarboxylate cements. Composite resins should never be placed over COPAL–BASED VARNISHES (natural resins). It may be necessary to apply several layers of varnish depending on the case.

12.4 CAVITY CEMENT BASES

A base is essentially a replacement or a substitute for the dentin that has been destroyed or removed. It encourages the recovery of the injured pulp and protects it against thermal, mechanical and chemical trauma.

There are a variety of materials that can be used as bases, depending on the individual situation. *Low–strength* liners such as calcium hydroxide, NON–REINFORCED ZINC OXIDE–EUGENOL (TYPE IV ZOE) and light–cured glass ionomers (e.g., Vitrebond) can be used as bases by building them up in layers to give them strength. *High–strength* bases such as zinc phosphate, REINFORCED ZINC OXIDE–EUGENOL (TYPE III ZOE) (e.g., IRM), zinc polycarboxylate and self–cure glass ionomers (e.g., Ketac–Bond) are more commonly used.

ZINC PHOSPHATE is the oldest and best known cement base and consists of ZINC OXIDE with a little manganese oxide and other trace elements. It is mixed with 55% ORTHOPHOSPHORIC ACID until the desired consistency is achieved. Varnish must be used under zinc phosphate to protect the pulp from the orthophosphoric acid. Although, if less than 0.5 mm of dentin is covering the pulp, a liner of CaOH should be applied instead of the varnish. Zinc phosphate has a high compressive strength, acts as a thermal insulator, and can be placed under composite restorations and over gutta–percha.

REINFORCED ZINC OXIDE–EUGENOL (TYPE III ZOE) (e.g., IRM) is a commonly used base. Although ZOE helps to sedate the pulp, it should never be placed directly on the exposed pulp because it can set up an inflammatory reaction. Calcium hydroxide should always be placed first on exposed pulp to stimulate reparative dentin. Cements containing eugenol should never be placed under composite resins, since the eugenol interferes with the curing process. Cements containing eugenol should not be used with cavity varnishes.

ZINC POLYCARBOXYLATE is not as strong as zinc phosphate but has a milder effect on the pulp. It also bonds somewhat to calcium in the dentin. The working time is about 2.5 minutes (half that of zinc phosphate).

GLASS IONOMERS (TYPE III) (e.g., Ketac Bond) are excellent as bases because they have good compressive strength (similar to zinc phosphate) and are less irritating to the pulp than zinc phosphate (although CaOH is still recommended for pulp exposures within 0.5 mm). Glass ionomers also bond to dentin, release fluoride, can be used over endodontically treated teeth and under composite restorations, and can be acid–etched.

12.5 RESTORATIVE MATERIALS

Restorative materials are used for the *conservative* restoration of teeth, including core build–ups. A restorative material is most commonly used when a defect in the enamel and dentin has to be repaired. This is often called a "FILLING." When used to cover a large defect, such as a lateral slab fracture, it may be called a "RESTORATION."

There are three materials that are used as restorative materials. These are *amalgam, composite* and *glass ionomer*. Since their properties and uses vary, it is important to have a good working knowledge of these materials. Information on their application is described in Chapter 6 (see amalgam fillings, 6.7, composite fillings, 6.8 and treatment of "neck" lesions, 6.10).

12.6 AMALGAM

AMALGAM has been the classic tooth filling material since the beginning of the century, replacing previously used cohesive gold and lead fillings. The word "amalgam" is a general term for any mixture of a metal or metals with mercury. Dental amalgam is a SILVER AMALGAM consisting of approximately silver 65% (min.), lead 29% (max.), copper 6% (max.), zinc 2% (max.), mercury 3% (max.). The silver alloy is provided in the form of either shavings or spheres, and the mercury is pure.

These metals are packaged in a capsule, with the mercury in a separate compartment of the capsule. Just before use, the mercury is released from its compartment by pulling, pushing or twisting the capsule. The capsule is then placed in an amalgamator, which is an electric mixing device, and mixed for 10–15 seconds. The alloy partially dissolves in the mercury to form a thick mixture similar in consistency to a good snowball. If the mixture is too dry, the filling will be too weak.

As the cavity is filled, a small amount of mercury is expressed, but this is reabsorbed into the next layer. This is part of the reason why a cavity should always be overfilled and the excess then removed. If the filling is too wet it will shrink and begin to "creep" after a year or so. The mercury reacts with the alloy particles forming a metal mixture that sets after about 10 minutes. After the amalgam filling has been condensed into the cavity, the mercury continues to react with the alloy particles until an optimal mixture has been achieved, producing a hard filling after about 24 hours. At this time there should be no more free mercury and therefore little danger from mercury poisoning. There is much controversy at the present time concerning this possibility.

12.7 COMPOSITE (ACRYLIC RESINS)

COMPOSITE RESTORATIVE MATERIALS (COMPOSITE) are used to restore teeth that, for esthetic reasons, must be filled with a tooth–colored filling material. Composite restoratives consist of 60–70 percent volume of FILLER PARTICLES dispersed in an ACRYLIC RESIN MATRIX. The filler particles (POLYMER) are commonly produced by grinding or milling crystalline quartz or lithium glass ceramics. There are three classifications of composites based on the size of the filler particles:

Microfill. The *particle* size is 0.02 – 0.04 microns. The *average* size is 0.04–0.4 microns (the large 0.4 size is due to agglomeration or sticking together of the small 0.04 micron particles).

Macrofill. The *particle* size is 1.5 – 100 microns. The *average* size is 8–12 microns. Also referred to as "conventional" composite.

Hybrid. The *particle* size is 0.6 – 1.5 microns. The *average* size is 1.0 micron.

HYBRIDS are a mixture of two kinds of filler particles (usually colloidal silica and glasses containing heavy metals) and have characteristics of both the microfill and macrofill. They are excellent for veterinary dentistry. The ACRYLIC RESIN (MONOMER) that is commonly used is the BIS–GMA (BISphenol–a–Glycidyl MethAcrylate).

ACRYLIC RESINS are available in two types, TYPE I the pure "UNFILLED" RESIN and TYPE II the "FILLED" RESIN. Type I liquid resin is generally used in restorative dentistry to *coat* the prepared and usually etched surface, prior to placing the type II filled resin paste (composite), both layers being either light–cured or self–cured. This adhesive layer of monomer creates a MECHANICAL BONDING (locking) into the ETCHED PORES (TUBULES) of the dentin and enamel (Photo 39), and a CHEMICAL BONDING to the overlaying filled resin (see acid–etch technique, 6.6).

The filler particles are bonded to the resin matrix by COUPLING AGENTS, those most commonly used being ORGANOSILANES.

Some composite restoratives are polymerized (or cured) chemically (e.g., Adaptic, Concise). These SELF–CURED composites are dual paste systems and have to be spatulated together in equal amounts. Others are LIGHT–CURED (e.g., Caulk/Dentsply's APH) and are packaged in either compules or syringes as a ready–mixed paste. A photo initiator and amine activator are contained in the paste. Light–cured composites require a special light source to ACTIVATE and CURE or HARDEN them. Although these instruments were formally ULTRAVIOLET LIGHT SYSTEMS, they had problems because of the limited penetration depth into the resin and lack of penetration through tooth structure.

The new VISIBLE LIGHT–ACTIVATING (LIGHT–CURING) SYSTEMS have totally replaced the ultraviolet light systems. The light source of the visible light–activating system is usually a tungsten halogen light bulb. WHITE LIGHT that is generated by the bulb passes through a filter that removes the infrared and visible spectrum for wavelengths greater than about 500 nanometers. Because of this, most instruments produce a BLUE LIGHT which is in the 400–500 nanometer range. It is worth the investment of a light–activating system, since you only have to wait 20–40 seconds for the composite to harden in shallow restorations before trimming and finishing. However, the most common cause of composite restoration failure is insufficient cure time. If there is any depth to a composite restoration, light–curing should be carried out for one minute plus. The only disadvantage of light–cured composites is that they can only be cured to a depth of 2 mm. To overcome this, composite should be built up and cured in layers.

12.8 GLASS IONOMERS

Glass ionomers are so named because the powder is ground *glass* and the setting reaction and adhesive bonding involves *ionic* bonds.

The powder (polymer) is an acid–soluble calcium fluoroaluminosilicate glass, having particle sizes from less than 15 microns up to 50 microns, depending on the type. The liquid (monomer) is polyacrylic acid, copolymerized with iticonic, maleic or tricarballylic acid. Glass ionomers are classified under types depending on their composition:

Type I Luting (sealing and cementing). Particle size is 15 microns or less.
Type II Restoration and core build–up. Particle size is 20–50 microns.
Type III Liners and bases. Particle size is 20–50 microns, with adjusted handling characteristics.

Glass ionomers as RESTORATIVES (e.g., Ketac–Fil) are mostly used in veterinary medicine for feline "neck" lesions (Class V cavities). These type II glass ionomers can also be used for Class III cavities, selected Class I cavities, carious lesions, restorations of deciduous teeth, repair of crown margins, bases under restorations and core build–ups. Glass ionomers are better than amalgam and composite for restoring these lesions, *unless strength is required,* because they CHEMICALLY BOND to enamel and dentin. They also release fluoride (reducing tooth sensitivity and secondary decay); save tooth structure (because drilling is not usually necessary); prevent microleakage by providing a tight marginal seal, as long as they are well placed (their coefficient of thermal expansion is similar to tooth structure); and they are biologically compatible (BIOCOMPATIBLE) with the pulp. *Success of glass ionomers as restoratives,* depends on:

1. Conditioning the tooth surface.
2. Proper mixing and handling.
3. Protection during setting.

CONDITIONING of the tooth surface (dentin and often cementum in "neck" lesions) starts with the cleansing of the area of plaque and debris. A fluoride or a glycerin–based paste should not be used since it will leave a film on the surface of the tooth that prevents good bonding of the glass ionomer. A PUMICE WASH should be used instead of paste, followed by a five– to ten–second swabbing with 10% POLYACRYLIC ACID. The goal is to remove the SMEAR LAYER but still leave a collagenous plug in the dentinal tubules, which acts as a barrier to penetration of the constituents of the cement and preserves the hydrodynamics of the dentin.

The SMEAR LAYER is a thin layer of fused residue of mineralized dentin matrix and bacterial debris, approximately five to ten microns thick, found on the eroded or the cut surface of the tooth. Although this smear layer can prevent proper bonding, it may provide additional protection to the dentin and pulp from a potential irritant. There is still controversy as to whether to remove or to leave the smear layer, however current research and opinion suggest removal of this layer.

In classic Class III or V cavities or lesions the smear layer should be removed in order to achieve maximum adhesive bonding to the dentin. All deep areas should be protected first with CaOH.

With light–cured glass ionomer liners, conditioning the dentin with polyacrylic acid is not required.

The smear layer on deep, cut or instrumented surfaces (which is different in composition from that on eroded surfaces) should not be removed, but left intact to act as a barrier to stop penetration of the tubules by the acid component of the cement. All deep areas should be protected first with CaOH.

Thus, if the dentin exposed is within 0.5 mm of the pulp, it is probably best to leave the smear layer, place a CaOH liner, then remove the smear layer from the rest of the exposed dentin. If there is more than 0.5 mm of dentin over the pulp, then remove the smear layer from the exposed area.

Following "conditioning," the area is rinsed with water, then lightly dried but not dehydrated.

Correct mixing of type II glass ionomers is important (carefully follow the manufacturer's instructions). Some are packaged as powder and liquid, which have to be mixed by hand, and others are packaged in premeasured capsules of powder and liquid (e.g., Ketac–Fil), which are mixed in an amalgamator. Although both have their advantages, when mixing the powder and liquid by hand, inaccuracies with amounts and technique can easily occur. This can lead to failure of the restoration due to expansion, shrinkage and/or reduced strength. Hand mixing should be done on a *cold* glass slab, which lengthens the working time. Once the cement is mixed, it should be placed on the tooth with a plastic placement instrument.

It is important to keep blood and saliva out the operating field. A layer of varnish should be placed gently over the cement, while it is hardening, as well as after it has been shaped and polished. This prevents desiccation and CRAZING (the appearance of minute cracks on the surface of the glass ionomer).

12.9 METAL REINFORCED GLASS IONOMERS

Metal filler particles can be added to glass ionomers to improve the strength, fracture toughness, and resistance to wear. A SILVER ALLOY ADMIX ("Miracle–Mix") is made by *mixing* spherical silver amalgam alloy powder with type II glass ionomer.

A CERMET (Ketac–Silver capsules and Chelon–Silver powder and liquid) is made by *fusing* silver particles to the glass powder.

12.10 LUTING CEMENTS

"LUTING" is defined as *sealing* a joint and *cementing* two substances together.

Luting cements in veterinary dentistry are used for cementing *orthodontic bands, brackets, buttons* and *hooks, pins, posts, cores,* and *cast metal crowns.*

Examples of luting cements include *zinc oxyphosphate* (e.g., Tenacin), *zinc silicophosphate* (e.g., Fluoro–thin), *zinc polycarboxylate* (e.g., Durelon), *zinc oxide–eugenol* (e.g., Fynal), *glass ionomers* (e.g., Fuji ionomer, Ketac–Cem) and *resin cements* (e.g., Comspan, Panavia).

These products all have different properties and the choice of which one to use depends on the situation involved. For most veterinary needs, the *glass ionomers* and *resin cements* will suffice.

It is important to follow the manufacturer's instructions carefully. Use a cool glass slab and mix the powder to the liquid quickly and thoroughly to the desired consistency. Make sure that there are no air bubbles and make sure that all surfaces are clean and dry, and hold the item to be luted firmly in place until the cement sets. Be sure to store the cements as directed on the label and discard them if they become cloudy, crystallized or outdated.

No one system suits all needs so it is wise to have several different types of luting cements available.

12.11 ABSORBENT PAPER POINTS

Following irrigation and prior to obturation of the root canal, residual moisture should be removed by means of sterile absorbent paper points. Complete drying of the canals is necessary for proper adhesion of the sealing cement to the canal walls.

Absorbent paper points are uniformly tapered (0.2 mm/mm), smooth–sided paper points to which a binder such as starch has been added to prevent unraveling and provide stiffness. Paper points are packaged sterilized in different sizes and lengths. Sizes are available in *standardized* sizes (ISO 15 – 140), or *conventional* (non–standardized) (sizes XX–fine, X–fine, fine, medium, coarse and X–coarse). The sizes, according to the new specifications, correspond with sizes for standardized and conventional gutta–percha points. Lengths are available in a standard length of 25 mm, or a veterinary length of 55 mm (Photo 42).

12.12 ROOT CANAL FILLING MATERIALS

Root canal filling and sealing materials should completely and hermetically seal the apex, accessory canals and the dentinal tubules of the root canal of the treated tooth. The ideal material for filling and sealing a root canal should have the following properties:

1. Non–irritating (to both tooth structure and periapical tissues).
2. Harmless.
3. Bactericidal or bacteriostatic.
4. Non–resorbable.
5. Slow–setting.
6. Remain permanently hard after placement.
7. Free of porosity.
8. Provide a good seal (laterally and apically).
9. Insoluble in tissue fluid.
10. Easy to introduce into the root canal.
11. Easy to remove from the root canal.
12. Sterile (or easy to sterilize).
13. Radiopaque.
14. Should not shrink after being inserted.
15. Should not stain the tooth structure.

None of the 150 or so root canal filling and sealing materials currently available fulfill all of the above criteria, so only a few of the most practical materials needed for the veterinarian will be discussed.

Root canal filling materials are divided into, PASTE, SEMI–SOLID and SOLID types.

PASTE–TYPE FILLING MATERIALS include *zinc oxide–eugenol cements* with various additives, *zinc oxyphosphate, zinc oxide* and *synthetic resins, polycarboxylate cements, epoxy resins, polyvinyl resins, acrylic, polyethylene, silicone rubber* and *chloro–percha*.

SEMI–SOLID FILLING MATERIALS include *gutta–percha, acrylic* and *gutta–percha composition points.*

SOLID FILLING MATERIALS include *silver points, vitallium points, chrome–cobalt points, silver amalgam, metal reinforced glass ionomers and metal reinforced composites.*

In young dogs with very wide pulp chambers, *amalgam, metal reinforced glass ionomers* and *metal reinforced composites* may be used to strengthen the thin–walled tooth against fracture. *Zinc–free amalgam, glass ionomers* and *IRM* are used to retrofill the apex of a tooth following apicoectomy.

Most semi–solid and solid filling materials consist purely of inert substances whose purpose is to mechanically fill the root canal. They do not completely fill and seal the canal by themselves. Consequently they are used in conjunction with paste–type filling materials that act as sealing agents. Most of these FILLER–SEALER materials are slow setting, taking several hours to set or harden. These materials also act as a lubricant that aids in the *seating* of the semi–solid and solid points or cones.

The paste–type root canal filler–sealer material (cement) is placed in the canal and made to flow and seal the apex, multiple apical foramina, accessory canals and dentinal tubules of the canal. Any minor discrepancies and irregularities in the canal walls will also be filled. This process is accomplished with the aid of lateral and vertical condensation of the semi–solid filling materials.

The most widespread root canal filling material is gutta–percha used in combination with filler–sealer materials (e.g., AH–26, zinc oxide–eugenol). Gutta–percha and AH–26 used together come close to meeting all the properties listed previously for root canal filler materials.

Some filler–sealer materials contain medication. They may be subdivided into anti–bacterial, anti–inflammatory, and mummifying. Their purpose is to prevent reinfection and inflammation in a root canal that has been cleaned, but in which sterility cannot be guaranteed (i.e., non–traumatic pulp exposure that is to be treated and filled in one sitting). These materials include *AH–26* (bismuth and epoxy resin), *zinc oxide–eugenol*, and *Diaket* (bismuth and polyvinyl resin). *Ledermix* (cortisone and tetracycline), *Endomethasone* (cortisone and paraformaldehyde), *Formocresol* (formaldehyde and cresol) and *Glutaraldehyde* are medications used in treating the canal prior to filling. Endomethasone has been widely used in human dentistry in Europe, is normally well tolerated, effective and easy to use, and has its place in veterinary dentistry. In human dentistry the use of Endomethasone is controversial at the present, since inadvertent overfilling of the root apex has in some cases caused necrosis of nervous tissue in the mandibular canal and the mucosal lining of the sinuses.

ZINC OXIDE–EUGENOL (ZOE) is easy to use, has a mild antibacterial action and is economical. However, it has a slow setting time and resorbs over time. It is also mildly irritating to periapical tissue should it leak through the apex. It is not compatible with composite, requiring a base over it before restoration with a composite.

AH–26 is an epoxy resin containing a non–toxic hardener. Its radiopacity is due to bismuth. It is strongly adhesive although contracts slightly while hardening, and is well tolerated by the periapical tissues (Photo 43).

GUTTA–PERCHA is the standard to which other obturating materials are compared. It has been used for over 100 years. The composition of gutta–percha used in endodontics is approximately 20% gutta–percha, 66% zinc oxide (filler), 11% heavy metal sulfates (radiopacifier) and 3% waxes or resins (plasticizer).

Gutta–percha points are packaged sterilized in different sizes and lengths. Sizes are available in *standardized* sizes (ISO 15 – 140) or *conventional* (non–standardized) (sizes X–fine, fine–fine, fine–medium, medium–fine, medium, medium–large and large). The STANDARDIZED POINTS are designed to have the same size and taper as standardized endodontic instruments (see root canal instruments, 3.20). The CONVENTIONAL (non–standardized) POINTS have a tip of one size and a body of another size. Although these shapes and sizes are not always uniform, it probably is not too important since the canal shapes are also variable. Lengths are available in a standard length of 25 mm, or a veterinary length of 45 mm.

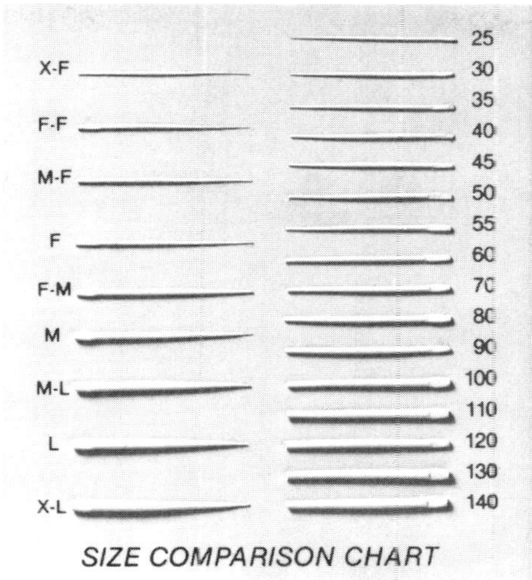

Figure 149. Gutta percha points (Hygenic Corp.).
Left — non–standardized points. Right — standardized points.

Gutta–percha itself is a tough rubber–like substance extracted from the latex of MAZERWOOD TREES (also called the PALAGIUM TREE and the GUTTA–PERCHA TREE), which are indigenous to Indonesia, South America, and the islands of Malaysia. Gutta–percha becomes deformable at temperatures above 48 degrees centigrade, or it can be softened with chloroform. THERMOPLASTICIZING GUTTA–PERCHA instruments are available (e.g., Obtura II), which temporarily liquefy the gutta–percha enough to be injected into the root canal through fine silver needles. Thermoplasticized gutta–percha can create an almost perfect sealing and filling of the canal, providing the canal is large enough to accept the injection needle tip (ISO size 40 or wider), and providing that the technique is accurate.

12.13 CORE BUILD–UP MATERIALS

There are several materials available for core build–up. Those most commonly used in veterinary medicine are type II metal reinforced glass ionomers (e.g., Ketac–Silver and Chelon–Silver and "Miracle Mix"). Other materials such as Core Paste (Denmat), composite resins (both light– and self–cured) and amalgam have been used.

A new product called "TI–CORE" (Essential Dental Systems) holds much promise, being a TITANIUM–REINFORCED self–cure COMPOSITE (Photo 65). TITANIUM is a highly biocompatible filler that adds strength and resilience, providing a strength equal to that of dentin. Although developed as a core build–up material for crowns, it shows promise in reinforcing and filling the large pulp cavities of endodontically treated canine teeth in young dogs. Ti–Core Flexi–flow is a two–paste system that can be introduced into the canal with a special syringe (Centrix, "speed slot" with needle tubes).

12.14 PINS (PARAPULPAL)

PARAPULPAL PINS, such as TMS PINS (Coltene/Whaledent), are often used for additional mechanical retention of restorative materials to the dentin of the tooth, as well as for increased stability and anti–rotational purposes during post and core procedures.

TMS (Thread Mate System) pins are small self–threading pins made of gold–plated stainless steel. Pins made of titanium alloy, which is highly biocompatable with tooth material, are also available. The TMS pins are made in three different *series* of pins, which describe their shape and method of insertion (TMS, TMS Link and TMS Link Plus). TMS and TMS Link series are available in four sizes, which denote the length and diameter of the pins. These are MINUTA, MINIKIN, MINIM and REGULAR. TMS Link Plus series are available in Minim and Regular sizes. BONDENT and MAX pins are more recent developments and have a greater ability to retain build–up material.

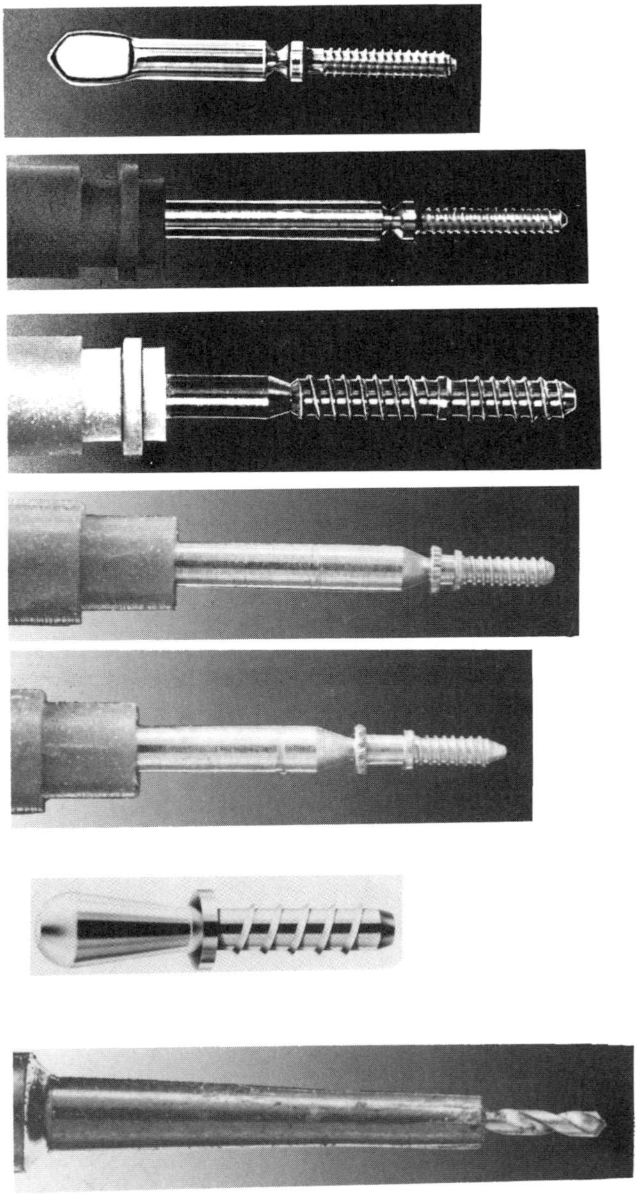

TMS (Minikin)

TMS Link (Minikin)

TMS Link Plus (Regular)

Bondent (short)

Bondent (long)

Max

Drill

Figure 150. Parapulpal pins (Coltene / Whaledent).

TMS series pins are pins designed for manual insertion with a pin holder/wrench.

TMS Link series pins are pins attached to a shaft with a plastic hub. They are designed for insertion with a low–speed handpiece.

TMS Link Plus series pins represent the next generation of pin design. They are similar to the Link series, but have a small shoulder built into the threaded part of the pin, at the insertion depth. This prevents overinsertion of the pin. Their depth of insertion has been shown to provide optimum retention of the restoration.

Bondent Dentin Bonding pins are also attached to a shaft and plastic hub, but have a double shoulder at the shear point. This prevents overinsertion of the pin as well as assisting in the retention of build–up materials.

Max Restorative pins are the latest generation of pins and are a combination of all the best features of the other pins. The head has been redesigned and is better for retention of build–up materials. Max pins also provide the lowest level of insertion stress, making it the safest pin available.

	PIN DIAMETER	DRILL DIAMETER	PIN LENGTH	DRILL LENGTH
TMS Minuta	0.375 mm (0.015")	0.350 mm (0.0135")	1.25 mm (0.050')	1.30 mm (0.051")
TMS Minikin	0.50 mm (0.020")	0.425 mm (0.017")	2.25 mm (0.090")	1.50 mm (0.060")
TMS Minim	0.60 mm (0.024")	0.525 mm (0.021")	5.0 mm (0.200")	2.0 mm (0.080")
TMS Regular	0.775 mm (0.031")	0.675 mm (0.027")	5.625 mm (0.016")	2.0 mm (0.080")
BONDENT (short)	0.50 mm (0.020")	0.425 mm (0.017")	2.0 mm (0.080")	1.875 mm (0.075")
BONDENT (long)	0.50 mm (0.020")	0.425 mm (0.017")	2.5 mm (0.090")	1.875 mm (0.075")
MAX (017)	0.50 mm (0.020")	0.425 mm (0.017")	2.5 mm (0.100")	1.90 mm (0.075")
MAX (021)	0.60 mm (0.024")	0.525 mm (0.021")	3.625 mm (0.145")	2.40 mm (0.095")

TABLE 2. Measurements of Parapulpal pins and matching drills (Coltene/Whaledent).

These pins are all manufactured as single–shear pins (except some of the TMS series), which means that when they are screwed into the dentin to the preset drill depth (Photo 38), the main shaft shears off from the pin. The Minim and Regular sizes are also made as double–shear pins, which provides two self–shearing pins on one shaft. The TMS pin kit includes pins, a drill (with a slightly smaller diameter than the pins), and a pin wrench. Bending tools, which enable the TMS series pin to be bent into the most desirable position to afford maximum retention, are also available.

TMS pins should be inserted into the dentin no less than 0.5 mm from the dentino–enamel junction and in the direction of the long axis of the tooth (Photo 37). The depth of insertion is preset by the drill. Pins should be placed so there is room for at least 1.5 mm of restorative material to cover them. If the pin is too close to the surface of the restorative material, it may be visible through the material. Care must be taken not to perforate or come close to the pulp in a vital tooth. After drilling the hole, the pin is screwed in manually using the pin wrench, or with a low–speed handpiece, until the shaft automatically shears from the pin. The pin can then be bent if necessary with the bending tool, so as to leave it in the most retentive or most anatomical position (Photo 38). Two pins bent towards each other will give better retention of the restorative material than if they are parallel to each other.

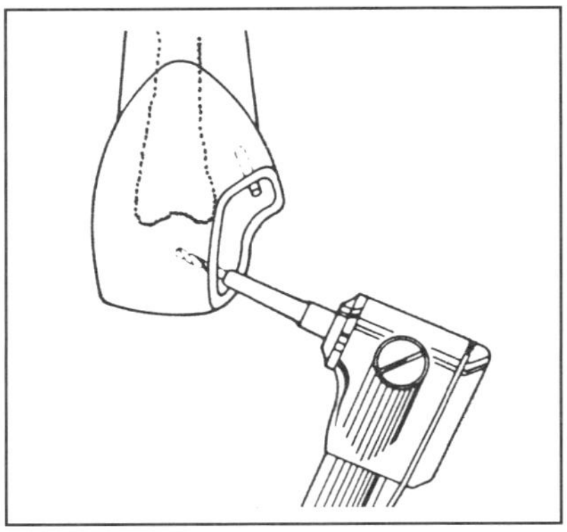

151 A.

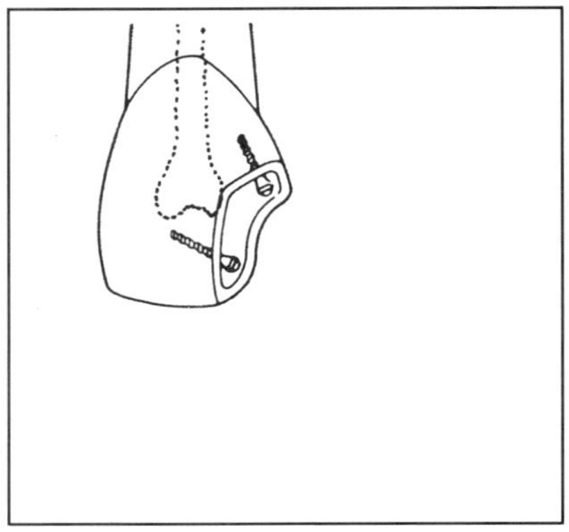

151 B.

Figure 151 A–B. Placement of parapulpal pins.

151 A. Drilling the hole with a special drill with stop.
151 B. Pins in place.

Although all these pins can be used in veterinary dentistry, the most useful sizes are the Minikin and the Regular. Bondent and the new Max pins are also excellent if additional retention of the restorative material is needed (e.g., lateral slab fractures).

Other manufactures of parapulpal pins include PCR and FO pin systems (Brassler), Filpin system (Vivadent) and Stabilok dentin pins (Fairfax).

ZETNER and *RABITSCH* (1986) have demonstrated a further interesting use for these pins, by using them to attach a plastic beak prosthesis to the remaining beak stump of a blackbird. *ZETNER* has also used these pins in a cat to fix the lower jaw after a fracture of the mandible. After pins were placed in the maxillary and mandibular canine teeth, the mandible and maxilla were placed in the correct occlusion. Composite material was then placed over the pins to lock the teeth together. The rostrally stabilized mandible was then able to heal together, similar to intermaxillary fixation in humans. Food was given in liquid form by syringe into the cheek pouches, until healing was complete. The pins and composite were then removed (see interarcade fixation, 10.7).

12.15 POSTS (PULPAL)

PULPAL POSTS or ENDO POSTS, such as the PARA–POST SYSTEM (Coltene/Whaledent), are used for retention of core build–up material and for adding strength to the remaining tooth structure. They are designed to be inserted into the root canal of the tooth following endodontic treatment. Para–Posts are SERRATED or

PASSIVE POSTS made of stainless steel. Posts made of titanium alloy are also available. Serrated or passive posts are not the same as *self–threading* posts. SELF–THREADING or ACTIVE POSTS are designed to be threaded into the canal, cutting a retentive thread into the dentin. A self–threading post has a spiral cutting thread with a slightly larger diameter than the matching drill. Passive posts have serrations, grooves or retention ledges, but their diameter is similar to the diameter of the matching drill. Retention with passive posts is obtained by the cement locking into the grooves or ledges. Some posts are completely smooth. These have very little retention and are not recommended.

The Para–Post system is a kit of posts with five different diameter sizes and five matching drill sizes. The sizes of these posts and drills are: 0.9 mm (0.036"), 1.0 mm (0.040"), 1.25 mm (0.050"), 1.5 mm (0.060"), 1.75 mm (0.070"). The length of each post is 20 mm (0.80").

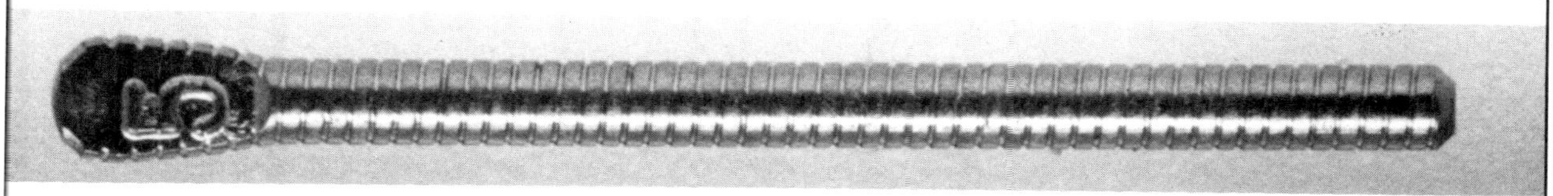

Para post

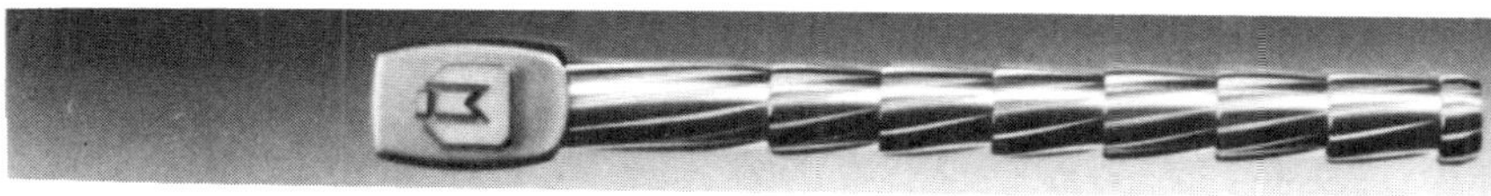

Para post plus

Figure 152. Pulpal posts (Coltene / Whaledent).

The smallest size of Para–Post drill that fits the canal should be used to commence drilling of the canal. Successively larger sizes are then used to enlarge the canal to the desired diameter. The depth of drilling and insertion should be about half the length of the root, or equal to approximately the length of the crown. This depth must be determined by measurement of the drill depth or with the aid of a radiograph.

After the canal has been drilled sufficiently to accept the post, the post is inserted then shortened and bent as necessary. Although bending of a post is not recommended, since it weakens the metal, bending a post is often necessary for the long curved canine teeth. Stainless steel posts can be bent, but titanium posts should not be bent. Titanium is very hard to bend, but once bent becomes brittle at that point.

Para–Posts have a VENTING GROOVE along one side of the length. This groove allows the excess cement to escape as the post is inserted, preventing a plunger–like compression of the cement at the apex of the canal.

PARA–POST PLUS is the next generation post featuring retention ledges to enhance overall retentiveness, and has nine spiral flutes around the post for easier venting of excess cement.

In order to obtain additional retention and to prevent rotation of the core build–up, TMS pins may be inserted into the dentin around the post. The pins may have to be bent into the most desirable position to afford maximum retention and anatomical shape.

Para–Posts are useful in small teeth for strengthening a core build–up, but cannot be used in large teeth (e.g., large canine teeth) because the canal length is too long. In young dogs the canal diameter is also too large. If posts are needed for large teeth they have to be custom made. STAINLESS STEEL SCREWS from the hardware store are adequate and a selection of different diameters and lengths should be kept available.

Although Para–Posts are commonly used there are other excellent post systems available. Other brands include Flexi–Post (Essential Dental systems), Radix Anchor system (Caulk/Dentsply), Kurer Anchor system (Teledyne Getz) and Dentatus Classic post system (Weissman Technology).

As an alternative to posts and screws, K–WIRES and small INTRAMEDULLARY (I.M.) PINS can be used as posts. Additional retention can be obtained by scoring the surface of the wire or the pin with a drill or a saw, or by tapping them with a thread. It is important to make a chamfer around the circumference of the end of these screws, K–wires and I.M. pins. Any right–angled end may cause fracture of the tooth at this point, if sufficient stress is applied.

12.16 IMPRESSIONS AND STONE MODELS

Impressions of the teeth are required when it is necessary to fabricate cast crowns, to prepare wire, metal, and acrylic appliances, and for forensic cases. There are several impression materials available, such as *alginate, silicone, polysulfide,* and *polyether rubber*. Although human impression trays can be used, correctly designed ANIMAL IMPRESSION TRAYS are now available (Photo 55) (Figure 153), or can be custom made by a dental laboratory.

ALGINATE is an inexpensive IMPRESSION MATERIAL that is commonly used to make working models of the dentition and occlusion. If extremely accurate impressions are required, such as for the fabrication of cast crowns, the rubber–like elastomeric materials should be used, since alginate is not dimensionally stable. The raw material of alginate is obtained from brown algae (seaweed), and is provided in powder form, consisting of alginate, calcium alginate, calcium carbonate, sodium salts as retarders, and other additives. The powder is mixed with a measured amount of water in a rubber bowl using a smooth "figure–of–eight" motion, and loaded in the impression tray. Alginate has two disadvantages. If it is left in too moist an atmosphere it will absorb water and expand, or if it is left in too dry an atmosphere it will lose water and shrink. Therefore, to produce an accurate stone model from an alginate impression, the stone should be poured immediately, although if wrapped in a damp cloth an alginate impression may be stored for an hour or two.

ELASTOMERS or ELASTOMERIC IMPRESSION MATERIALS, such as silicone, polysulfide and polyether rubber, have the ability to retain their shape for several weeks, and are useful if the veterinarian wishes to have the dental laboratory pour the stone model. They are also more accurate and produce finer detail than alginate. However, they are much more expensive than alginate.

Elastomers contain large molecules with weak interaction among them, tied together at certain points to form a three–dimensional network, then when released they snap back to their relaxed entangled state. These materials are usually two–component systems with polymerization and/or cross–linking occurring either by a condensation reaction or an addition reaction.

There are three basic types of elastomers, POLYSULFIDES, SILICONES and POLYETHERS. The most commonly used impression material is SILICONE or POLYSILOXANE. Although these impression materials are more expensive than alginate, their convenience, longer storage time, ability to make multiple models and their ease of use make them a good choice. These materials consist of highly polymerized silicone oxide chains with an inorganic filler. They are supplied as a highly viscous paste with a separate liquid catalyst, usually in a tube. When these are mixed, they cure within a few minutes, to form a rubber–like compound with very good reproductive properties. An important property of an impression material is its elasticity. This is the ability of a material to completely recover its original shape after being deformed as it is removed from the tooth. Silicone rubber is very good in this respect.

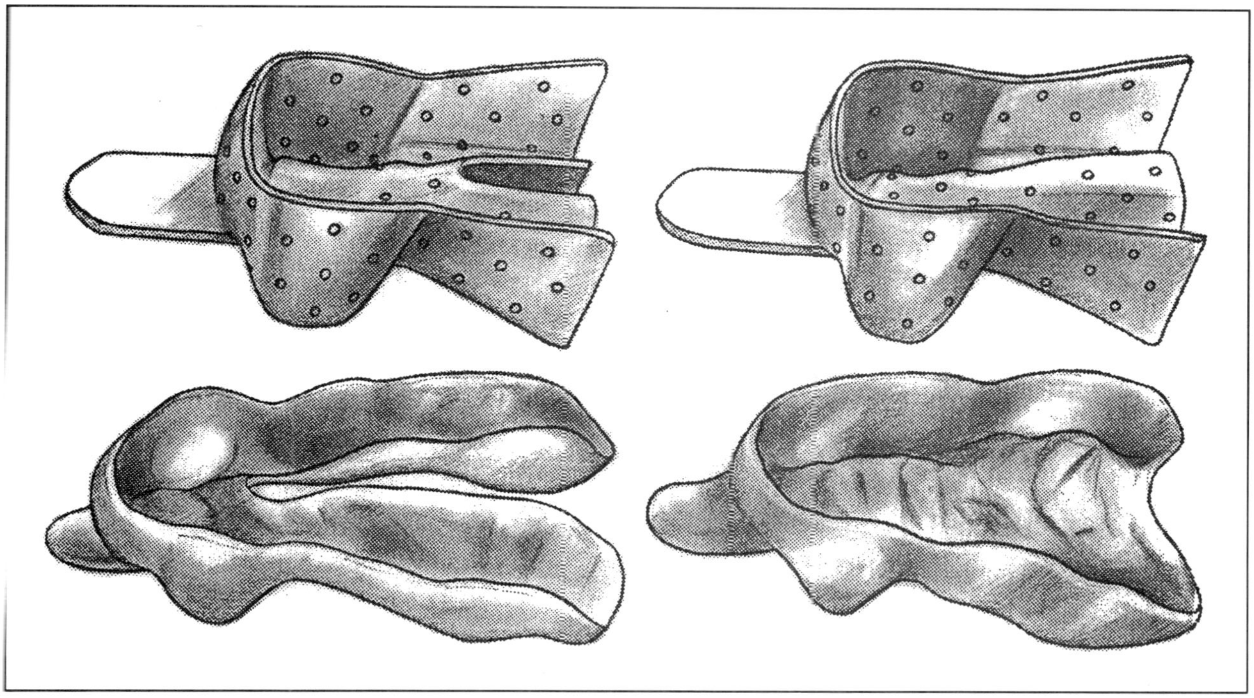

Figure 153. Animal impression trays.

Some of the better known impression materials are Permlastic (polysulfide), Impregum (polyether) and President, Imprint, Optosil, Silasoft and Permagum (silicone). Polyether rubber materials are often better when there is a bleeding impression field, since they are hydrophilic.

DENTAL STONE is a gypsum product (principally calcium sulfate hemihydrate) which when mixed with water forms a *positive* model from the *negative* impression. The *mixing time*, when hand spatulating, is generally about one minute. The *working time*, which is the time available as a workable mix, is about three minutes. The final *setting time*, when the stone is "ready for use" is about 30 minutes, although it is wise to wait one hour or more to be safe. Factors that affect these times are the particle size of the hemihydrate, the water to powder ratio, the method of mixing, the temperature and the addition of either retarders or accelerators. Trapping of air in the mix must be avoided by use of an electric vibrator, debubbling solutions in the tray, or a vacuum mixing device.

It is important to find a dental laboratory that shows a special interest and has experience in veterinary dentistry (e.g., Precision Ceramics, Montclair, California, U.S.A.). Since impressions, crowns and appliances can be sent via the mail or other delivery companies, it is not necessary to find a laboratory in your hometown.

12.17 METALS FOR CROWNS (CAPS)

Cast metal crowns are made of alloys that are a combination of two or more metals. The types of metals used fall into three categories: precious, semi–precious and non–precious. Many combinations are possible and the choices are usually dictated by the dental laboratory preparing them. Those suitable for veterinary dentistry are often based on cost, strength and corrosion resistance.

Non–precious or base metal alloys consist primarily of nickel (60–80 percent) and chromium (12–20 percent). Hundreds of combinations exist with varying amounts of minor elements such as carbon, molybdenum, aluminum, manganese, tungsten, niobium, boron, silicon and beryllium. Their structural properties and corrosion resistance vary, thus the metal best suited for each particular case should be considered.

Non–precious metal alloys are generally harder, stronger and stiffer than precious or semi–precious alloys. Although most non–precious metals are poorly corrosion resistant in vitro, the clinical significance of this is not known, and long term studies of intraoral corrosion are needed. Allergic reactions to nickel have been reported in some sensitive humans.

CHROME–COBALT–MOLYBDENUM ALLOY is often used to make cast metal crowns. It is non–irritating, very hard, corrosion resistant and hypoallergenic (because it is nickel–free). It has a melting point of 1350 degrees centigrade, which means that special equipment is required for casting.

STAINLESS STEEL is an alloy of iron, carbon, nickel and chromium. It is strong, non–irritating, inexpensive but poorly corrosion resistant for long term use in the mouth. It has been commonly used in the past for veterinary dental cast crowns (Photo 67).

GOLD (19 carat), alloyed with platinum, is highly corrosion resistant and non–irritating (Photo 69). It melts at a temperature of 900 to 1000 degrees centigrade, so it can be easily cast, annealed and hardened. It is also relatively expensive. Gold alloy can be used as a base for PORCELAIN FUSED TO METAL CROWNS, The manufacturing process for such crowns is very complex, requiring temperatures of 1250 degrees centigrade, and is naturally expensive. Porcelain fused to metal crowns are not well suited for most dogs, since there is a tendency for the facing to splinter and break. However, the cosmetic effect is outstanding.

SILVER–PALLADIUM ALLOYS are an excellent choice for veterinary dentistry, exhibiting high strength and corrosion resistance, as well as reasonable working properties.

TITANIUM ALLOY crowns are now being made by some dental laboratories that have the necessary equipment. They are extremely strong, very light and highly biocompatible. Also, they can be ANODIZED to look similar to gold (Photo 66) or to stainless steel.

When deciding on the type of metal to be used over a metal–filled core build–up, it is important to match the ELECTRICAL POTENTIAL of the metals (GALVANIC EFFECT) as closely as possible. For example, a titanium crown would obviously be a good match with a titanium core build–up material (e.g., Ti–Core). However, a gold crown would not be a good match with an amalgam core build–up, or a stainless steel crown with a silver filled build–up. Although a cast metal crown is generally insulated from the post core build–up by the cement, there are always potentially areas that may have some contact. Also, metal crowns that have contact with each other should have compatible electrical potentials.

Regardless of the alloy chosen, the surface finish should be smooth and highly polished. Rough areas will abrade opposing teeth and entrap oral fluids and debris. This can cause subsequent plaque accumulation and possible tarnishing or discoloring of the alloy. If adjustments are made to exterior surfaces of a cast restoration, the affected area should be smoothed with a rubber wheel and repolished.

SILICOATING is a recent development that involves the fusion of a SILICONE DIOXIDE LINER to the inside of the crown. This CERAMIC INTERFACE increases the bond strength of the metal to the luting cements by creating a mechanical and chemical bond. The equipment required to carry this out is expensive and is not available at all dental laboratories. Since the forces applied to crowns in animals can be severe, silicoating should be considered, and a laboratory found that performs this service.

12.18 ORTHODONTIC WIRES, ELASTICS, BRACKETS AND HOOKS

For those venturing into the field of veterinary orthodontics, the amount of materials and equipment needed is not great, but it is important to have the correct ones. The following is a list of orthodontic equipment and materials that are needed to perform most veterinary orthodontic procedures:

1. ORTHODONTIC (and intraoral) WIRES. Dead soft stainless steel ligature wire in gauges 16, 18, 20, 22, 24, 26, 28, 30.
2. STRAIGHT WIRE. Round, 14" – lengths.
3. ARCH WIRES. (Sizes – soft 0.635 mm and 0.762 mm.)
4. ELASTIC (ENERGY) POWER CHAIN. (Sizes – closed / medium / narrow.)
5. BULK ELASTICS. (Weight – 1–3 oz.)
6. TUBULAR ELASTIC TIE THREAD.
7. ELASTIC LIGATURE THREAD. (Strength – light / medium / heavy weight.)
8. ELASTOMERIC LIGATURES.
9. STAINLESS STEEL BRACKETS. Mandibular central bracket, with edgewise straight slot for a 0.022 arch wire. (The mandibular central base – smallest human bracket base.)
10. LINGUAL BUTTONS. Stainless steel with mesh backing on the base.
11. LINGUAL BUTTONS. Molded plastic, direct bond.
12. LINGUAL HOOKS. Stainless steel with mesh backing on the base.
13. EXPANSION SCREWS. Spring loaded and conventional type. Stainless steel. Length 10–15 mm. Width 8.6 mm. Thickness 4 mm. Expansion capacity 4–6 mm.
14. PISTON SCREWS. Housing serrated piston screws (Sizes – short – 4 mm, medium – 6 mm, long – 8 mm.)
15. PISTON SCREW REAMER.
16. MINI SCREWDRIVER (Jewelers' type).
17. INSERT KEY.
18. PLIERS:
    - Wire bending pliers (Angle).
    - Wire cutters (Belzer).
    - Three–jaw pliers (Aderer).
    - Tweed arch pliers.
    - Bird–beak pliers.

Three–stage loop–forming pliers.
Clasp adjusting pliers.
Band/bracket removing pliers, with nylon tip.
Long nose pliers.
Light wire pliers.
Lingual arch forming pliers.

There are many other products to choose from. It is wise to seek the advice of a veterinary or a human orthodontist to assist you. An orthodontic catalog can also be of great assistance (e.g., Rocky Mountain Orthodontics (RMO), Denver, Colorado, U.S.A.).

Another excellent source of help is your dental laboratory. They will be able to produce many fixed and removable orthodontic devices that you may need and guide you as to what to do.

12.19 ACRYLIC (FOR INTRAORAL SPLINTS)

Plastic orthodontic appliances and plastic oral splints are made of a self–curing acrylic (chemical–curing acrylic, cold–curing acrylic or auto–curing acrylic) material called POLY–METHYL METHACRYLATE (ACRYLIC). This is similar to the heat–curing acrylics, but is not as strong or as durable. It is much more convenient to use, requiring little or no special experience. Wires to hold the appliance in place, and active elements such as springs and screws, are imbedded in the acrylic during its construction (see acrylic splints, 10.6).

The acrylic material is supplied as a powder (polymer) and a liquid (monomer). The liquid is often colored, pink for human dentures, and gray for veterinary use. The liquid is poured into a porcelain, a glass or a rubber vessel, and the powder added until the desired consistency is reached. Normally, this is when all the powder is just wetted and a thin film of dry powder remains on the surface. The mixture is then stirred together and formed to the desired shape. In practice, if you mix too much monomer (liquid) to the polymer (powder), the excess monomer will evaporate in the course of the next few days.

The curing process takes only a few minutes, and is an exothermic reaction, so the mixture may become quite warm. If the acrylic is to be formed in the mouth, the heat produced can damage the oral tissues, setting up severe inflammation and even necrosis. Oral tissues under the splint should be coated with Vaseline or an antiinflammatory ointment to minimize damage. If it is practical to remove the splint from the mouth as soon as it is hard, further heat production can be dissipated by placing it in warm water for 10–30 minutes. When the exothermic heat reaction has stopped, it can be replaced in the mouth.

To avoid the problem of heat completely, acrylic splints can be made on a dental model and placed in the mouth when the heat has dissipated. However, because this requires additional anesthesia time, impression taking and model production, it is not usually practical in many cases.

Chronic inflammation caused by a splint usually regresses spontaneously as soon as the splint is removed. A light–curing acrylic splinting material (Dentsply's "TRIAD") is made in pliable sheets. It is especially useful to help stabilize jaw fractures (see acrylic splints, 10.6).

CHAPTER 13

MARKETING

Advanced dentistry for small animals is still not widely practiced, but is spreading rapidly. Good teaching at the University level in this subject is in its infancy, although there is enormous growing interest in general practice, as indicated by an increasing number of articles and local, national and international lectures and congresses on this subject.

Two veterinary schools in Europe, University of Berlin (Germany) and the University of Vienna (Austria), are currently teaching advanced dentistry. In the U.S.A., the University of Pennsylvania, the University of Missouri and Colorado State University are also teaching advanced veterinary dentistry. The University of Illinois and Auburn University are beginning veterinary dental programs. The University of California is opening a "state of the art" dentistry suite with four operatories, in 1992. Hopefully all veterinary schools will eventually teach this subject, so that full dental services will be a routine part of veterinary practice in the future.

Since approximately 80 percent of all patients coming into small animal practices have something wrong with their teeth or their gums, this subject has to be addressed at the student and practicing veterinarian level. Although cleaning teeth, treating gum disease and teeth extractions account for a large part of these cases, it is important that veterinarians and their technicians know how to do this correctly. Each tooth in the mouth should be treated as a separate entity, and thoroughly cleaned and inspected for problems. Proper instruments, techniques and knowledge of animal dentistry are extremely important. By not having the proper skills and not offering the client all the options, we could be verging on negligence and even malpractice. Nobody wants to allow that to happen. Veterinarians have already been sued for improper teeth cleaning and extractions, and inadequate dental care.

If you have a technician or a trained staff member doing your prophys, always inspect the mouth yourself before and after treatment. Periodically spot check the prophylaxis by using some plaque disclosing solution on the teeth. Always check the pocket depth of suspicious looking areas with a periodontal probe and chart all your findings. All teeth extractions and any advanced dental procedures must be performed by the veterinarian, and any broken roots properly removed. The veterinarian is ultimately responsible (and liable) for any dental work performed.

Veterinary dentistry allows a practitioner an opportunity to expand the practice and to provide a service either for a special clientele (guard, hunting, show, breeding and police dog owners), or those who just want the best for their pets. This will lead to increased referrals and business. Even if you have the knowledge, skills, and equipment to perform advanced dentistry, you must market this service. Clients have to know about you and realize the importance of good dentistry.

13.1 RECEPTION ROOM

The reception room, where clients often spend a good bit of time, is an excellent place to begin to educate and motivate the pet owner. Good close-up color photographs of different procedures (e.g., teeth before and after cleaning, fractured teeth before and after crown restoration, etc.), should be hung on the wall or kept in a photo album. Color posters and dental pamphlets promoting home care can also be placed in the reception room, along with samples and displays of home dental care products. Use products labeled specifically for animal use. Any free pamphlets and samples, or products sold, should have a stamp or a label indicating your hospital name, address and telephone number. This opportunity for free advertising should not be missed. Anything else that is unusual, such as stone models, orthodontic devices or even a photograph of your dental equipment can be displayed in the reception room to help to motivate the client.

The staff should be thoroughly versed in your services and encouraged to talk to the clients enthusiastically about dentistry and home care. Let your staff watch you doing different procedures so that they have a better idea of what you really do. Videos on animal dentistry are available, and you or your staff should take every opportunity to educate clients while they wait.

One thing that all clients have in common is the teeth of their pets. Clients in the reception room talk about "their" cases, and will be impressed by the wide range of dental procedures that you offer.

13.2 EXAMINATION ROOM

Once the client is in the examination room, you have a captive audience to discuss pets' teeth. Be basic and brief unless you feel the client is showing an interest that would justify further discussion. Most clients only retain about 10 percent of what you say. Every pet seen should receive a *thorough* examination of the mouth and teeth. Statistics indicate that about 80 percent of all pets seen have something wrong with the teeth or the gums. If the problems are *not* being mentioned to the owner and *not* being recorded on the pet's chart, then you are *not* practicing good medicine, and could be verging on negligence. Preventive care is always preferable to curative care.

Dentistry is generally easy to market for two reasons. *Firstly,* most of the hard work in marketing has been done for us by the human dental profession. Just about everybody has been to the dentist and already knows the basics of dentistry. Advertisements in magazines and on television constantly promote dental care and services. *Secondly*, you have the pet in front of you to show the client the problem. Once the condition is pointed out the client cannot deny its existence.

Teeth are teeth, no matter what species, and are taken care of the same way. It is rare that a client will let their pet suffer with conditions that can be corrected, unless it is a matter of economics. To demonstrate what services are available, your color photographs will be useful again. Keep a photo album in the examination room of all the procedures that you can do, showing before, during and after treatment. Photographs of the results will usually convince the client that treatment is necessary. If you do not have good pictures of your own, use the photos in this text. Some form of visual demonstration helps the client retain your comments.

Models showing the normal dentition of dogs and cats are very useful in veterinary dentistry. They can be used to show clients their pets' dental problems as well as how the suggested treatment will be performed. Although real skulls with teeth can be used, most clients do not like to see an animal skull. Plastic models are available, including new TRANSPARENT MODELS called VISI-MODELS (Dr. Shipp's Laboratories). These models show the full dentition as well as the roots of the teeth embedded in a transparent plastic base. Once the client sees the dentition and the root structure, they are better able to understand some of the complicated problems and treatments that you are faced with. They may also better understand your fees.

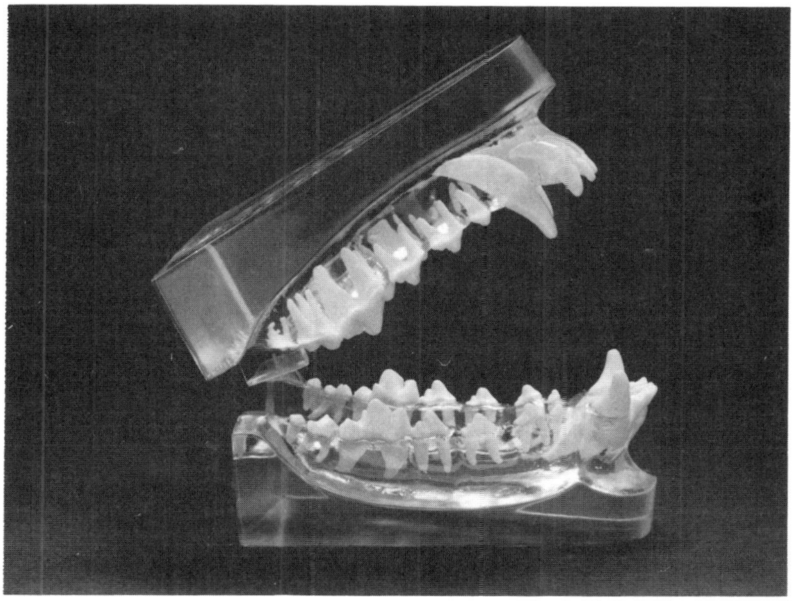

Figure 156. Visi-Model (Dr. Shipp's Laboratories).

Although the only dental problem may be the need for a prophylaxis, it is equally important to stress home dental care. Many clients will initially laugh at the idea of brushing their pets' teeth. Do not be put off and do not expect all clients to comply. However, at least you have done what your profession requires, and have suggested home care. Record this on your chart. Next time you see the pet and the teeth are still a problem, mention home care again. Many clients will eventually take you seriously and do something about it. Sometimes it takes two or three anesthetics, prophies and expenses to bring the point home. Pet dental care is a new field for most people and will take time to catch on. As a professional, you must keep encouraging pet dental care and eventually you will get results.

If the owner is willing to try home care, demonstrate on the owner's pet with an animal toothbrush (e.g., CET Animal Toothbrush), then let them try while you help hold the pet. For those who *do* comply, you are going to sell home dental care products. For those who *do not* comply, you are going to do more prophies. Either way you are in a winning situation. Always stress that dental procedures are in the best interest of the pets' health. Free puppy and kitten home care starter kits (e.g., VRx Products) are a good idea to encourage clients to start home care early. As for older pets, no animal is too old to start having its teeth brushed. Modern veterinary dentistry should offer the best information and techniques currently available. For instance one should not "scratch off a bit of this calculus," but instead try to inform the client of the damage that can occur if the condition is allowed to persist. It should be made clear that a thorough prophylaxis can only be completed properly under general anesthesia or sometimes sedation. This is because the *most important part of cleaning teeth is subgingival scaling, and no pet will tolerate this without chemical restraint.* Also, hard to reach areas, such as the lingual and palatal surfaces of the teeth as well as the posterior teeth, cannot be accessed without restraint. Gas anesthesia with intubation should always be used for animal dentistry, except for very mild or quick cases. When the pet is totally relaxed under general anesthesia, better access to all the teeth can be achieved. Due to the inflated cuff of the endotracheal tube sealing the trachea, calculus, debris and water spray cannot be inhaled into the lungs.

With the advent of new gas anesthetics (e.g., isoflurane), pets of all ages can be safely and successfully treated for dental problems, and worries by the owners can be allayed. Older animals usually need more dental treatment than younger animals, although the decision is often to extract seriously involved teeth in older pets with chronic periodontal disease. Since infection from the oral cavity can spread via the bloodstream to the rest of the body, it is important to take care of geriatric patients. Once treatment has been performed, home care should be encouraged. If this is not done, most pets will accumulate calculus within a year. Some small breeds may need their teeth cleaned again within three to six months, unless home care is performed.

13.3 EQUIPMENT AND DENTAL OPERATORY

Be proud of your dental equipment and operatory and let your clients see what is available for their pets' dental needs. A clean and well–organized work area will make a considerably better impression of efficiency than a handful of rusty dental instruments in an old shoe box.

The cost of equipment tends to vary. A dental or a veterinary supplier will be able to provide this information. The investment is not expensive compared to other investments, and the return is rapid. Second–hand equipment from human dentists is often out of date for them, but perfectly adequate for you to start with. You can always upgrade your equipment later. In the early stages it can pay to cultivate the friendship of dentists, and to buy certain items from them, as well as getting their assistance and cooperation in cases where you may need help. Dentists, especially those who are pet owners, are generally very willing to help you in any way possible.

It is good marketing to have all of your dental equipment neatly arranged in your surgery or your treatment area. A good investment is an instrument cabinet on wheels, second hand if necessary, which can be rolled into a corner when not in use. Dental units on wheels (e.g., VRx Products iM3 unit, Schein's Vet base) can be placed out of the way when not in use. Dental instruments need not be stored in sterile conditions, since most procedures (except oral surgery) take place in a relatively non-sterile environment. However, all instruments, burs and endo-files should be cold-sterilized after use on each patient.

Dental instruments and materials can be neatly arranged in drawers or on shelves in the dental area. Most people have never seen a veterinary dental operatory and will be very impressed. They will also be surprised how similar it seems to their dentist's office. It is often a good idea to show the client some of the instruments that will be used, and explain how the anesthetic machine and monitors work. Some clients will be interested in watching the procedure. Clients who watch are fascinated by what you are doing, and usually have no idea that such work could be done. Letting people watch should be totally acceptable and will be a topic of conversation with them for months and years to come. If the client has dropped the pet off for the dental procedure, it is good public relations to call the client immediately after the procedure has been performed, especially geriatric patients. The first thing to say is that everything went as planned, and that the pet is doing well. This is especially important if someone else answers the phone or there is a message machine. Many clients worry that something bad has happened when you leave a message to call them.

DENTAL CHARTS are very useful from the marketing viewpoint, apart from their medicolegal use. Make a copy of your diagnosis and treatment chart and give it to the client after the procedure. They will show it to their spouses, children, relatives, as well as keep it in their pet's medical file, if they have one. These charts will help clients to understand what you did and help you to justify your charges. Separate dental charts for cats and dogs should be available.

13.4 FOLLOW-UP CARE

Follow-up phone calls often produce more good public relations than the treatment you do. Either call the evening of the treatment or the next day to inquire how the pet is feeling. Clients are amazed at your concern and this will endear you to them forever.

The most important thing that clients seem to be concerned with is whether there will be any post–operative pain. This probably relates to their own experiences with the dentist. Luckily most animals do not exhibit much pain following dental procedures, but be sure to ask if the pet seems to have any pain. It is a good idea to give the pet a medication for pain following a major procedure. Be sure to tell the client upon discharge that you have done this. Counsel the client as to what to do if the pet shows pain, and prescribe medication if necessary. A follow-up phone call or a recheck should be done one to three weeks later.

As pets get older more frequent dental examinations are necessary. It is best to use a reminder system, such as cards or phone calls. Annual dental examinations can be done with vaccinations, or they can be scheduled separately. It is good to mention on the vaccination reminder card that a dental examination will be carried out. With puppies, tell the owner what to look for while the pet is teething. Set up an examination when the pet is about six to seven months of age, in order to check for retained deciduous teeth or for developing malocclusions. This gives the client an impression of thoroughness and enables you to discuss how home dental care is progressing.

13.5 BOOKING APPOINTMENTS

Although most dental appointments will be routine, there are times when clients may want to be present during the dental procedure. If your specialty is dentistry or you get referral cases who often travel some distance to see you, it can be advantageous to coordinate your examination followed immediately by the procedure. As soon as the animal has recovered, the client can leave and miss the rush hour traffic! Clients will appreciate this thoughtfulness and tell their friends. If you are a referral veterinary dentist, it is best to discuss the problem on the phone with the referring veterinarian and with the client before the case is scheduled. This not only reassures the veterinarian and the client of your knowledge, but gives you a chance to evaluate the case and plan the necessary time slot required.

It is a good idea to set aside blocks of surgery time that are reserved for dental cases. This saves on preparation time, since the instruments and materials are all set out for several patients.

13.6 FEES

The price of performing dental procedures is sometimes a major determining factor in whether the client will agree to your recommended treatment. Although money may be a problem with some of the clients, this does not mean that you should lower your fees to accommodate them. There may be a few hardship cases that you wish to help out, but you cannot run a business if you lose money. You could work out a payment plan if you trust the client, but the use of credit cards is better, providing the limit has not been exceeded. Although the cost of certain procedures can be high, it should not be the duty of the veterinarian to determine how much the client is prepared to spend. As long as the pet gets the correct and best possible service, the cost is often secondary. Invariably there is some relative or friend who will help if the owner does not have the money. Remember, banks are in the business of lending money not veterinarians. You work hard for your fee and should not take the risk of not getting paid.

Fees for veterinary services will obviously vary depending on many factors. However, the financial investment for continuing education in dentistry, equipment and materials is a real cost to you. Do not underestimate your competence and ability to perform a service that most veterinarians cannot do.

Prices for dental services should be on a variable scale, since the same procedure can be easy, average or difficult to perform. This applies especially to teeth cleaning and extractions. The variable fee is fair to both the client and the veterinarian, and will give you respect for your honesty. Variable prices for more complex procedures can be listed on your PRICE LIST as “A,” “B,” or “C.” The price for “B” is the average price, “A” for an easy procedure and “C” for a difficult procedure.

The fee for anesthesia should always be listed separately and based on the anesthesia time. If the price of general anesthesia for a human is compared with that for an animal, veterinarians are offering a very good deal. It is the one price that clients usually never question. Often the anesthesia fee is more than the procedure fee, but this is fully justified. After all, anesthesia is a highly skilled procedure and the fee should be appropriate.

It is a good idea to list all of your dental services individually on your printed INVOICE. Even if they do not apply to the case in hand, it is excellent advertising for all the services you perform (Table 3). Quoting exact fees can often be difficult. There are many times that you do not know what you will be faced with until the animal has been anesthetized, the teeth cleaned and radiographs taken. A general quote can be given, with the understanding that this may vary depending on what may have to be done. When quoting on the telephone for cases that you have not yet seen, only quote in very general terms. It is best to encourage an examination before being more specific. Often what the client thinks has to be done will be different to what really has to be done.

Some owners are skeptical about what can be done at first, but after proper counseling they are more prepared to accept the necessity for dental treatment for their animals and pay what it costs. Anybody who has a toothache wouldn’t wish the pain on their worst enemy’s dog, let alone their own. Conversely, there are many clients who are very sophisticated in their knowledge of what is now available to them, as far as veterinary dentistry is concerned. They treat their pets as though they were children or members of the family, and demand the very best care.

Clients have been known to drive hundreds of miles to obtain the services of a veterinary dentist. Do not underestimate the value of advanced dental services.

DENTISTRY		
Description		**Charges**
Teeth cleaning (cat) (curettage / root planing)	A / B / C	
Teeth cleaning (dog) (curettage / root planing)	A / B / C	
Extraction (deciduous tooth)	A / B / C	
Extraction (retained tooth)	A / B / C	
Extraction (incisor)	A / B / C	
Extraction (canine tooth)	A / B / C	
Extraction (premolar)	A / B / C	
Extraction (molar)	A / B / C	
Extraction (multiple teeth)	A / B / C	
Extraction (difficult tooth)	A / B / C	
Acrylic bridge / prosthesis / splint (preparation / removal / repair)	A / B / C	
Alveoloplasty	A / B / C	
Apicoectomy	A / B / C	
Biopsy (bone / tissue)	A / B / C	
Bite wing appliance	A / B / C	
Braces/retainers — (wire/elastic/synthetic)	A / B / C	
Bridge (permanent/temporary)	A / B / C	
Crown and crown preparation	A / B / C	
Crown reduction, pulp capping and restoration	A / B / C	
Crown reduction (rodent)	A / B / C	
Culture and sensitivity (aerobic/anaerobic)	A / B / C	
Electrosurgery / electrocautery	A / B / C	
Expansion appliance	A / B / C	
Filling tooth (amalgam/composite/glass ionomer)	A / B / C	
Flap surgery (double reverse/open/repositioned/sliding)	A / B / C	
Fluoride treatment	A / B / C	
Gingivectomy/gingivoplasty	A / B / C	
Hemisection/section — tooth	A / B / C	
Impacted tooth (exposure/removal)	A / B / C	
Implant (core/osseous/synthetic)	A / B / C	
Impression/stone model	A / B / C	
Inclined plane appliance	A / B / C	
Mandible/maxilla — fracture repair	A / B / C	
Odontoplasty/ostectomy/osteoplasty/osteotomy	A / B / C	
Oronasal/oroantral — fistula repair	A / B / C	
Orthodontic appliance (bracket/buttons/hooks)	A / B / C	
Pit/fissure — sealing	A / B / C	
Post/core build-up	A / B / C	
Pulpotomy, pulp capping and filling	A / B / C	
Reimplantation of tooth (acrylic/wire)	A / B / C	
Restoration of tooth	A / B / C	
Root canal (single/double/triple/canine tooth)	A / B / C	
Splinting (interdental/periodontal)	A / B / C	
Tumor/epulis/papilloma — removal	A / B / C	
Wiring (circumferential/interdental/interosseous)	A / B / C	
X-rays (mandible/maxilla/occlusal/periapical)	A / B / C	

TABLE 3. **Dental Invoice.**

Many new clients come in dissatisfied because the treatment they have received elsewhere has been superficial. Often the dog or the cat has suffered oral conditions for years, and treatment has been at best only palliative. Competent full service modern dentistry offers a wonderful opportunity to prove that you are an excellent and thorough veterinarian. It will usually bring in much new business because people talk to their friends about what you do to their pets.

Good dental treatment will not always work a miracle, but often there will be an immediate improvement in the pets' behavior and eating habits. Lack of bad breath will be instantly noticed by the client. Many owners are amazed at the increased physical fitness of their pet that often follows periodontal treatment. By removing the focal source of infection from the mouth, the generalized bacteremia, often infecting primarily the heart, will subside. Dramatic health improvements, such as increased vitality, activity and appetite are readily noticed by the owner and prove the success of the treatment. This will also justify, in the client's mind, that their money was well spent. Such results will be self-marketing for future care, not to mention additional cases from the friends that they tell. It will also be easier to convince the owner of the benefits of home dental care, or more regular dental check ups and prophies. Thorough dental care will also prove your competence as a veterinarian as well as showing your advanced level of practice.

13.7 ADVERTISING

Although some clients and veterinarians in your area may have heard that you perform advanced veterinary dentistry, there are probably many more who would like to use your services, but do not know about it.

Promoting the service will certainly boost your case load and income. It will also help numerous pets who would otherwise go without better dental care.

There are many ways in which this can be done. A professional advertisement in your local veterinary newsletter or magazine is probably the easiest way to let other veterinarians know what you offer. State which services you perform and that all referrals will be strictly dental only. Always send the veterinarian a written report of what you did, including a statement such as "thank you for the referral." Another way to reach your colleagues is to send them a mailer, including business cards and a map of your location.

Most local and state veterinary associations keep a list of doctors who specialize or have a special interest in different fields. Be sure to notify the association of your services.

Advertising (tastefully) in the yellow pages of the telephone directory may prove useful, but is not always cost effective.

Local and state veterinary organizations usually have meetings and lectures on a regular basis. These are excellent places to talk about dentistry and to give lectures. The use of good close–up photographs is imperative to show the different cases and procedures. Lecturing to kennel clubs and breeders also can prove very educational to these groups. They will pass the word around about your services.

Writing articles for local (as well as national) veterinary magazines will give you recognition in the field and inform other veterinarians of the advances in animal dentistry.

If you send a newsletter to your clients, this is an excellent way to inform your clients about pet dentistry. If you do not send a newsletter to your clients, make up a letter about your dental services, and have it professionally reproduced to mail to your clients.

Talking about animal dentistry on local radio and television, or getting an article written in a newspaper or magazine, are other ways of marketing your services and will help the profession in general. Many people are still unaware of what can be done to their pets in the field of dentistry. The more exposure we get as a profession the better the care will be for our four-legged friends.

Human dentists can be a source of spreading information about your services. Talk to them about what you offer for pets and often they will talk to their human patients who have pets. Dentists may even be willing to display information on animal dentistry in their reception rooms.

In all of your marketing, stress the need for home dental care. This is probably the most important, yet most neglected, area of our profession.

❖❖❖

Well, by now you should be well versed in the field of veterinary dentistry. We hope that this book will help you in your future practice. Our aim is to be of assistance to you, and should you have any comments or questions, feel free to contact either of us.

Good luck!

ANTHONY D. SHIPP
D.V.M., F.A.V.D.

Dr. Shipp's Animal Hospital
351 N. Foothill Rd.
Beverly Hills, CA 90210
U.S.A.
Tel. (310) 550–0101
Fax. (310) 550–1664

PETER FAHRENKRUG
Dr. med. vet., Dr. med. dent., F.A.V.D.

Kirschenallee 30
D–2087 HASLOH
Hamburg
Germany
Tel. 04106–60 200
Fax. 04106–60 300

Products and Manufacturers

PRODUCT	MANUFACTURER
Aerrane.	Anaquest.
AH–26.	De Trey / Dentsply.
Amalgambond.	Parkell Poducts.
APH.	Caulk / Dentsply.
Cavitron ultrasonic scaler.	Caulk / Dentsply.
Centrix speed slot with needle tubes.	Centrix, Inc.
CET Animal CHX 0.12% Chlorhexidine gel.	VRx Products.
CET Animal toothbrush.	VRx Products.
CET Animal toothpaste.	VRx Products.
CET Oral hygiene spray.	VRx Products.
CET Prophypaste.	VRx Products.
Chelon–Silver.	ESPE-Premier Dental Products Co.
Comspan.	Caulk / Dentsply.
Copanol–F.	Sultan Chemists, Inc.
Core–Paste.	Denmat, Inc.
Dental charts (dog and cat).	Dr. Shipp's Laboratories.
Dentatus Classic post system.	Weissman Technology International, Inc.
Diaket.	ESPE–Premier Dental Products Co.
Durelon.	ESPE–Premier Dental Products Co.
Dycal.	Caulk / Dentsply.
Fahrenkrug elevator.	Schein, Inc.
Filipin system.	Vivadent.
Flexi–Post.	Essential Dental Systems, Inc.
Fluoro–thin.	S. S. White Burs.
FO pin system.	Brassler U.S.A., Inc.
Fuji–ionomer.	G C America, Inc.
Fynal.	Caulk / Dentsply.
Geristore.	Denmat, Inc.
Hypocal.	Ellman International, Inc.

PRODUCT	MANUFACTURER
Impregum.	ESPE–Premier Dental Products Co.
Imprint.	3–M Products.
Inceram.	Vident.
Insta–Fix.	Microcopy.
Insta–Neg.	Microcopy.
Insta–Veloper.	Microcopy.
IRM.	Caulk / Dentsply.
Kerr–life.	Sybron Corp.
Ketac–Cem.	ESPE–Premier Dental Products Co.
Ketac–Fil.	ESPE–Premier Dental Products Co.
Ketac–Silver.	ESPE–Premier Dental Products Co.
Kurer Anchor system.	Teledyne Getz.
Ledemix.	Lederle Arzneimittel GmBH u. Co.
Miracle Mix.	G C America, Inc.
Mirage.	Chamelon Dental Products, Inc.
Obtura II.	Texceed Corp.
Optosil.	Miles, Inc. Dental Products.
Panavia.	Morita.
Para–Post.	Coltene / Whaledent.
PCR pin system.	Brassler.
Permagum.	ESPE-Premier Dental Products Co.
Permlastic.	Kerr Manufacturing Co.
President.	Coltene / Whaledent.
Profin Directional system.	Weissman Technology International, Inc.
Prophymatic.	Medidenta International, Inc.
Radix Anchor system.	Caulk / Dentsply.
Roto-Pro burs.	Schein, Inc.
Silasoft.	Dental Innovators, Inc.
Stabilok dentin pins.	Fairfax Dental, Inc.
Stieglitz fragment and root extraction forceps.	Schein, Inc.
Tenacin.	Caulk / Dentsply.
Ti–Core.	Essential Dental Systems, Inc.
Titan sonic scaler.	Star Dental.
TMS pins.	Coltene / Whaledent.
Triad.	Dentsply International Inc. (York).
Visi–Model.	Dr. Shipp's Laboratories.
Vitrebond.	3M dental products.

MANUFACTURER	ADDRESS • TELEPHONE NUMBER
Anaquest	3005 West Bell Highway Madison, Wisconsin 53713. (800) 225-5479
Beck and Co.	657 E. 9th Street , Costa Mesa, California 92627-0258 (800) 854-0153
Brassler U.S.A., Inc.	800 King George Blvd. Savannah, Georgia 31419 (800) 841-4522
Caulk / Dentsply (Division of Dentsply International, Inc.)	P.O. Box 359, Lakeview and Clarke Avenues Milford, Delaware 19963-0359 (800) 532-2855
Centrix, Inc.	30 Stran Rd., Milford, Connecticut 06460-3008 (800) 235-5862
Chamelon Dental Products, Inc.	200 N. 6th Street Kansas City, Kansas 66101 (800) 366-0001
Coltene/Whaledent	236 5th Ave., New York, New York 10001 (800) 221-3046
De Trey / Dentsply	Postfach 5346, De Trey Strasse 1, D-7750 Konstanz 12, Germany 49-7531-5830
Denmat, Inc.	P.O. Box 1729 Santa Maria, California 93456 (800) 433-6628
Dental Innovators, Inc.	717 East Chapman Ave. Orange, California 92666 (714) 538-6655
Dentsply International, Inc. (York Division)	570 W. College Ave. York, Pennsylvania 17405-0872 (800) 877-0020
Dr. Shipp's Laboratories	351 N. Foothill Rd. Beverly Hills, California 90210 (800) 442-0107
Ellman International, Inc.	1135 Railroad Ave. Hewlett, New York 11557 (800) 835-5355
ESPE - Premier Dental Products Co.	P.O. Box 111 Norristown, Pennsylvania 19404 (800) 344-8235

MANUFACTURER	ADDRESS ● TELEPHONE NUMBER
Essential Dental Systems, Inc.	89 Leuning Street, South Hackensack, New Jersey 07606 (800) 223-5394
Fairfax Dental, Inc.	2601 South Bayshore Drive, Suite 845, Miami, Florida 33133 (800) 233-2305
G C America, Inc.	3737 West 127th Street Chicago, Illinois 60658 (800) 323-7063
Hygenic Corporation	1245 Home Ave. Akron, Ohio 44310 (800) 321-2135
Kerr Manufacturing Co.	28200 Wick Rd. Romulus, Michigan 48174 (800) 537-7123
Lederle Arzneimittel GmbH u. Co.	Pfaffenrieder Str. 7, D-8190 Wolfratshausen, Germany 08171 212 02
Medidenta International, Inc.	39-23 62nd Street, P.O. Box 409 Woodside, New York 11377 (800) 221-0750
Microcopy	3120 Moon Station Rd., P.O. Box 2017 Kennesaw, (Atlanta) Georgia 30144-9017 (800) 235-1863
Miles, Inc. Dental Products	4315 S. Lafayette Blvd. South Bend, Indiana 46614 (800) 343-5336
Morita USA, Inc.	14712 Bentley Circle Tustin, California 92680 (800) 752-9729
Parkell Products	155 Schmitt Blvd., P.O. Box 376 Farmingdale, New York 11735. (800) 243-7446
Precision Ceramics Demtal Laboratory	9591 Central Ave. Montclair, California 91763 (800) 223-6322
RMO (Rocky Mountain Orthodontics), Inc.	P.O. Box 17085 Denver, Colorado 80217-0085 (800) 525-6375
S. S. White Burs	1145 Towbin Ave. Lakewood, New Jersey 08701 (800) 535-2877

MANUFACTURER	ADDRESS ● TELEPHONE NUMBER
Schein, Inc.	5 Harbor Park Drive Port Washington, New York 11050 (800) 872-4346
Star Dental Products	1816 Colonial Village Lane Lancaster, Pennsylvania 17601 (800) 275-3320
Sultan Chemists, Inc.	Englewood, New Jersey 07631 (800) 637-8582
Sybron Corporation	411 E. Wisconsin, 24th floor Milwaukee, Wisconsin 53202 (414) 274-6600
3M Dental Products	3M Center, Bldg. 275-2SE-03 St. Paul, Minnesota 55144-1000 (800) 733-8524
Teledyne Getz	1550 Greenleaf Ave. Elk Grove Village, Illinois 60007 (800) 323-6650
Texceed Corporation	3001 Redhill Ave., Bldg. 4 #104 Costa Mesa, California 92626 (800) 344-1321
Vident	5130 Commerce Drive Baldwin Park, California 91706 (800) 828-3839
Vivadent (Division of Ivoclar N. America)	175 Pineview Drive Amherst, New York 14228 (800) 533-6825
VRx Products	1656 240th Street Harbor City, California 90710 (800) 969-7387
Weissman Technology International, Inc. (Dentatus International AB, Sweden)	192 Lexington Ave. New York City, New York 10016 (800) 323-3136

BIBLIOGRAPHY

Aitchison, J. 1963. *Changing incisor dentition of bulldogs.* Vet. rec. 75. S. 153ff.

Albrecht, G. u. P. Hentschel. 1973. *Die Bedeutung der Zahnbehandlung bei Dienst-und Jagdhunden.* Monatsh. f. Vet. Med. 28, S. 615.

Alten, S. von. 1938. *Zahnkrankheiten bei Hunden.* Diss. Hannover.

Bartels, K. P. 1973. *Zahnbehandlung beim Hund.* Tierärztl. Praxis, 1, S. 437ff.

Barthold, K. P. 1987. *Zahnstein im Kleintiergebiss.* Der Praktische Tierarzt, 68, 5/87, S. 44.

Becker, E. 1959. *Über die Osteosynthese bei kleinen Haustieren und kl. landwirtschaftlichen Nutztieren mit Hilfe eines hierfür zusammengestellten Instrumentariums.* Dt. Tierärztl. Wschrift, 66, S. 345ff.

Becker, E. 1965. *Über Zahn-u. Kieferkrankheiten bei unseren Haustieren.* Zahnärztl. Praxis, 16, S. 143ff.

Bieniek, H., K. W. Bieniek u. U. H. Kurz. 1983. *Kunststoffaufbau des frakturierten Caninus beim Hund mit Hilfe der Tiefziehfolienform.* Kleintier-Praxis, 28, S. 342ff.

Bieniek, H., M. Sager u. Ch. Remmers. 1987. *Osteomyelitis der Kieferknochen beim Foxhound.* Der Praktische Tierarzt, 68, 5/87, S. 74ff.

Bieniek, K. W., H. Küpper u. H. Bienek. 1987. *Metallkeramische Kronen zur Prothetischen Behandlung des Hundecaninus.* Der Praktische Tierarzt, 68, 5/87, S. 85-87.

Bieniek, K. W .u. H. Küpper. 1988. *Hi-Ceram:Ein neues Verfahren zur prothetischen Rehabilitation von Hundezähnen. Kleintierpraxis.* 33, Heft 3, 1988, S. 93-98.

Bieniek, H. 1988. *Zur Verwendung von Zahnröntgenfilmen in der Kleintierpraxis.* Der Praktische Tierarzt, 69, 11/88, S. J 1ff.

Bieniek K. W. u. H. Küpper. 1988. *Zur Ätiologie und Therapie der Parodontopathien beim Kleintier unter besonderer Berücksichtigung von parodontalen Implantaten.* Der Praktische Tierarzt, 69, 11/88. S. 11ff.

Bigler, B. 1978. *Experimentelle und klinische Unters. zur Frage d. endodontischen Therapie des Hundegebisses.* Zbl. Vet. Med. 25, S. 794.

Bodingbauer, J. 1947. a. *Vergleichende Betrachtungen über das Vorkommen der Karies beim Menschen und beim Hunde.* Z. Stomatologie 44, S. 333ff.

Bodingbauer, J. 1947. b. *Neuerlicher, erweiterter Vorschlag für eine einheitliche, vereinfachte Bez. der Hundezähne.* Wien: Tierärztl. Monatsschrift, 34, S. 277ff.

Bodingbauer, J. 1947. c. *Zahnfrakturen beim Hund.* Wien. Tierärztl. Monatsschrift 34, S. 442ff.

Bodingbauer, J. 1948. *Wurzelspitzenresektion beim Hund.* Wien. Tierärztl. Monatsschrift, 35, S. 49ff.

Bodingbauer, J. 1955. *Zahnkaries beim Hund.* Wien. Tierärztl. Monatsschrift 42, S. 177ff.

Bodingbauer, J. 1958. *Zähne, in: Wirth, D: Lexikon der praktischen Therapie und Prophylaxe für Tierärzte.* 2. Aufl., Vlg Urban & Schwarzenberg, Wien.

Bohmer, E. 1988. *Zahnerkrankungen bei Hasenartigen und Nagern.* Der Praktische Tierarzt, 69, 11/88, S. 37ff.

Bojrab, M. J. and M. A. Tholen. 1990. *Small Animal Oral Medicine and Surgery.* Philadelphia: Lea and Febiger.

Brass, W. 1976. *Zur Korrektur von Zahnstellungs- und Kieferanomalien des Hundes mit Dehnungs- Platten und durch kieferchirurgische. Massnahmen.* Kleintier-Praxis, 21, S. 75ff.

Bundesverband der Deutschen Zahnärzte e. V. (BDZ) 1984. *Information über zahnärztliche Arzneimittel.* Köln.

Bundgaard, A. 1978. *Tandregulering (orthodontisk behandling) hos hund.* Dansk Vet. Tidskr. 61, S. 8ff.

Carranaza, F. A. 1990. *Glickman's Clinical Periodontology.* 7th ed. Philadelphia: W. B. Saunders Co.

Christoph, H. J. 1960. *Abriss der Klinik der Hundekrankheiten.* Fischer Vlg Jena.

Cohen, S. and R. C. Burns. 1991. *Pathways of the Pulp.* 5th ed., St. Louis: Mosby Year Book.

Dicks, F. u. W. Zöllner. 1988. *Glasionomerzement für einen praktikablen Einsatz in der Tierzahnheilkunde.* Der Praktische Tierarzt, 69, 11/88, S. 32ff.

Dürr, U. 1968. *Zum Kalzium- und Phosphorgehalt in den Zähnen der Haustiere.* Berl. u. Münch. Tierärzt. Wschrift, 81, S. 221ff.

Dürr, U. u. P. Reichart. 1978. *Gingivitis der Katze, medikamentöse und chirurgische Therapie.* Kleintier-Praxis, 23, S. 231-235.

Eichner, K. 1980. *Zahnärztliche Werkstoffe und ihre Verarbeitung.* 3. Auflage, Huethig-Vlg. Heidelberg.

Eisenmenger, E. and K. Zetner. 1985. *Veterinary Dentistry.* Philadelphia: Lea and Febiger.

Eisenmenger, E. 1971. *Konservierende Behandlung von Zahnfrakturen des Hundes* Wien. Tierärztl. Monatsschrift, 58, S. 30ff.

Eisenmenger, E. 1974. *Schwerpunkte und Fortschritte der tierärztlichen Zahnheilkunde.* Kleintier-Praxis. 19, S. 181ff.

Eisenmenger, E. u. K. Zetner. 1982. *Tierärztliche Zahnheilkunde.* Lehrbuch; Paul Parey Verlag.

Ellenberger-Baum, 1974. *Handbuch der vergleichenden Anatomie der Haustiere* 18. Auflage Reprint, Springer-Vlg Berlin, Heidelberg, New York.

Emily, P. and S. Penman. 1990. *Handbook of Small Animal Dentistry.* Oxford, England: Pergamon Press.

Emmel, L. 1938. *Die Herkunft des Schmelzes der erwachsenen Nager, mit Untersuchungen über den Nagezahn von sciurus vulg.* L. Z. wiss Zoologie, 150, S. 538ff.

Fahrenkrug, P. 1982. *Stand und Möglichkeiten der Zahnheilkunde bei Haustieren.* Diss. med. dent. Hamburg.

Fahrenkrug, P. 1987. *Kieferorthopädische Behandlungsmöglichkeiten im Hundegebiss.* Der Praktische Tierarzt, 68, 5/87, S. 30ff.

Fahrenkrug, P. 1987. *Neue Instrumente für die Zahnbehandlung in der Kleintierpraxis.* Der Praktische Tierarzt, 68, 5/87, S. 48ff.

Fahrenkrug, P. 1987. *Die Abdrucknahme im Hunde-/Katzengebiss.* Der Praktische Tierarzt, 68, 5/87, S. 5ff.

Fahrenkrug, P. 1988. *Tierzahnheilkunde-quo vadis? Versuch einer Standortbestimmung und Zukunftsperspektive.* Der Praktische Tierarzt, 69, 11/88, S. 5ff.

First Annual Eastern States Veterinary Conference, Jan. 16-18. 1984. *Canine Dentistry, Symposium Proceedings.* Princetown Junction, New Jersey: Veterinary Learning Systems.

Fraguglione, D. 1957. *Das Milchgebiss des Feldhasen.* Z. Jagdwissenschaft, 3, S. 141ff.

Frost, P. 1986. *The Veterinary Clinics of North America, Small Animal Practice, Vol 16, Number 5.* Philadephia: W. B. Saunders Co.

Frost, P. 1982. *Canine Dentistry, A Compendium.* Day Communications.

Frost, P. 1990. *Canine Dentistry.* 3rd ed., Day Communications.

Gabka, J. 1979. *Indikationen und Ergebnisse des extraoralen Schraubenschienenverbandes nach Becker (eine 20-jährige Bilanz).* Der prakt. Tierarzt, 59. 9/1979, S. 726ff.

Gabka, J. u. H. Harnisch, 1982. *Operationskurs für Zahnmediziner.* Thieme-Verlag Stuttgart, 2. Auflage, 1982.

Gardner, A., B. Drake, and G. Keary. 1962. *Dental caries in domesticated dogs.* J. Am. Vet. Med. Assoc., 140, S. 433ff.

Greck, J. H., Kraft u. P. Kunath. 1976. *Überkronung von Eckzähnen bei Fleischfressern.* Tierärztl. Praxis, 4, S. 507ff.

Grossman, L. I., S. Oliet and C. E. Del Rio. 1988. : *Endodontic Practice.* 11th ed. Philadelphia: Lea and Febiger.

Haack, D., F. Korbner u. B. Hertsch. 1987. *Zahnkaries und Zahnfrakturen der Oberkieferbackenzähne beim Pferd.* Der Praktische Tierarzt, 68, 5/87, S. 59ff.

Habermehl, K. H. 1975. *Die Altersbestimmung bei Haus- u. Labortieren.* 2. Aufl. Vlg Paul Parey, Berlin u. Hamburg.

Harlan, K. 1975. *Kieferorthopädische Behandlung bei Hunden.* Der prakt. Tierarzt, 56, S. 156ff.

Harvey, C. E. 1988. *Die radikalchirurgische Resektion maxillärer und mandibulärer Läsionen bei Hund und Katze.* Der Praktische Tierarzt, 69, 11/88, S. 6ff.

Harvey, C. E. 1985. *Veterinary Dentistry.* Philadelphia: W. B. Saunders Co.

Harvey, C. E. and H. S. Orr. 1990. *Manual of Small Animal Dentistry.* Chettenham: British Small Animal Veterinary Association.

Hauck, E. 1942. *Untersuchungen über die Form und Abänderungsbreite des Hundegebisses.* Wien. Tierärztl. Monatsschrift, 29, S. 249, 273ff.

Hawkins, B. J. 1989. *Proceedings from Veterinary Dental Symposium.* New Orleans.

Heilmann, M. und P. Fahrenkrug. 1987. *Zur Kieferorthopädie im Hundegebiss.* Der Praktische Tierarzt, 68, 5/87, S. 24ff.

Hoffman-Axthelm, W. 1978. *Lexikon der Zahnmedizin.* Quintessenz-Vlg, Berlin.

Holmstrom, S. E., P. Frost and R. L.Gammon. 1992. *Veterinary Dental Techniques.* Philadelphia: W. B. Saunders Co.

Ishikawa, G. and C. A.Waldron. 1987. *Color Atlas of Oral Pathology.* St. Louis: Ishiyaku EuroAmerica.

Jablonski, S. 1982. *Illustrated Dictionary of Dentistry.* Philadelphia: W.B. Saunders Co.

Jänicke-Lorenz, J. u. R. Lorenz. 1988. *Zur Anwendung von Dynexan A-Gel in der Kleintierpraxis.* DpT., 69, 5/88, S. 40.

Joest, E. 1967. *Handbuch der speziellen pathologischen Anatomie der Haustiere.* Band V., Digestionsapparat Teil l, Zähne bearbeitet von Becker, E., Parey-Vlg., Berlin.

Jüde, H. D., W. Kühl u. A. Rossbach. 1979. *Einführung in die zahnärztliche Prothetik.* Köln 2. Auflage.

Kaplan, B. u. S. Marx. 1967. *Restoration of the maxillary canine teeth of a dog with enamel and dentin hypoplasia.* J. Am. Vet. Med. Assoc., 150, S. 603ff.

Kealy u. J. Kevin. 1981. *Röntgendiagnostik bei Hund und Katze.* Enke-Verlag, Stuttgart.

Keil, A. 1949. *Über die Frage des natürlichen Vorkommens und der experimentellen Erzeugung echter Zahnkaries bei Tieren.* DZZ, 4, S. 694ff.

Keil, A. 1966. *Grundzüge der Odontologie.* 2.Aufl., Borntraeger-Verlag, Berlin.

Kind, R. and F. Mays. 1976. *Use of an inclined plane for correction of ectopic mandibular canine tooth in a dog.* Vet. Med., Small Animal Clinician, 5/76, S. 52ff.

Kinoshita, S. and R. Wen.1985. *A Color Atlas of Periodontics.* St. Louis: Ishiyaku EuroAmerica.

Kirk, R. W. 1989. *Current Veterinary Therapy X, Small Animal Practice.* Philadelphia: W. B. Saunders Co.

Kittel, R. 1972. *Der Goldhamster.* Neue Brehm-Bücherei, Wittenberg.

Klein, H. 1979. *Vergleich verschiedener Überkronungstechniken am künstlich frakturierten Caninus des Hundes.* Diss., Hannover.

Klein, H. 1980. *Metallgusskronen mit zentralem Wurzelstift zur prothetischen Versorgung frakturierter Canini.* Kleintier-Praxis, 25, S. 197ff.

Körber, K. 1979. *Zur Parodontopathia beim Hund.* Kleintier-Praxis. 24, S. 179-166.

Krüger, E. 1979. *Lehrbuch der chirurgischen Zahn-,Mund- und Kieferheilkunde.* Band 1, Band 2, Band 3 Quintessenz-Vlg., Berlin.

Lange, D. E. 1981. *Parodontologie in der täglichen Praxis.* Berlin. Quintessenz-Vlg.

Langlais, R. P. and M. J. Kasle. 1985. *Exercises in Oral Radiographic Interpretation.* 2nd ed., Philadephia: W.B. Saunders Co.

Langland, O.E., F. H. Sippy and Langlais R. P. 1984. *Textbook of Dental Radiology.* 2nd ed., Springfield, Illinois: Charles C. Thomas.

Lehmann, K. M. 1985. *Einführung in die Zahnersatzkunde.* 5. Aufl., Urban & Schwarzenberg, München.

Lengnick, H. D. 1981. *Fallbericht zur Caninusfehlstellung infolge eines persistierenden Caninus.* Kleintier-Praxis, 26, S. 311ff.

Leopold, S. and D. J. Spinella. 1964. *A technique for canine root canal restoration.* Vet. Med., Small Animal Clinician. 59, S. 29, ff.

Levine, N. 1986. *Current Treatment in Dental Practice.* Philadelphia: W.B. Saunders Co.

Lindhe, J. 1985. *Textbook of Clinical Periodontology.* Philadelphia: W.B. Saunders, Co. (Munksgaard).

Manfra-Maretta, S. 1990. *Problems in Veterinary Medicine, Vol 2, Number 1.* Philadephia: J. B. Lippincott.

Manfra-Marretta, S. 1988. *The diagnosis and treatment of oronasal fistulas in three cats.* J. Vet Dent., Vol.5, 1,3/88, S. 4-6.

Marxkors, R. 1977. *Propädeutik der zahnärztlichen Prothetik.* Hüthig-Verlag, Heidelberg.

Meyer, G. 1978. *Zahnanomalien bei Meerschweinchen.* Kleintier-Praxis 23, S. 81ff.

Miller, M., G. C. Christensen and H. E. Evans. 1964. *Anatomy of the dog.* Philadelphia and London. W. B. Saunders Co.

Nachtsheim, H. 1936. *Erbliche Zahnanomalien beim Kaninchen.* Züchtungskunde, 11, S. 273ff

Neumann,W. 1988. *Rekonstruktion frakturierter Zähne beim Hund mit verschiedenen Kunststoffmaterialien.* Der Praktische Tierarzt, 69, 11/88, S. 26ff.

Nickel, R., A. Schummer u. E. Seiferle. 1967. *Lehrbuch der Anatomie der Haustiere.* Band 2, Parey-Verlag, Berlin.

Page, R.C. and H. E. Schroeder. 1982. *Periodontitis in Man and Other Animals.* Basel, Switzerland: Karger.

Pfeifer, E. G., M. Kämpfer u. H.Neu. 1988. *Die Behandlung der chronischen Gingivitis der Katze.* DpT, 69, 2/88, S. 29-32.

Phillips, R. W. 1991. *Skinner's Science of Dental Materials.* 9th ed., Philadelphia: W.B. Saunders.

Pollock, S. 1968. *Restoration of a broken canine tooth.* Vet. Med., Small Animal Clinician, 1/68. S. 27ff.

Prieur, W. D. 1976. *Zahnsteinentfernung mit dem Ultraschallgerät.* Praktischer Tierarzt 30, S. 20-23.

Proffit, W. R. 1986. *Contemporary Orthodontics.* St. Louis: Mosby.

Ramy, C. T. and V. A. Segreto. 1967. *Apicectomy and root canal therapy for exposed pulp canal in the dog.* J. Am. Vet. Med. Assoc. 150, S. 977ff.

Reichart, P. u. K. Apelt. 1977. *Technik der Überkronungen im Kleintiergebiss.* Tierärztl.-Praxis. 5, S. 481ff.

Reichart, P. 1978. a. *Kariestherapie im Hunde- u. Katzengebiss.* Tierärztl-Praxis. 6, 8 S. 361ff.

Reichart, P. 1978. b. *Die Extraktion im Hunde- u. Katzengebiss.* Fachpraxis. Nr. 2, S. 40 ff. Fa. Albrecht. Aulendorf.

Reichart, P. 1978. c. in: Kraft. W. u. U.M. Dürr, Hrsg. 1978. *Katzenkrankheiten.* Schaper-Vlg. Hannover. S. 223ff.

Reichart, P. 1979. d. *Trauma im Kleintiergebiss.* Fachpraxis. Nr. 2, S. 56, Fa. Albrecht. Aulendorf.

Rhodes, J. 1960. *Insertion of an amalgam filling into the lower canine tooth of a dog.* Vet. Rec. 72, S. 538ff.

Robin, Y. 1961. *Pose d'une couronne en or sur une incisive de chien.* Rec. Med. Vet. 112, S. 503ff.

Ross, D. L. and U. W. Myers. 1970. *Endodontic therapy for canine teeth in the dog.* J. Am. Vet. Med. Ass. 157, S. 1713ff.

Sauerwein, E. 1976. *Zahnerhaltungskunde.* Stuttgart: Thieme-Vlg.

Schebitz, H. u. H. Wilkens. 1977. *Atlas der Röntgenanatomie von Hund und Katze.* Verlag. Paul Parey, Berlin und Hamburg. 3. Auflage.

Scheffler, K. H. 1979. *Restitution des dens caninus beim Diensthund.* Monatshefte für Veterinärmedizin, 34, S. 504-507.

Scheffler, K. H. 1979. *Restitution des dens caninus beim Diensthund.* Monatshefte für Veterinärmedizin, 34, S. 504-507.

Schmidt, H. 1984. *Altersbedingte Veränderungen der Pulpenanatomie im Gebiss des Beagle-Hundes.* Diss. Med. dent., Hamburg.

Schmidt, H. u. P. Fahrenkrug. 1987. *Altersbedingte Pulpenveränderungen im Hundegebiss.* Der Praktische Tierarzt. 68, 5/87, S. 12ff.

Schroeder, H. 1982. *Orale Strukturbiologie.* 2. Auflage, Thieme-Verlag, Stuttgart.

Schulze, W. u. H. Conrad. 1965. *Zur konservierenden Zahnheilkunde in der Hundepraxis.* Berl. u. Münch. Tierärztl. Wschrift, 68, S. 338, ff, 369ff.

Schwenzer, Norbert. 1981. *Zahn-, Mund-, Kieferheilkunde.* Thieme Vlg., Stuttgart: Band 1.

Selhorst, F. 1964. *Orthodontische und kieferorthopädische. Behandlungen an Hunden.* Diss. München.

Shafer, W. G., M. K. Hine and B. M. Levy. 1983. *A Textbook of Oral Pathology.* 4th ed., Philadelphia: W. B. Saunders Co.

Shipp, A. D. 1991. "Crown Reduction —Disarming of Biting Pets." *J. Vet. Dent.,* Vol 8, No. 3, 4ff.

Spannbrucker, D. u. H. O. Schmidtke. 1977. *Anomalien der Backenzähne bei Zwergkaninchen und Meerschweinchen.* Kleintier-Praxis, 22, S. 331ff.

Stülpnagel, M. u. B. Becker. 1978. *Zur Technik des Beschleifens von Backenzähnen bei Nagern.* Kleintier-Praxis, 23, S. 395ff.

Stülpnagel, M. 1979. *Konservierende Zahnbehandlung bei kleinen Haustieren.* Collegium veterinarium. S. 74ff.

Theile, H. 1960. *Korrektur einer abnormen brachygnathia superior beim Boxer durch Unterkieferkürzung.* M. H. Vet. Med., 15, S. 864ff.

Tholen, M. A. 1983. *Concepts in Veterinary Dentistry.* Edwardsville, Kansas: Veterinary Medicine Publishing Co.

Triadan, H. 1972. *Tierzahnheilkunde: Zahnerhaltung (Füllungstherapie mit composite materials und Endodontie bei Affen und Raubtieren.* Schweiz.Archiv Tierheilkde., 114, S. 292ff.

Triadan, H. 1973. *Tierzahnheilkunde: Parodontologie bei Affen und Raubtieren.* Schweiz. Archiv Tierheilkde. 115, S. 401ff.

Triadan, H. 1987. *Verschiedene Füllungsmethoden für Hundezahndefekte*. Der Praktische Tierarzt. 68, 5/87, S 5ff.

Ueberberg, H. 1965. *Beobachtung einer sog. Anodontie bei einer Hauskatze*. Zbl. Vet. Med. A 12, S. 193ff.

Verstraete, F. J. 1989. *Zur Therapie der Mandibulafraktur beim Hund*. Der Praktische Tierarzt. 70, 1/89, S. 18ff.

Walton, R. E. and M. Torabinejad. 1989. *Principles and Practice of Endodontics*. Philadephia: W. B. Saunders Co.

Ward, H. L., M. Simring u. H. Spranger. 1976. *Parodontologisches Praktikum*. Hanser Verlag, München. Wien.

Weber, W. u. P. Fahrenkrug. 1987. *Oro-nasale Fisteln nach Caninusverlust im Oberkiefer des Hundes*. Der Praktische Tierarzt. 68, S. 83ff.

Wegner, W. 1975. *Kleine Kynologie*. Terra-Vlg. Konstanz.

Wegner, W. 1987. *Genetisch bedingte Zahnanomalien*. Der Praktische Tierarzt, 68, 5/87, S. 19ff.

Wissdorf, H. 1984. *Beitrag zur Zahnentwicklung und deren Störungen beim Hund*. Report, Nr. 18., Effem-Forschung, S. 9ff.

Zetner, K. 1974. *Tierzahnheilkunde: Kunststoffbrücke zur Fixierung einer Oberkieferfraktur beim Hund*. Kleintier-Praxis. 19, S. 166ff.

Zetner, K. u. J. Trcka, 1975. *Tierzahnheilkunde: die antibakterielle Wirksamkeit von Chlorhexidinimprägnierten Composites*. Wien-Tierärztl. Monatsschrift, 62, S. 383ff.

Zetner, K. 1976. *Die prothetische Versorgung von Zahnfrakturen mit Adhäsivkunststoffen*. Kleintier-Praxis. S. 271, 2ff.

Zetner, K. 1984. *Fortschritte in der Tierzahnheilkunde*. Report, Nr. 18, Feb. 84, Effem-Forschung, S. 9ff.

Zetner, K. u. A. Rabitsch. 1986. *Beitrag zur Technik der Schnabelprothetik bei Kleinvögeln. Kleintier-Praxis*. 31, S. 251ff.

Zetner, K. u. A. Gaspar. 1987. *Diagnostik und Therapie des Pemphiguskomplexes in der Mundhöhle*. Der Praktische Tierarzt, 68, 5/87, S. 66ff.

INDEX

A

B

C

D

E

F

G

H

I

J

K

L

M

N

O

P

Q

R

S

T

Dental abnormalities

Photo 1.

Chronically retained deciduous canine teeth. Gingival recession, periodontal disease and heavy calculus deposits. Note the typical position of retained deciduous canine teeth. Maxillary — caudal to permanent. Mandibular — lateral to permanent.

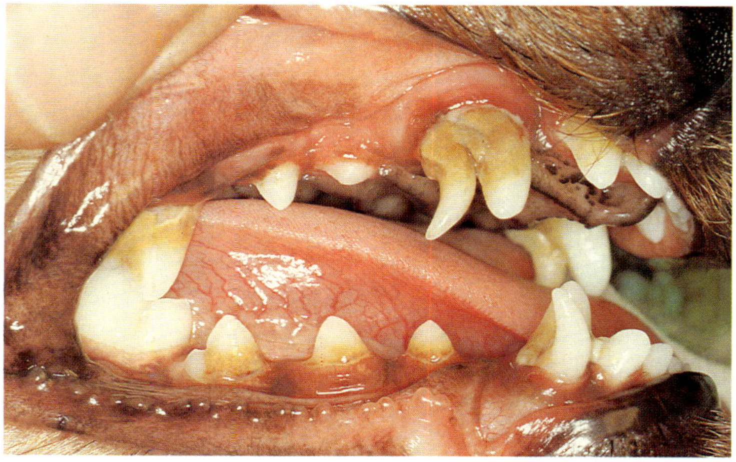

Photo 2.

Gingival flap and osteotomy over root of retained deciduous canine tooth. Double–ended curved Fahrenkrug elevator facilitates removal of long deciduous root.

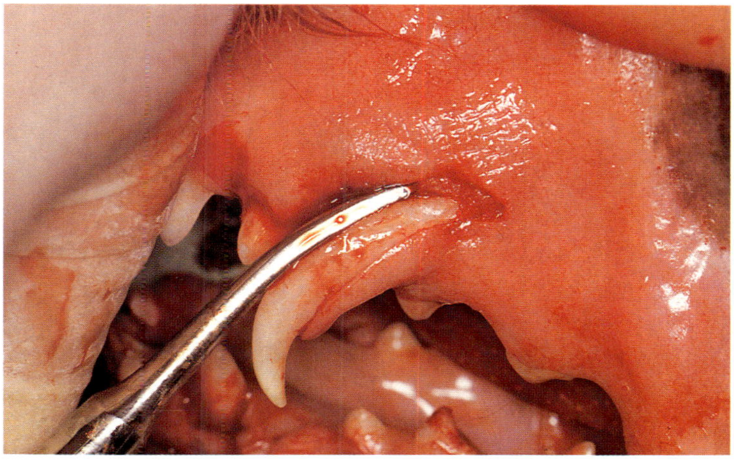

Photo 3.

"Distemper mouth." Severe enamel hypoplasia due to virus infection when young. The porous exposed dentin is stained by food debis, pigments and plaque. Severe prognathism and crowding is also evident.

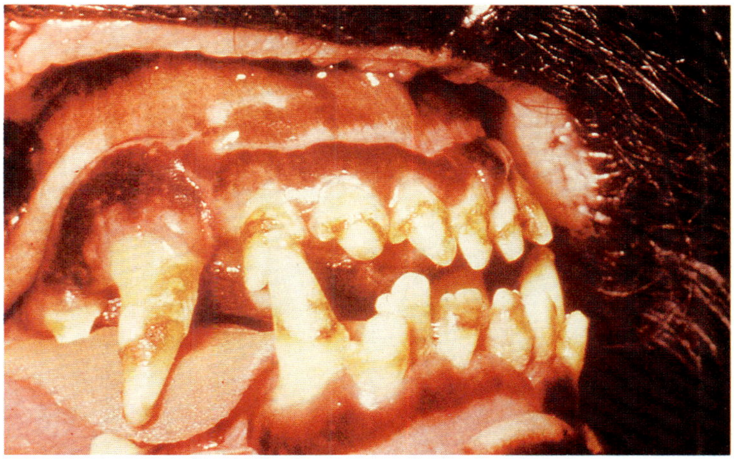

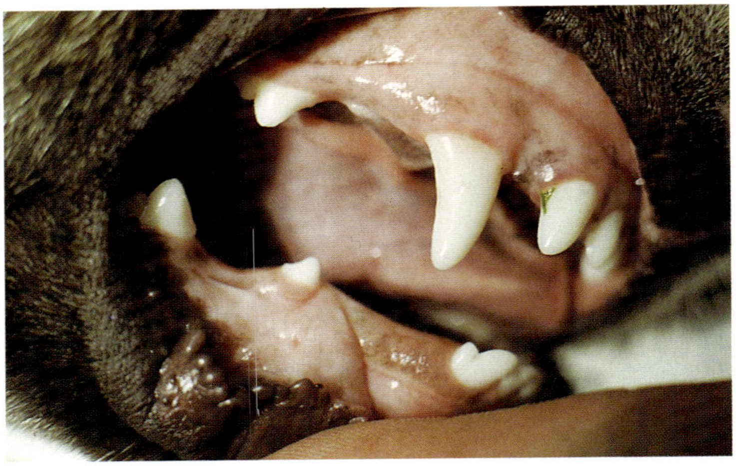

Photo 4.

Mandibular canine tooth not visible. Tooth may be totally absent or impacted (see below).

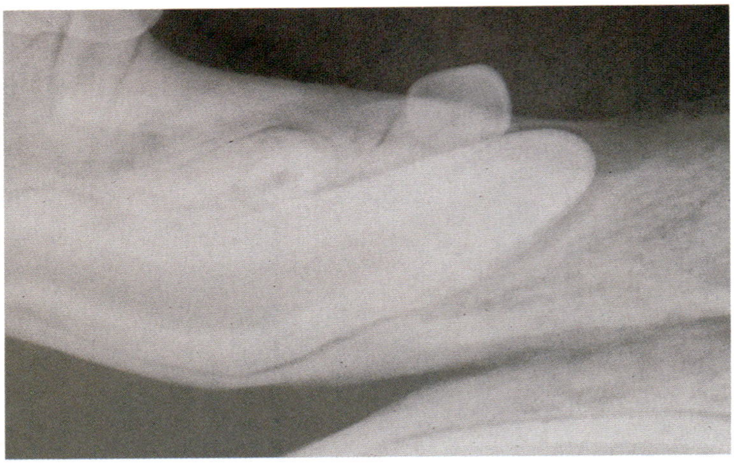

Photo 5.

Radiograph of photo above shows fully developed impacted mandibular canine tooth.

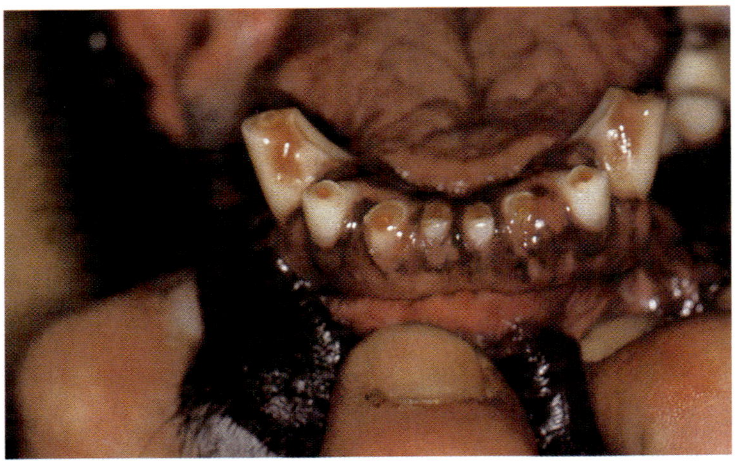

Photo 6.

Severe attrition of anterior teeth, caused by chronic chewing on hard objects. Brown staining of exposed dentin. Rings in center of teeth show stained reparative dentin over the exposed pulp.

Photo 7.

Sectioning of maxillary 1st molar tooth with carbide bur through the furcation area. All three segments of the tooth are then extracted separately.

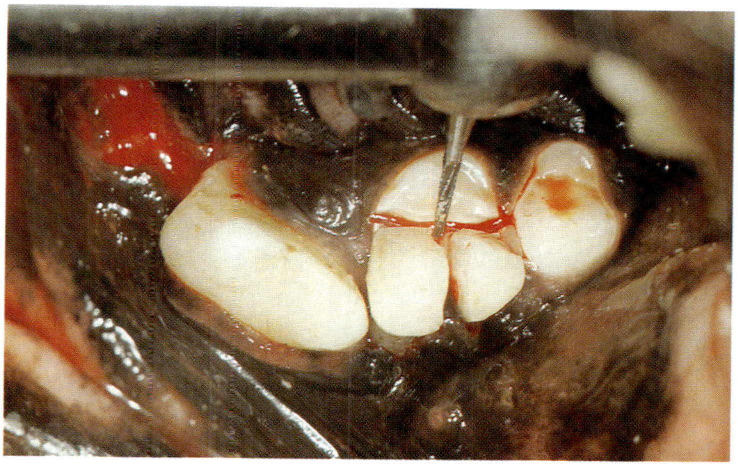

Photo 8.

Correct method of elevating a tooth, using the contacting tooth (or segment) as a fulcrum.

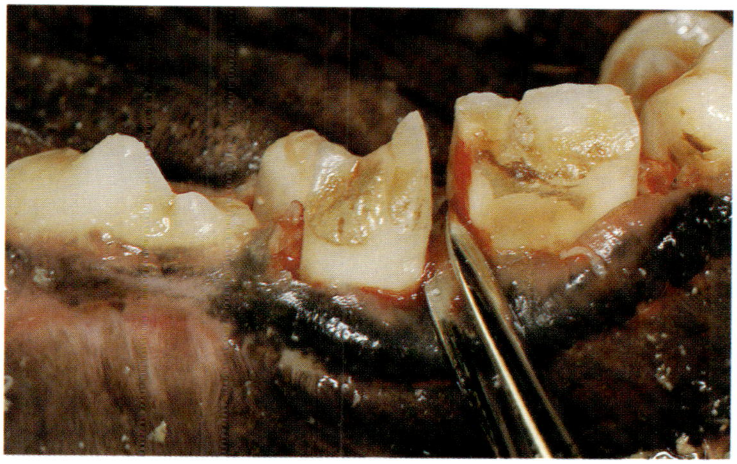

Photo 9.

Hemisection of maxillary fourth premolar in a cat. Drilling some of the tooth structure (odontoplasty) and alveolar bone (alveoloplasty) assists in removing the tooth.

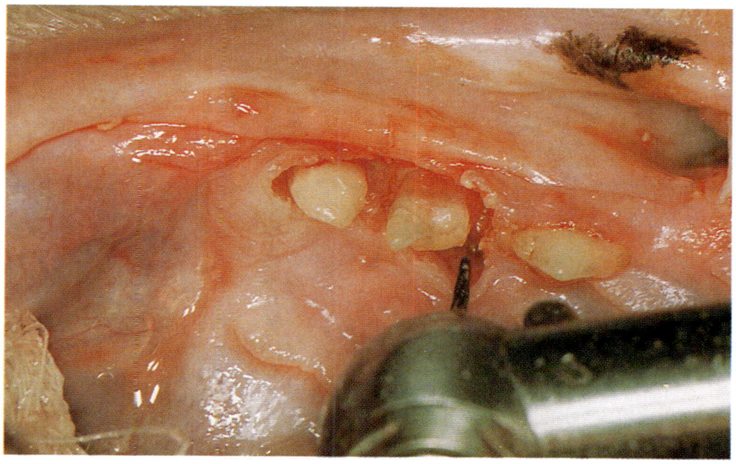

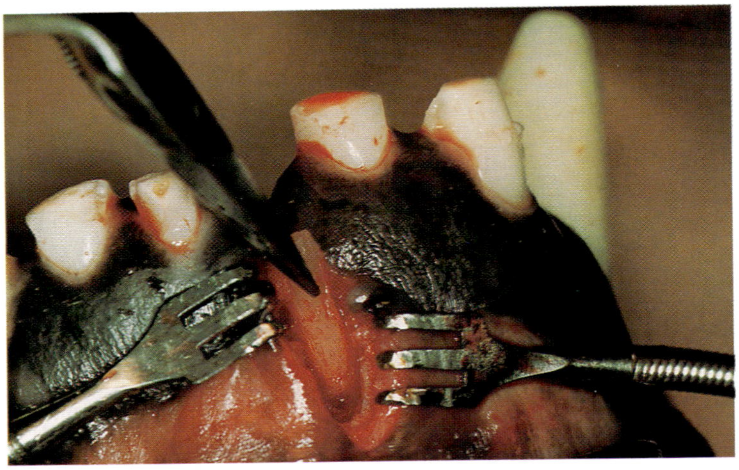

Photo 10.

Gingival flap and extraction of broken root of central incisor, with Stieglitz root and fragment extraction forceps.

ORONASAL FISTULA

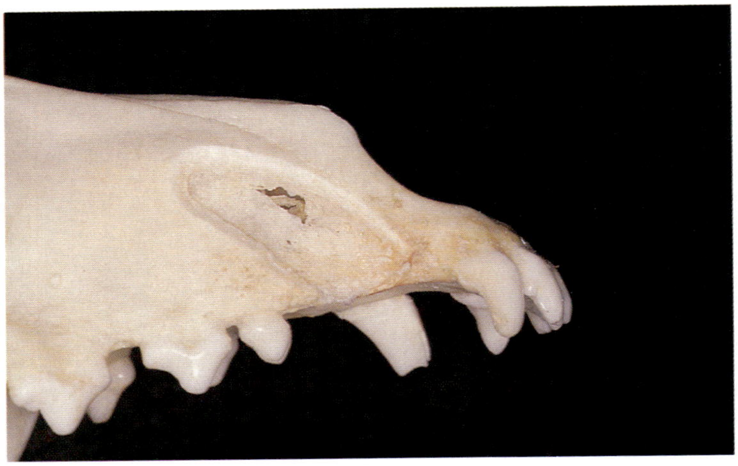

Photo 11.

Alveolar wall medial to the maxillary canine tooth is very thin and easily damaged during luxation and extraction of a canine tooth.

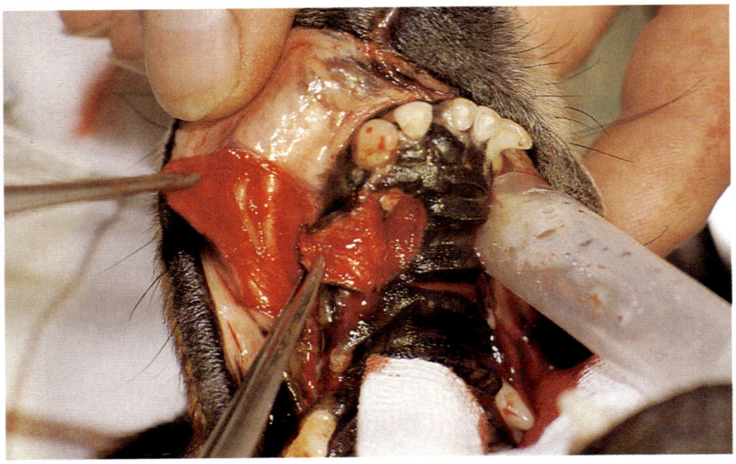

Photo 12.

Double flap technique to close oronasal fistula. Palatal flap prepared to cover defect. Second mucosal flap raised to cover palatal flap and donor site.

Photo 13.

End result of chronic periodontal disease due to gun shot injury. Severe calculus build–up has been removed.

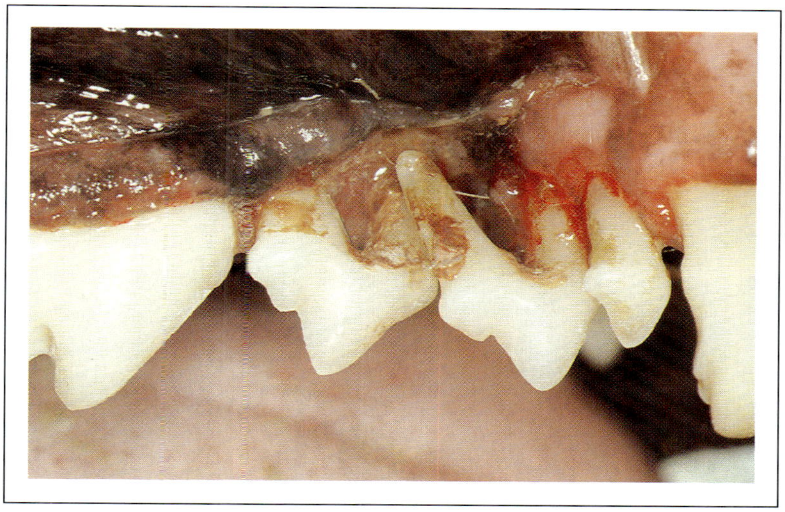

Photo 14.

Removal of first three maxillary premolars revealed combined *oroantral* and *oronasal* fistula. Mucogingival flap raised to cover defect, after removal of necrotic material and food debris from cavity.

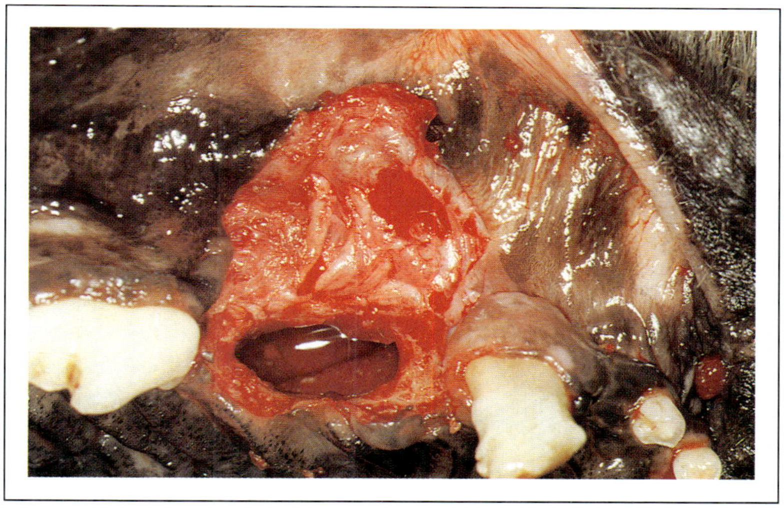

Photo 15

Surgical site after closure. Note deformed maxillary canine tooth.

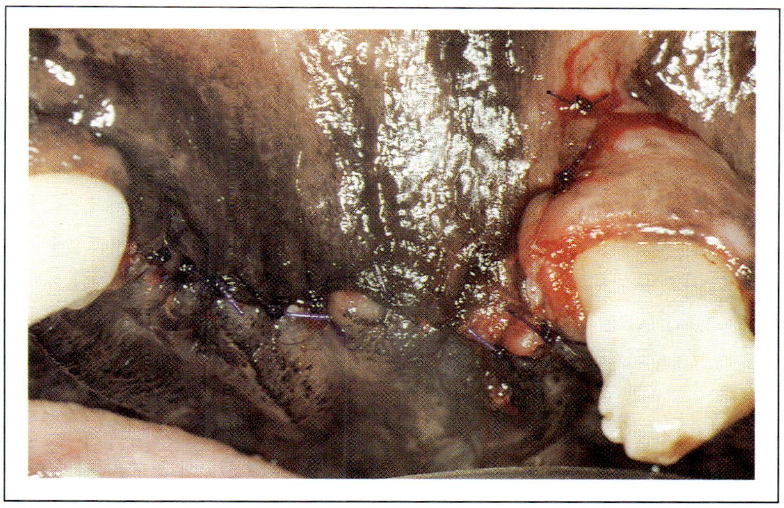

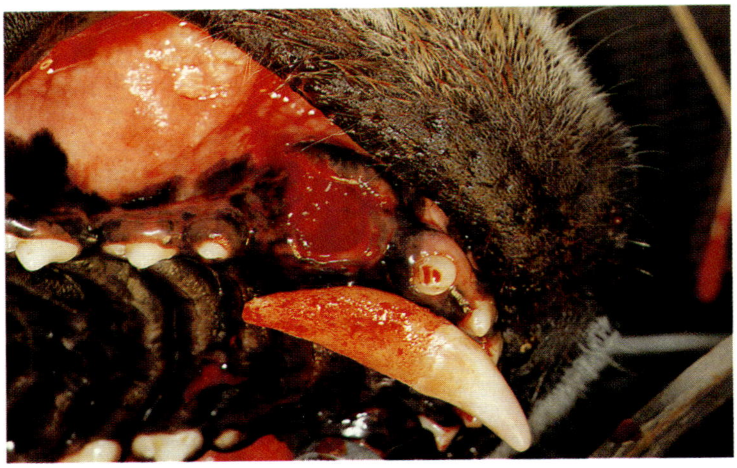

Photo 16.

Completely avulsed right maxillary canine tooth.

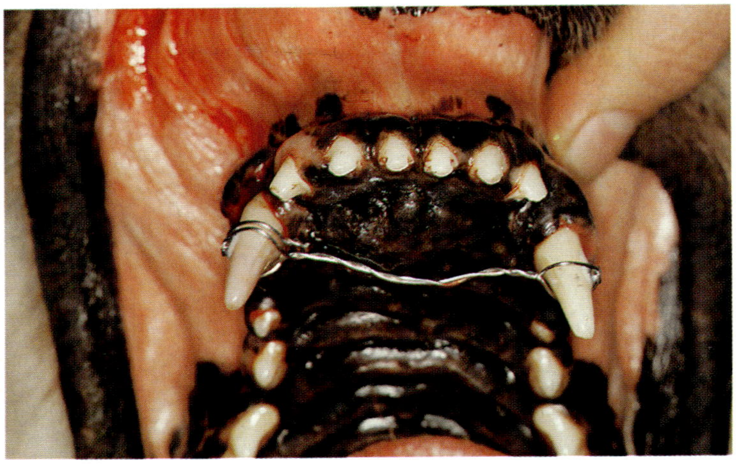

Photo 17.

Slotted brackets bonded on to buccal surface of canine teeth, prevent wire from slipping off. The wire is twisted across the palate, stabilizing the avulsed tooth and reinforcing the acrylic splint.

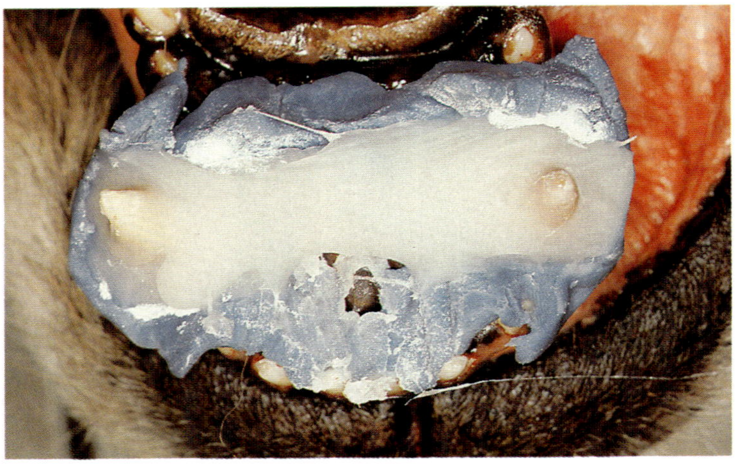

Photo 18.

Trough of Playdough for forming the acrylic splint.

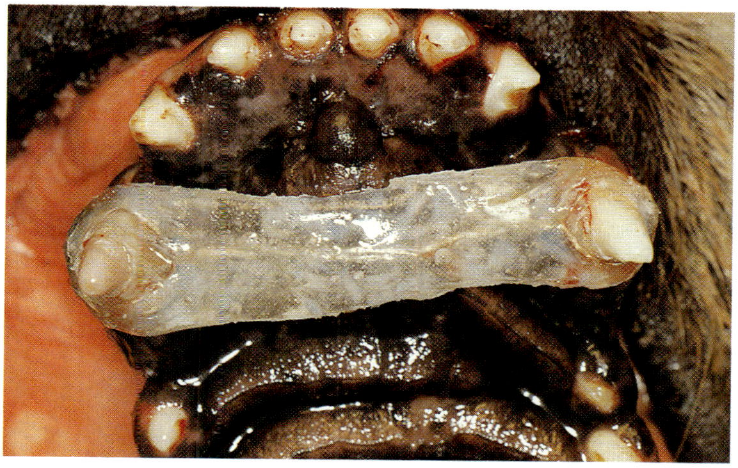

Photo 19.

Acrylic splint incorporating wire, after removal of Playdough and shaping with acrylic trimming bur.

Periodontology

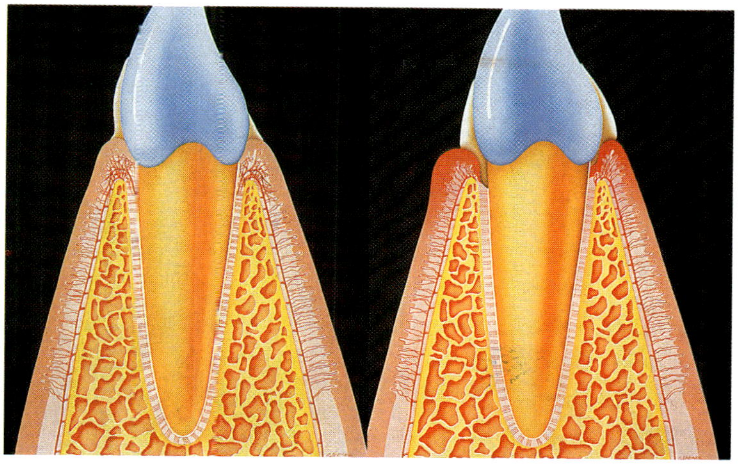

Photo 20.

Left. Calculus deposits on crown of tooth. Gingiva appears normal, with a pinkish color.

Right**.** Calculus deposits on crown and in periodontal pocket. Early stage of periodontal disease. Gingiva inflamed and swollen creating pseudo–pockets (both stages reversible). (Courtesy Blend–a–med–Forschung, Mainz, Germany.)

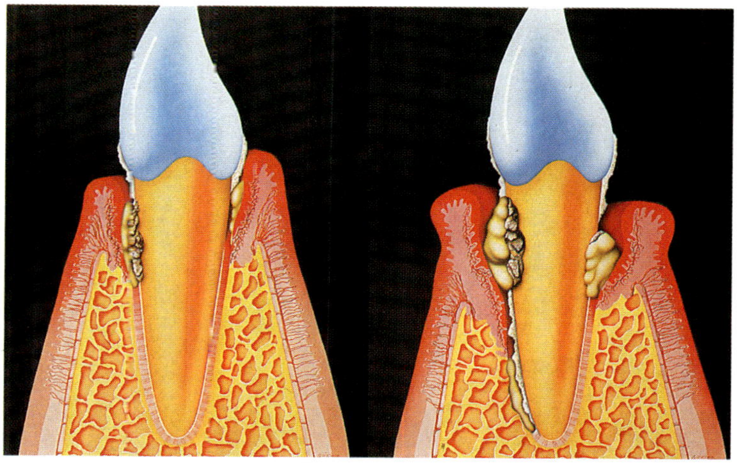

Photo 21.

Left. Moderate subgingival calculus (concretion), deep pockets, loss of epithelial attachment. Horizontal alveolar bone loss. Severe gingivitis. Advanced periodontal disease.

Right**.** Heavy concretion deposits. Deep pockets. Severe horizontal and vertical bone loss. Chronic periodontal disease. (Both stages irreversible). (Courtesy Blend–a–med–Forschung, Mainz, Germany.)

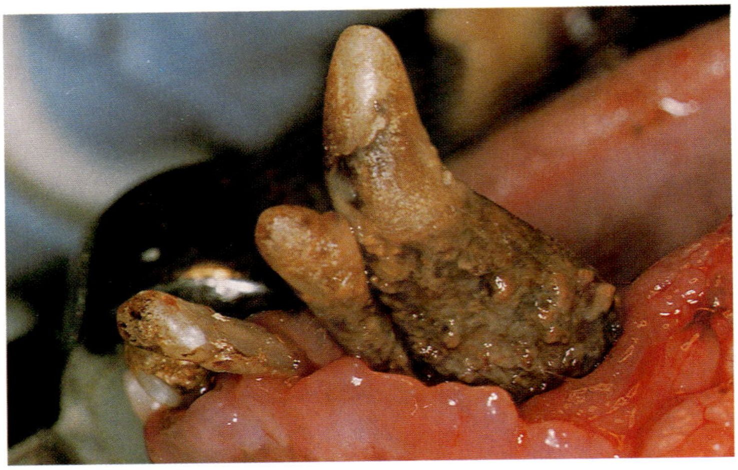

Photo 22.

End stage of severe chronic periodontal disease. Gingiva bleeding, inflamed, hyperplastic and regressed. Teeth are extremely mobile due to bone loss. Chronic infection of gingiva and bone. Extraction necessary at this stage.

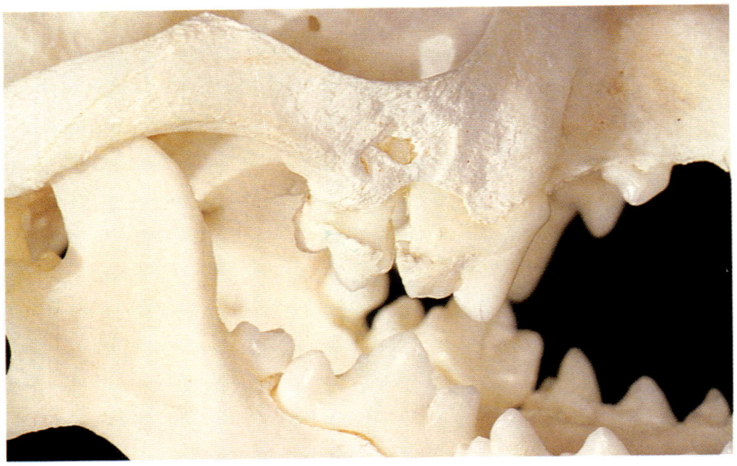

Photo 23.

Horizontal and vertical bone loss, with a fistula over the first molar mesio–buccal root apex. End result of chronic periodontal disease.

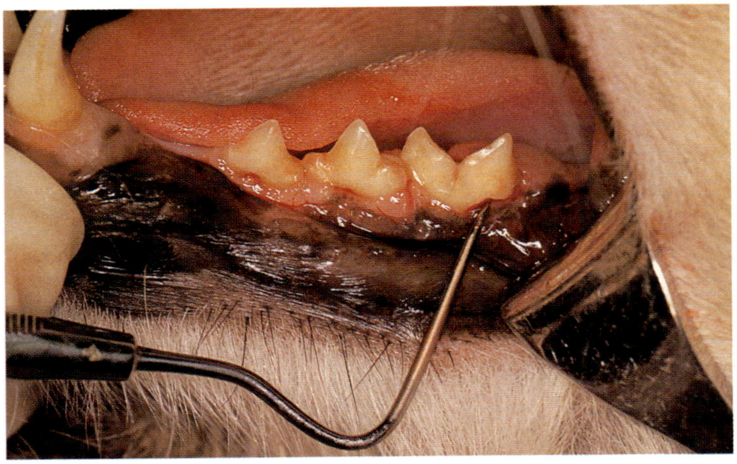

Photo 24.

"Neck" lesion of distal root of mandibular first molar in a cat. Probing is necessary to detect extent of lesion.

Photo 25.

Severe generalized LPGS showing very red glossy hyperplastic bleeding gingiva. (Courtesy Dr. Ken Lyon.)

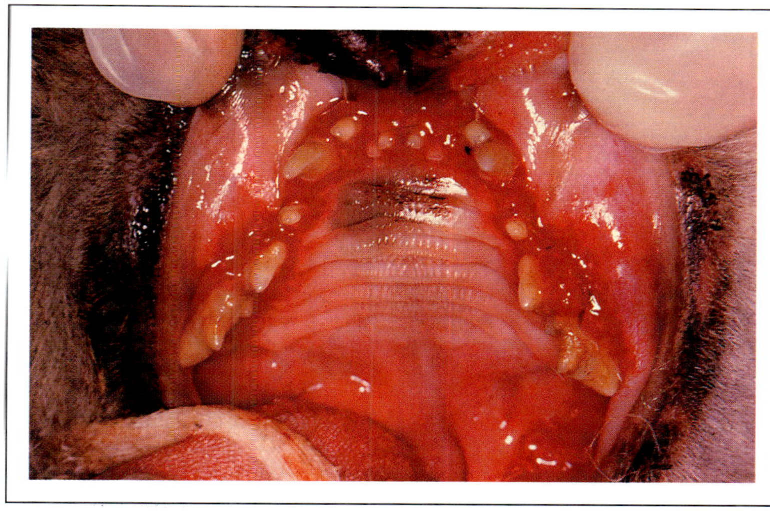

Photo 26.

Full mouth extraction of above case results in almost complete healing of gingiva, two months post–operatively. (Courtesy Dr. Ken Lyon.)

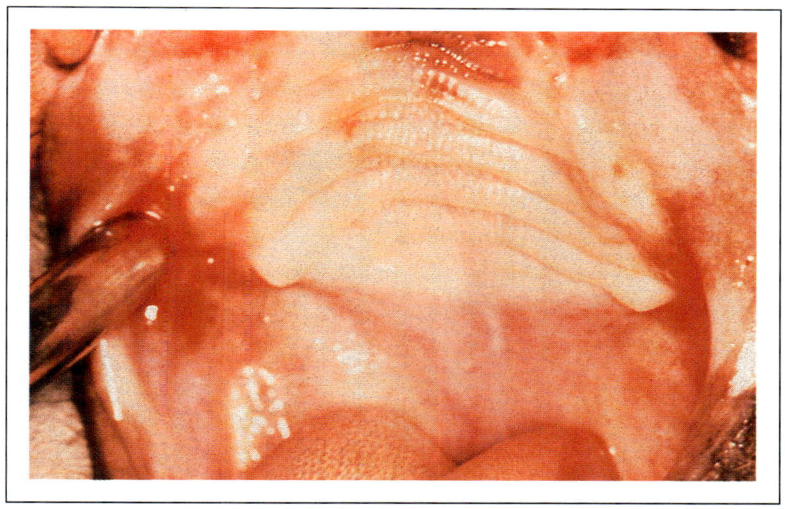

Photo 27.

Alveoloplasty and osteoplasty of exposed mandibular bone following extraction of caudal teeth. All sharp edges, irregular protuberances and infected bone are removed with a round bur.

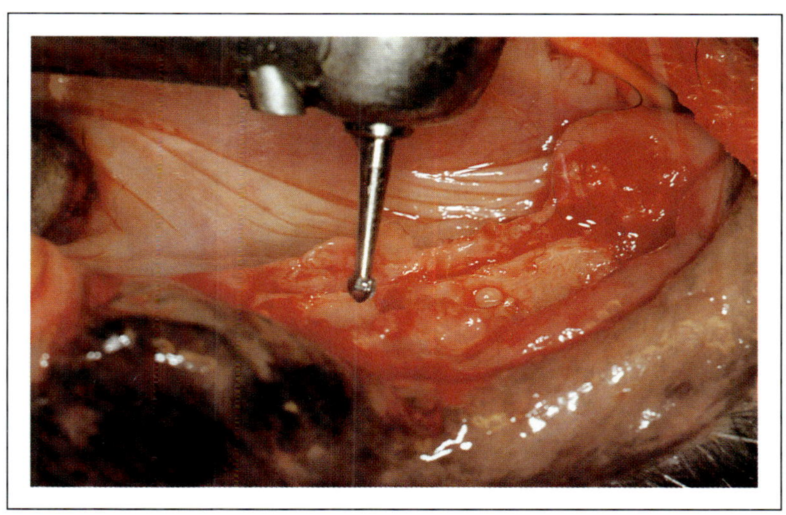

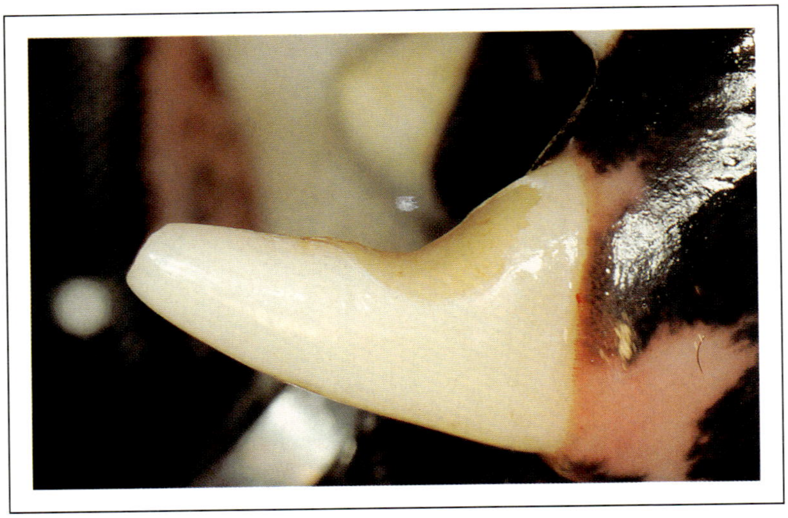

Photo 34.

"Cage–biter" syndrome. Enamel and dentin attrition on distal surface of canine tooth. Exposure of dentin will encourage further wear and weaken the tooth.

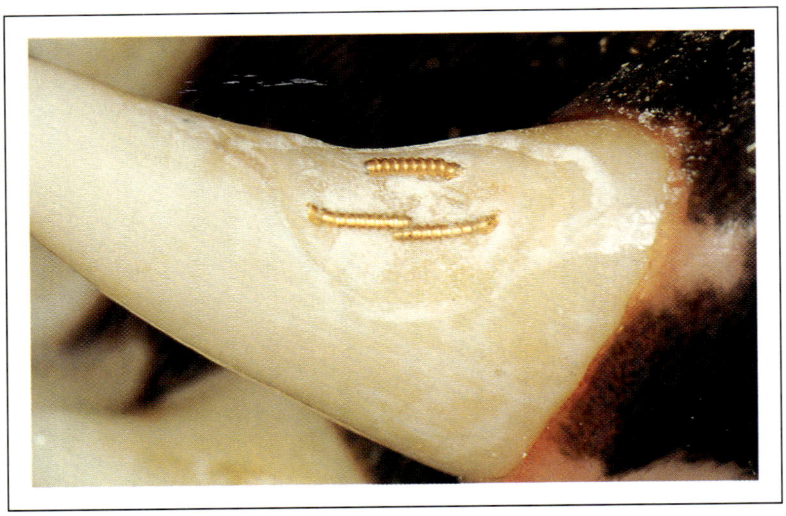

Photo 35.

Parapulpal pins in dentin for additional retention of restorative material.

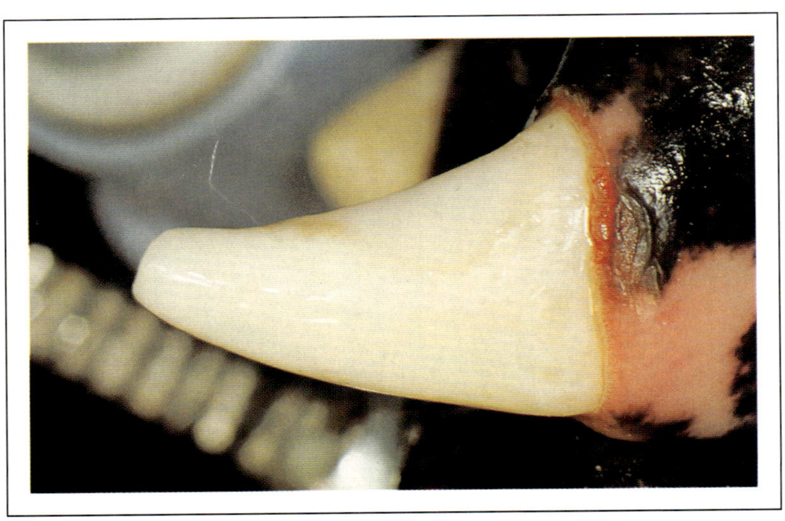

Photo 36.

Completed composite restoration incorporating the parapulpal pins.

Photo 37.

Parapulpal pins in dentin of fractured canine tooth, to aid in retention of restoration material. Base material has been placed in pulp chamber following endodontic treatment. Note position of pins for maximum retention of restorative material. Position also avoids penetration of pulp chamber and damage to enamel

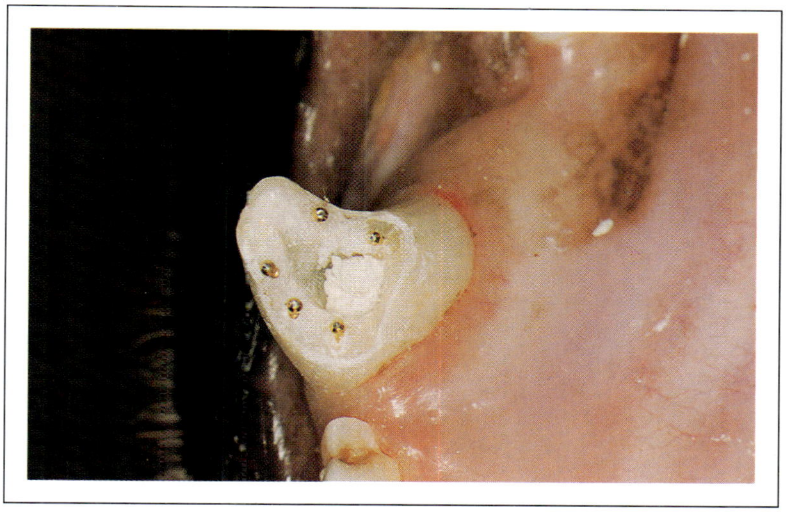

Photo 38.

Parapulpal pins in dentin of fractured maxillary fourth premolar. Drilling hole for placement of pin. Special drill presets depth. Pins bent to achieve maximum retentive and anatomical position.

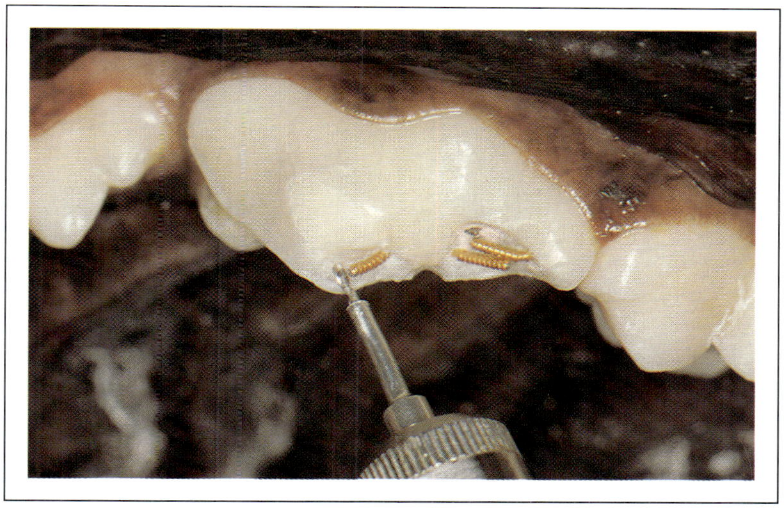

Photo 39.

Electro–micrograph of acid–etched enamel surface. Note: left side unetched, right side etched. Etching opens up enamel surface for mechanical retention of composite. (Courtesy ESPE GmbH, Germany.)

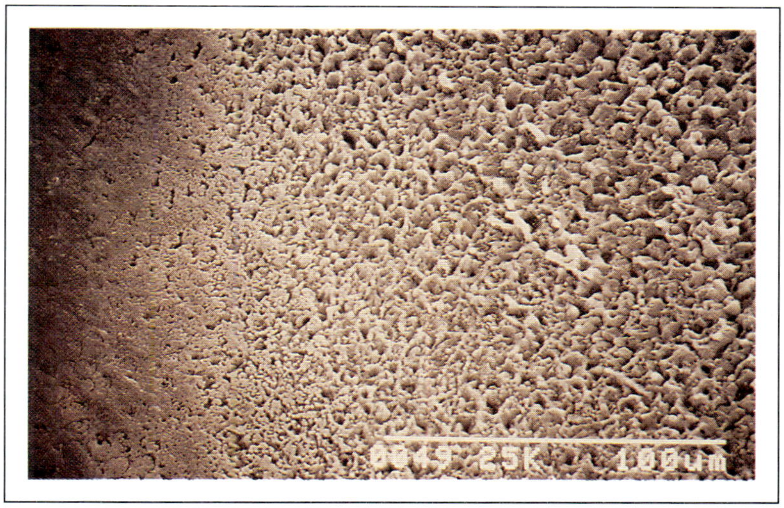

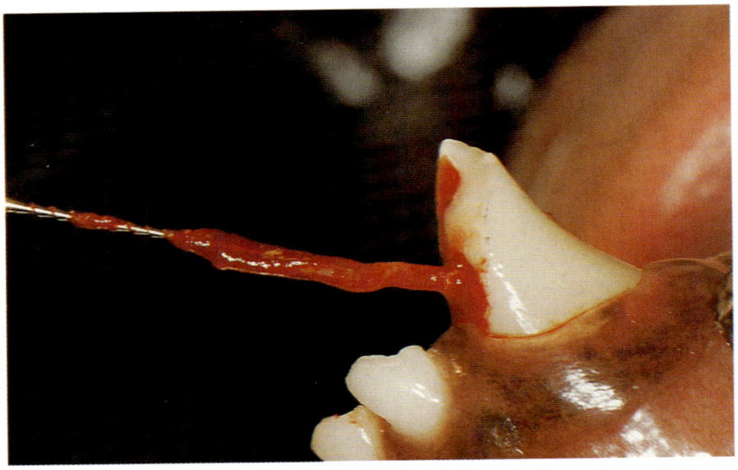

Photo 40.

Removal of intact pulp contents through coronal access hole of fractured mandibular canine tooth.

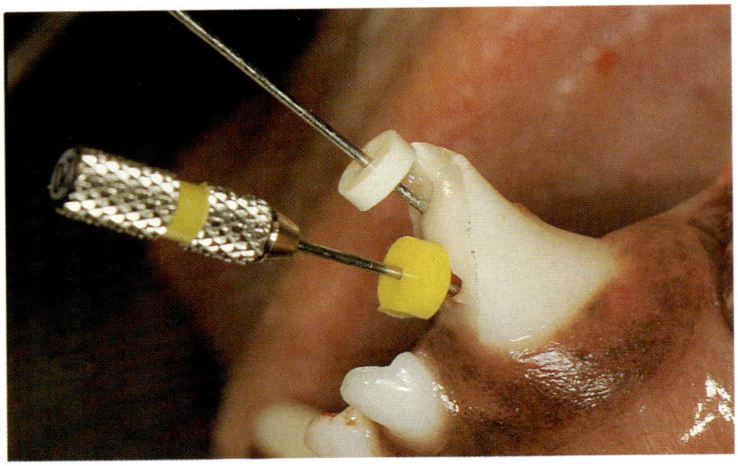

Photo 41.

Instrumentation of pulp cavity. Coronal access hole (white stop). Accessory access hole (yellow stop).

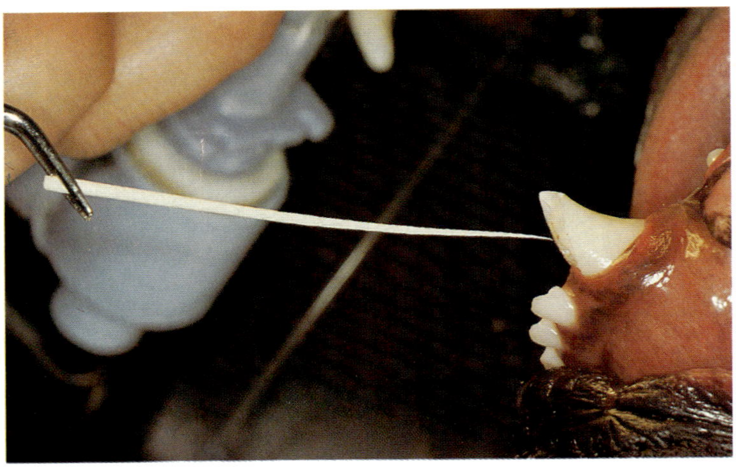

Photo 42.

Drying pulp cavity with 55 mm absorbent paper point following irrigation.

Photo 43.

Lentulo spiral filler introducing sealing cement (AH–26) from a spatula into the pulp cavity.

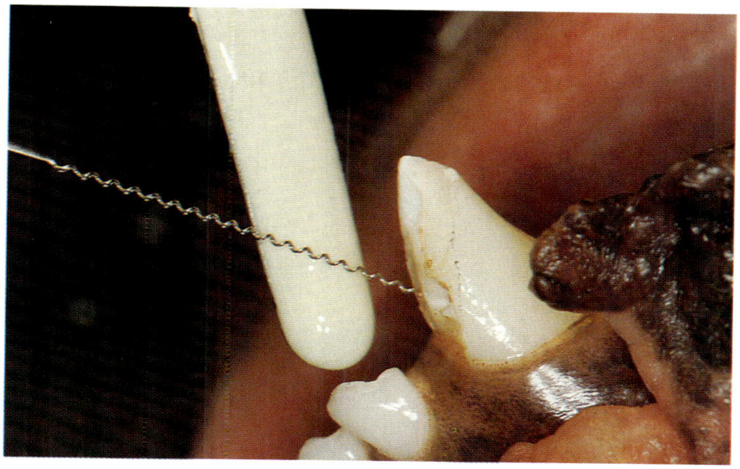

Photo 44.

Obturation of pulp cavity with gutta–percha points and sealer/filler.

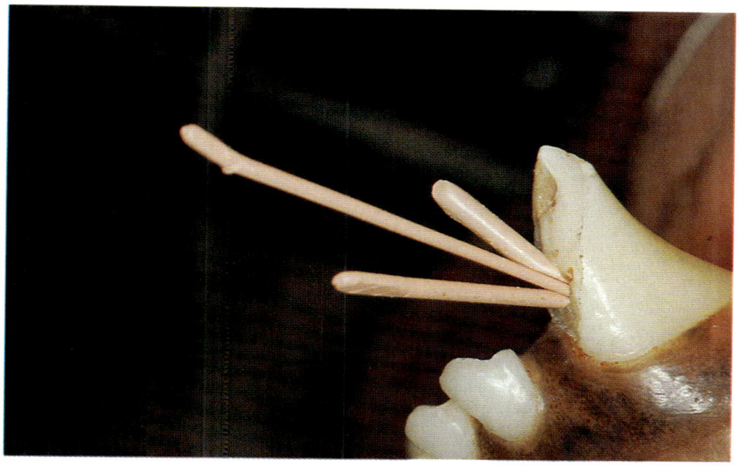

Photo 45.

Restoration finished with light–cured composite.

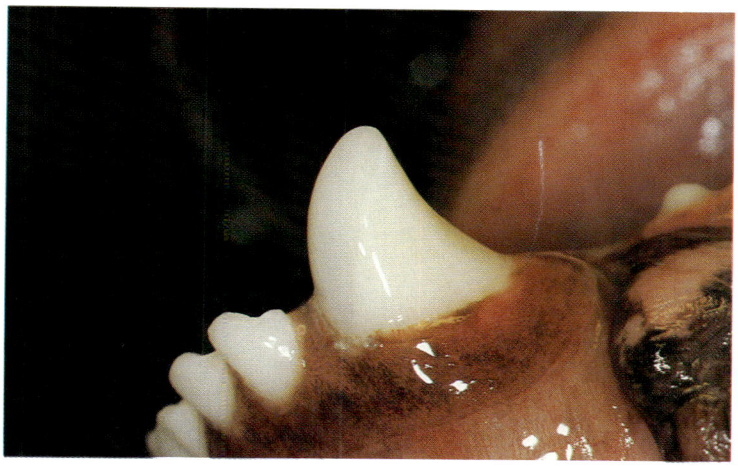

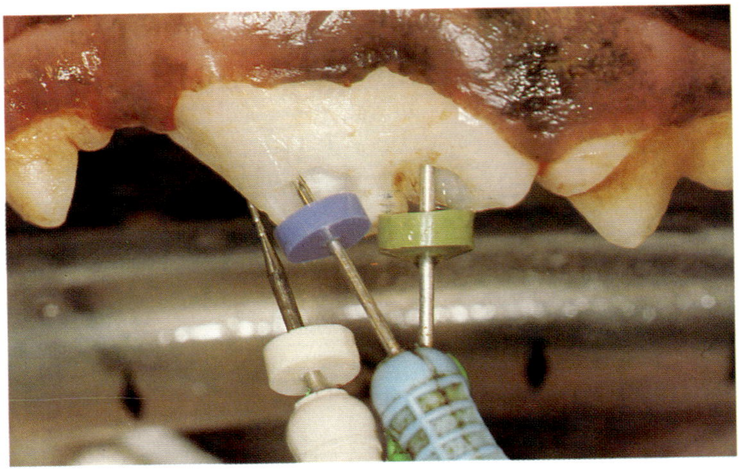

Photo 46.

Triple root canal of maxillary fourth premolar. Note Hedstrom files in *three* separate access holes.

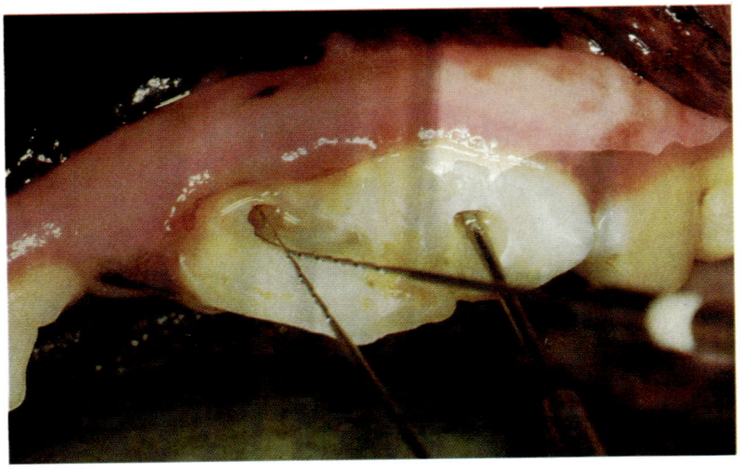

Photo 47.

Triple root canal of maxillary fourth premolar. Note Hedstrom files in *two* access holes. Transcoronal approach of mesio–palatal root.

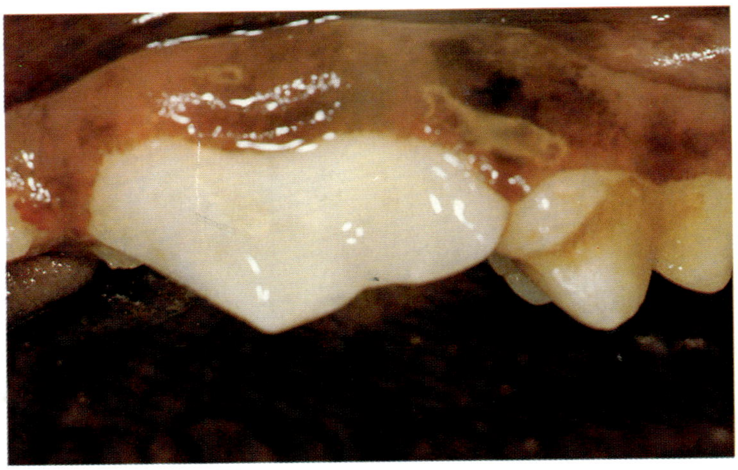

Photo 48.

Crown restored with light–cured composite following triple root canal procedure.

Photo 49.

Triple root canal of maxillary fourth premolar in a cat.

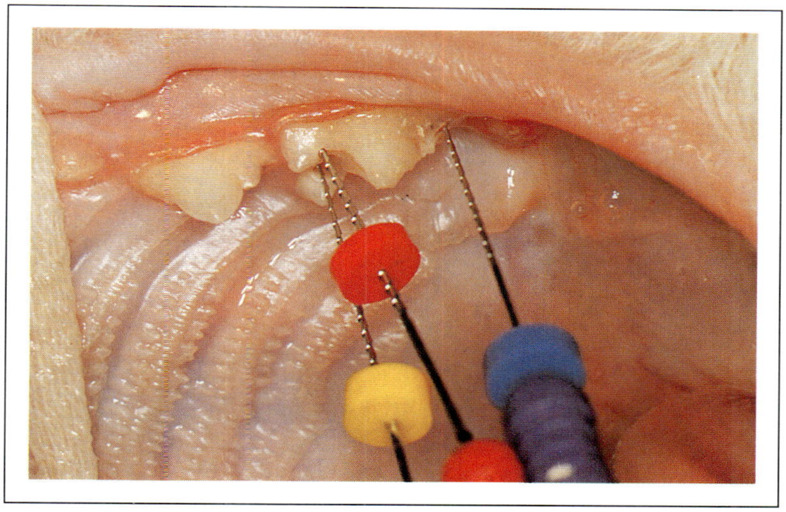

Photo 50.

Lateral slab fracture of maxillary fourth premolar of a dog. Bleeding from exposed pulp. Note loose buccal fragment retained by gingival attachment.

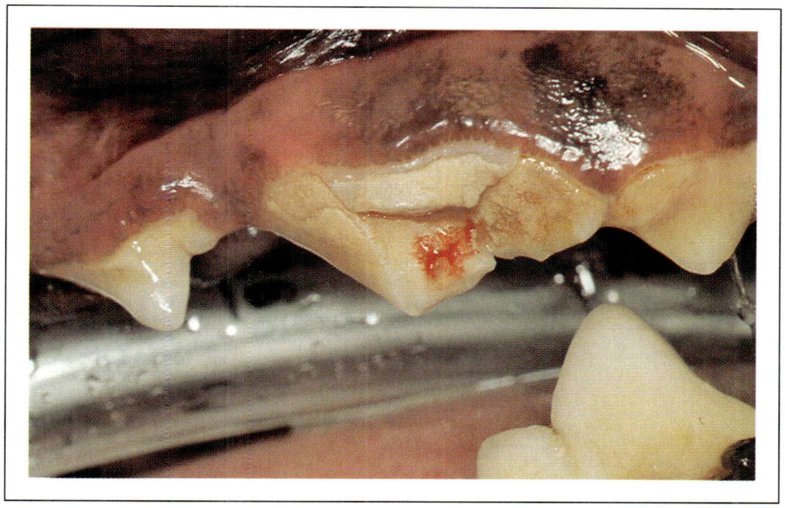

Photo 51.

Abscess below left eye. Result of fistula in infraorbital region due to abscessed maxillary fourth premolar

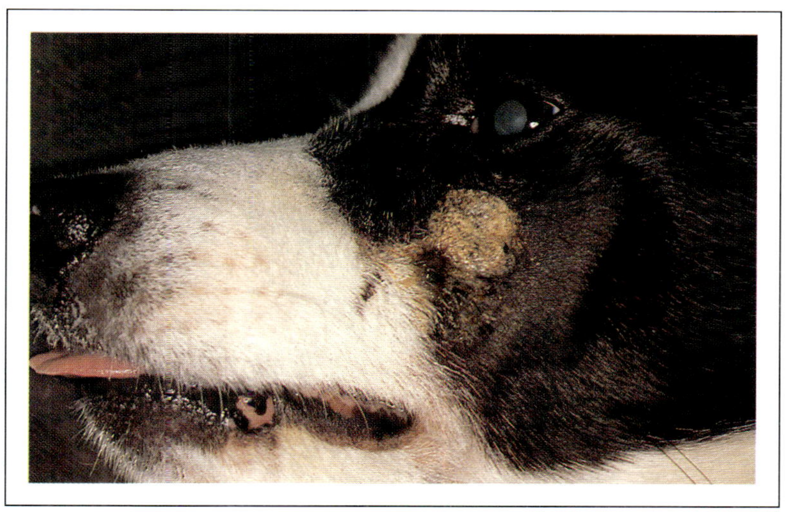

CROWN REDUCTION

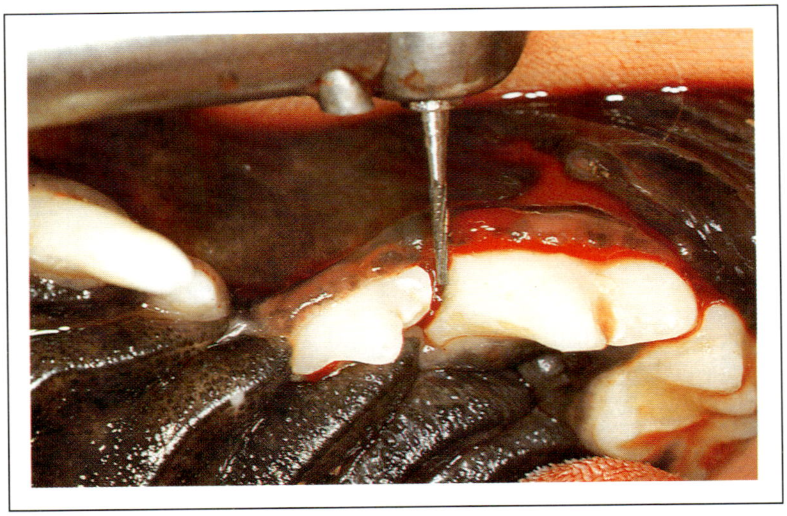

Photo 58.

Odontoplasty of contacting surfaces of teeth. The procedure aids in preventing food and debris impacting in this area.

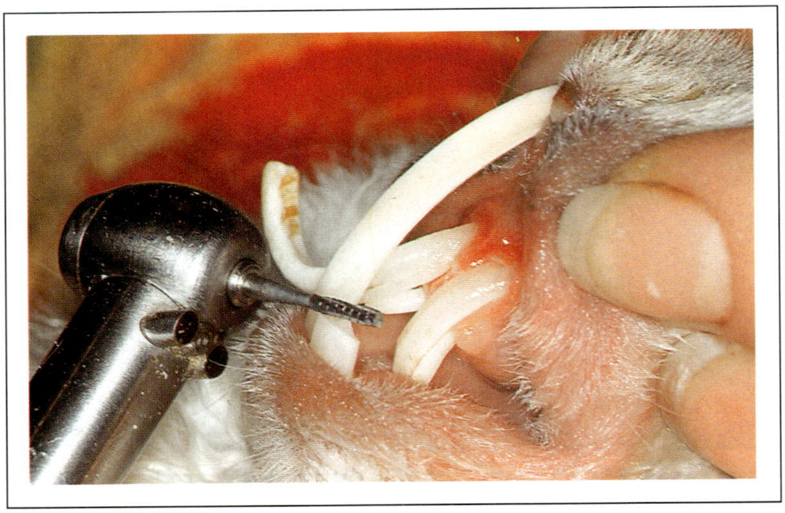

Photo 59.

Crown reduction of overgrown rabbit incisors. Note the direction in which the teeth overgrow. "Peg–teeth" visible just caudal to maxillary incisors.

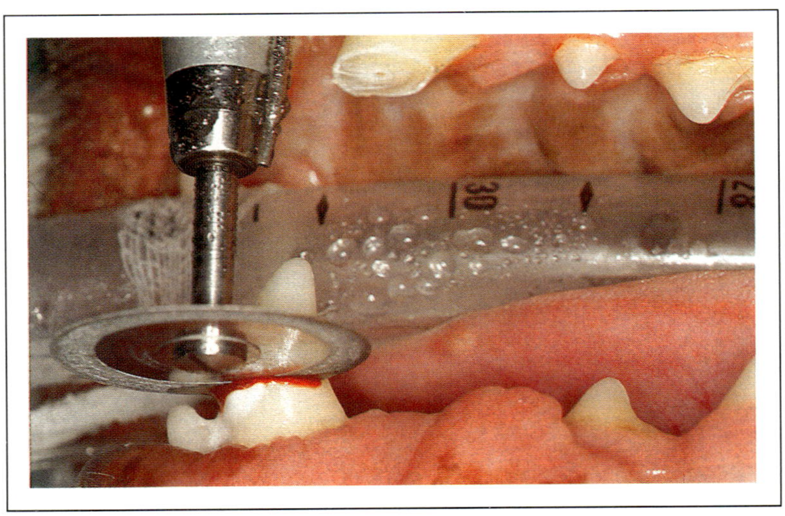

Photo 60.

Crown reduction of canine tooth for disarming a dog. Diamond disc in a low–speed handpiece.

Photo 61.

Inverted cone bur preparing cavity. Amputated vital pulp has been partially removed and capped.

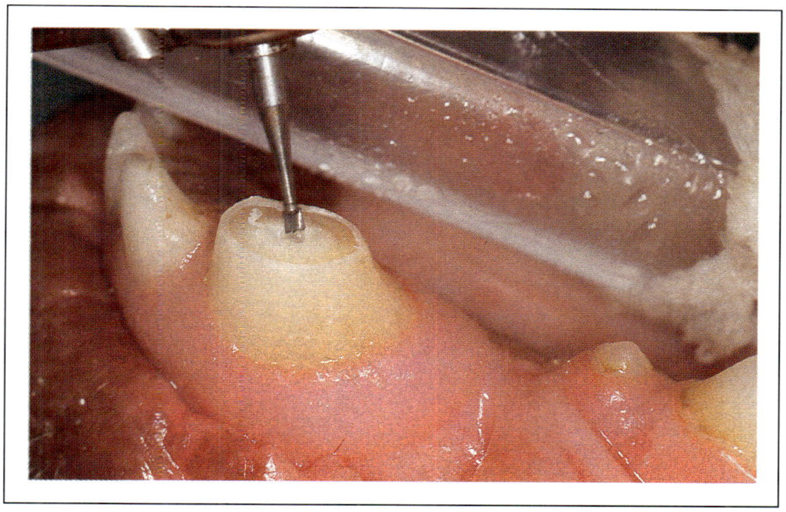

Photo 62.

Chamfering edge of reduced crown with fissure bur.

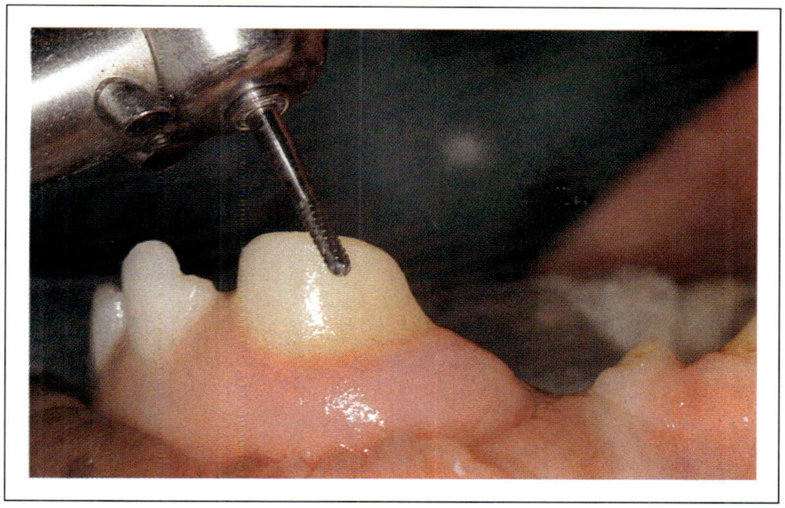

Photo 63.

Finished result of crown reduction of all four canine teeth. Composite restoration material covering surface of reduced crowns.

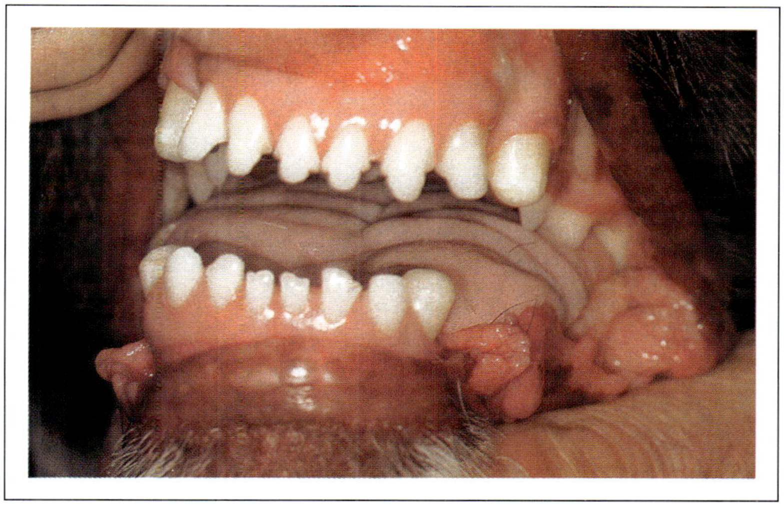

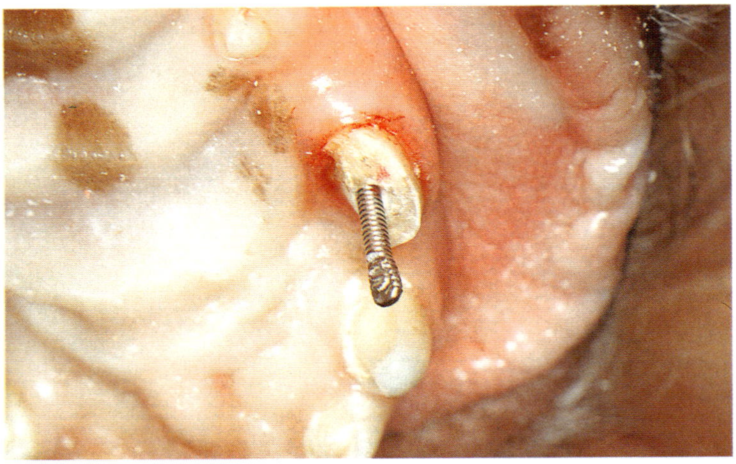

Photo 64.

Pulpal post in fractured canine tooth, following endodontic therapy.

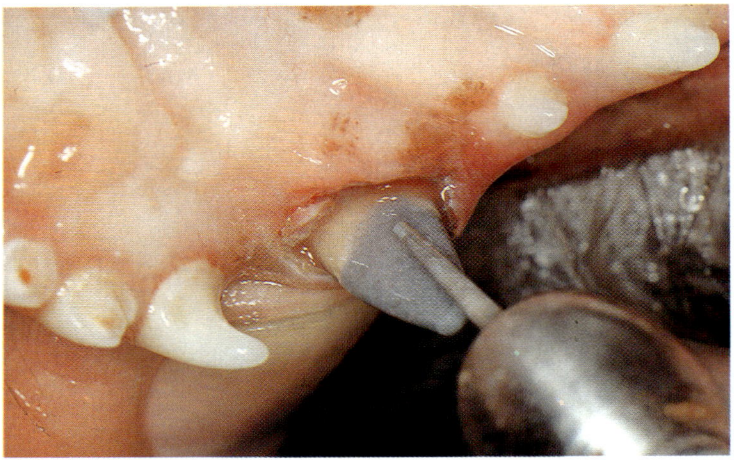

Photo 65.

Core build–up over pulpal post, using titanium composite (Ti–Core). Contouring with bur.

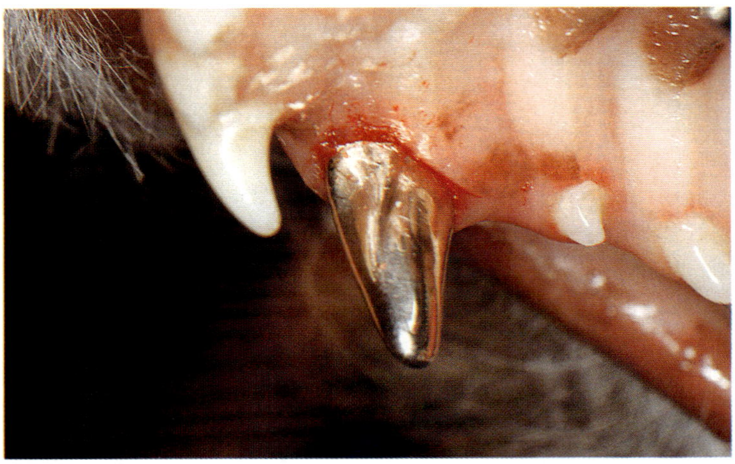

Photo 66.

Titanium alloy crown cemented in place. Crown has been anodized to look similar to gold.

Photo 67.

Stainless steel crown cemented on maxillary fourth premolar following slab fracture, endodontic treatment and crown preparation.

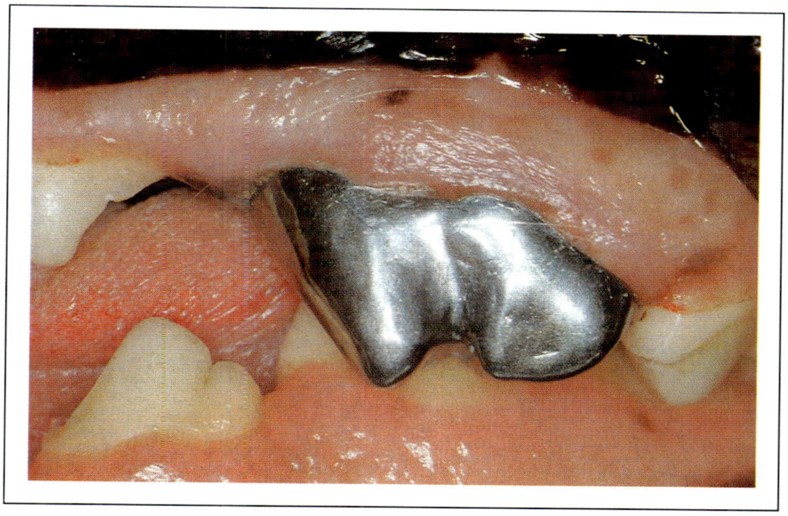

Photo 68.

Porcelain fused to metal crown on lateral maxillary incisor. Overgrown gingival margin has been contoured by electrosurgery.

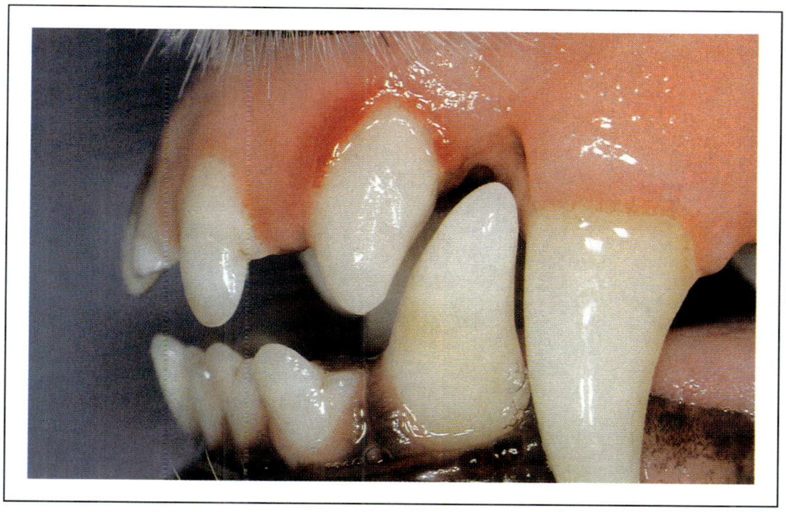

Photo 69.

Gold alloy crown cemented on maxillary canine tooth of a cat. Mirror image shows palatal surface and margin.

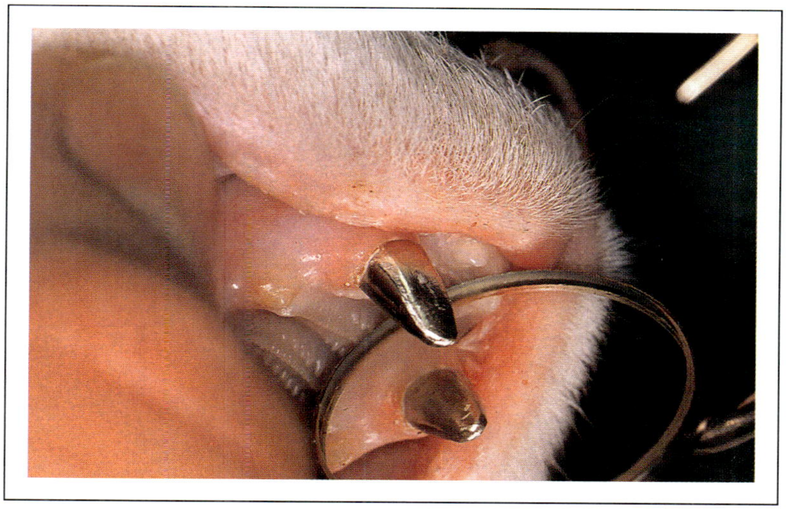

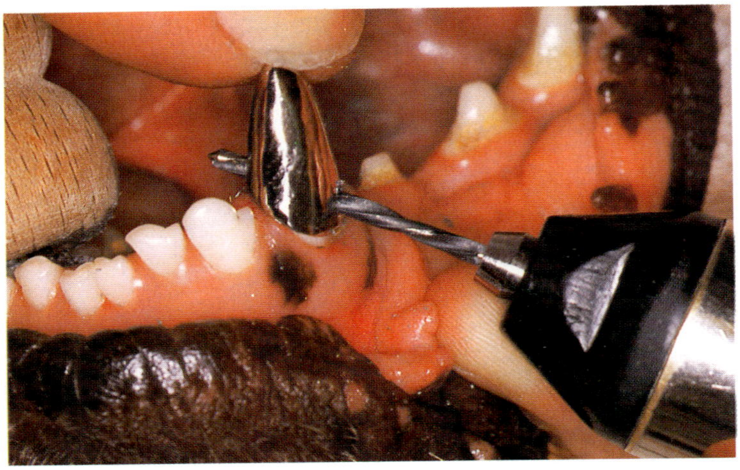

Photo 70.

Cross–pin crown technique (Fahrenkrug). Drilling hole through crown and "stump."

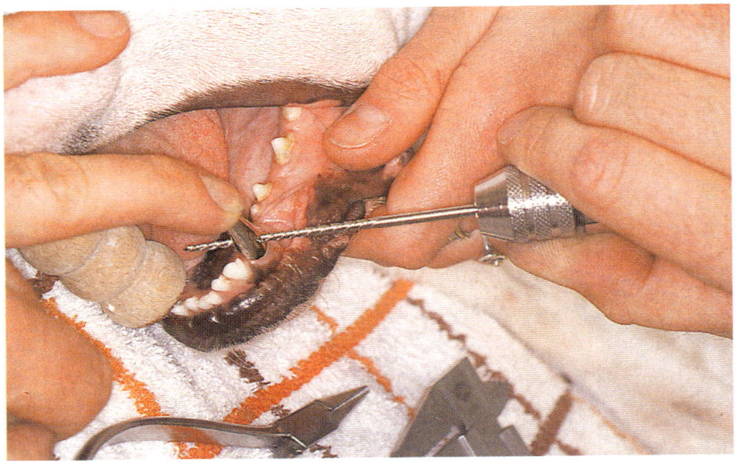

Photo 71.

Reaming of hole with conical shaped reamer.

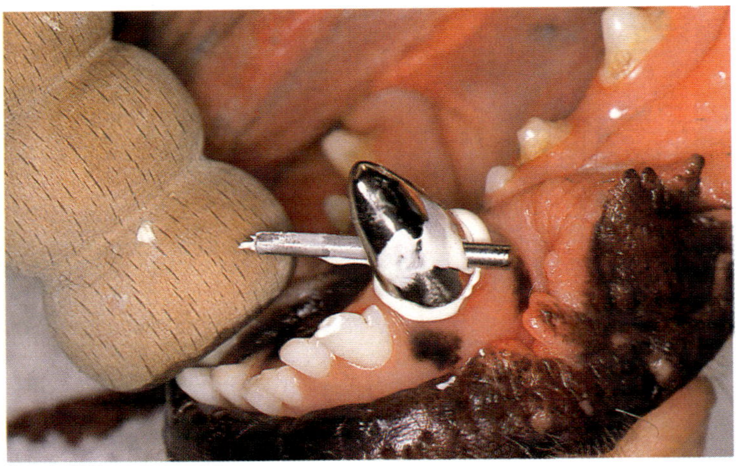

Photo 72.

Pin cemented in place through crown and tooth structure. After cement has set, protruding ends of pin are cut off, smoothed and polished.

Photo 73.

Finished result of cross–pin technique. Ends of pins cut flush to crown surface, smoothed and polished.

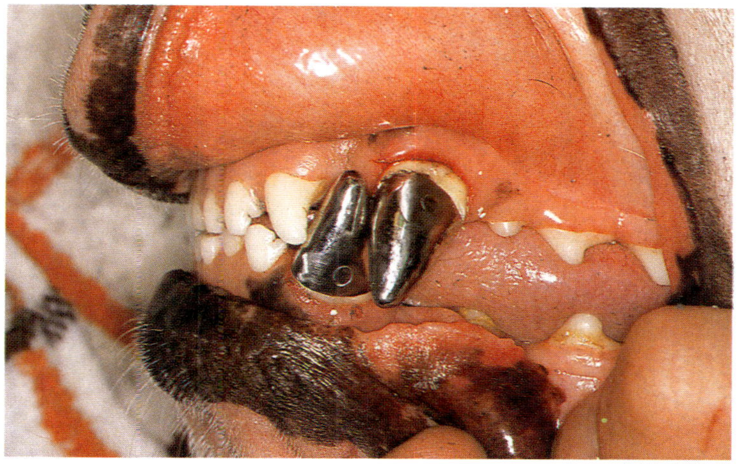

Photo 74.

Left. Cast crown and post unit showing integration of post and crown.
Right. Unit cemented in place. The crown is shorter than original tooth to reduce leverage forces.

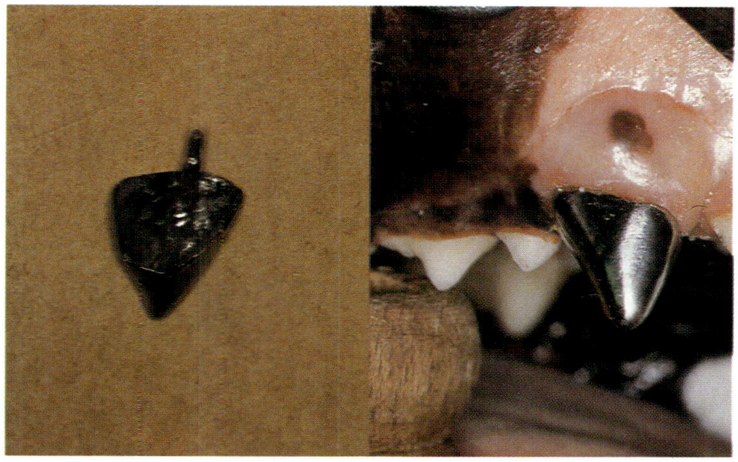

Photo 75.

Cast metal half–crown cemented on tip of canine tooth. Crown covers exposed dentin of fractured tip.

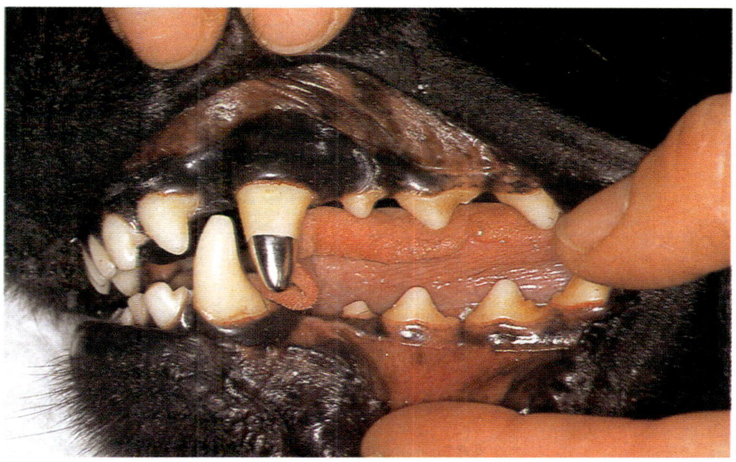

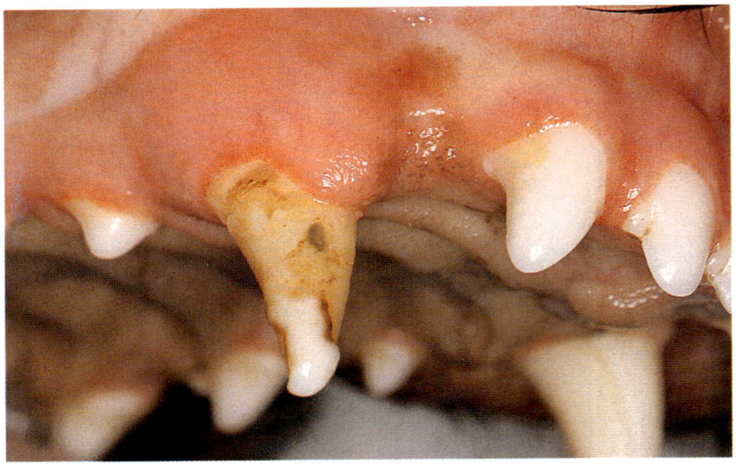

Photo 76.

Enamel hypoplasia of maxillary canine tooth. Pulp not exposed.

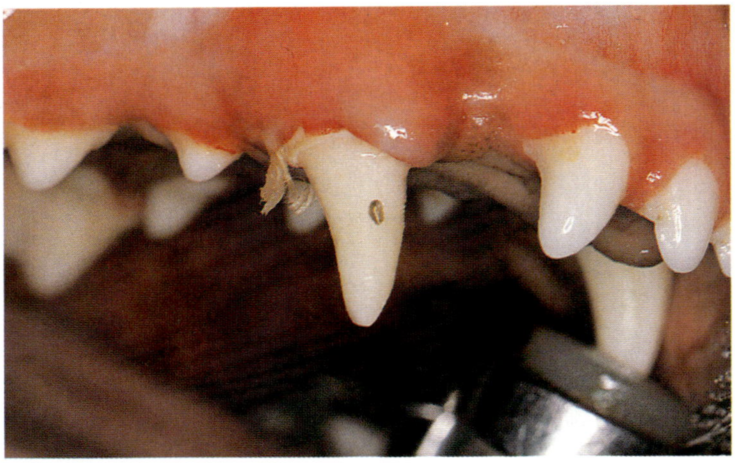

Photo 77.

Crown prepared and ready for impression. Note circumferential bevelling at gingival margin and retraction cord in sulcus.

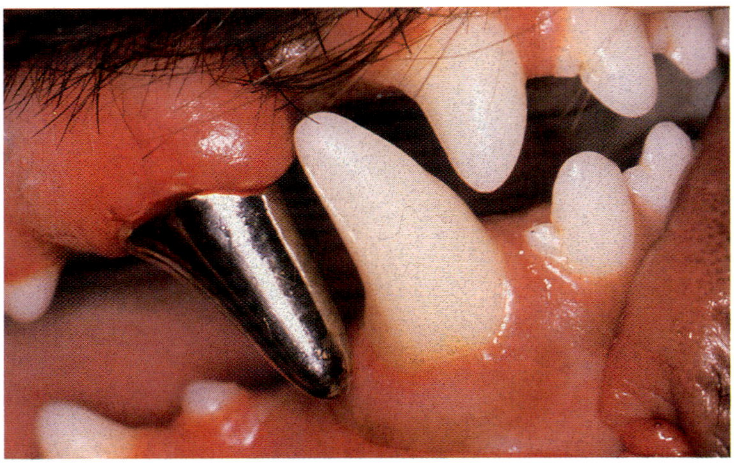

Photo 78.

Stainless steel crown on maxillary canine tooth. Crown is shorter than original crown and has a rounded tip to minimize leverage forces.

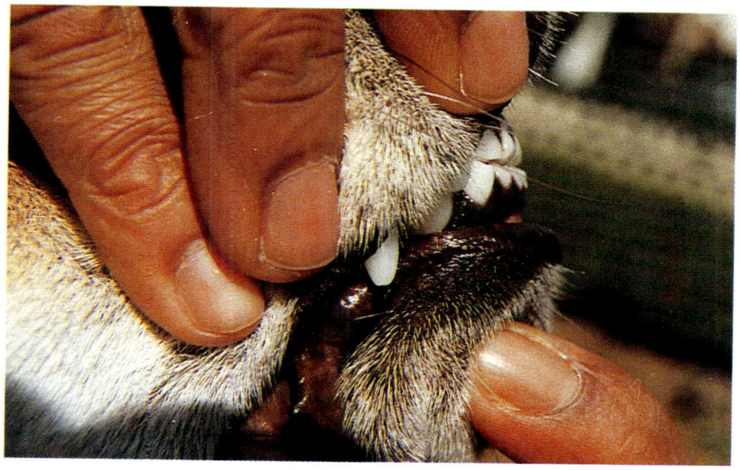

Photo 79.

Level (even) bite. Incisal edges meet end on end causing attrition.

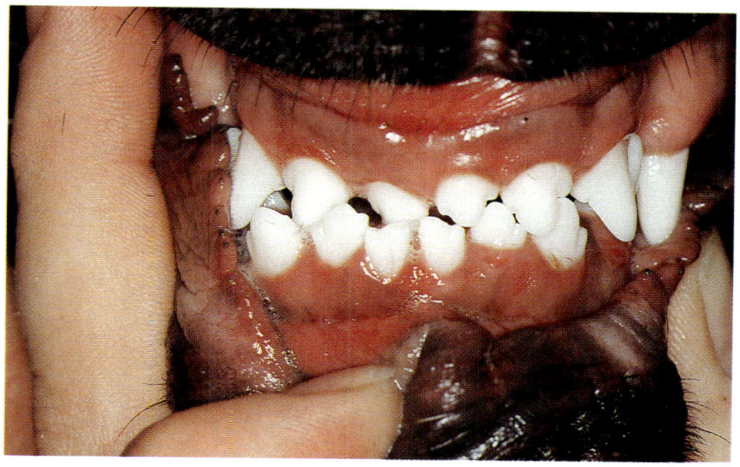

Photo 80.

Anterior crossbite. Note maxillary incisors on right of photo are in normal mesial occlusion. Maxillary incisors on left of photo are in abnormal distal occlusion.

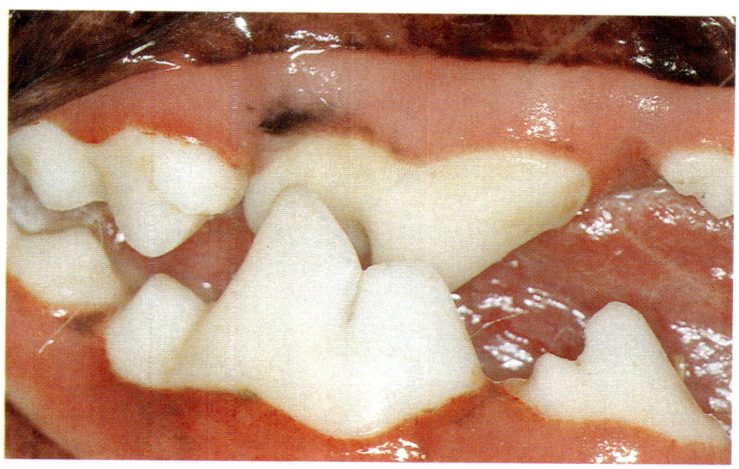

Photo 81.

Posterior crossbite. Mandibular first molar lies buccal to maxillary fourth premolar. This condition facilitates calculus build–up on the mandibular first molar. (Teeth cleaned prior to photo.)

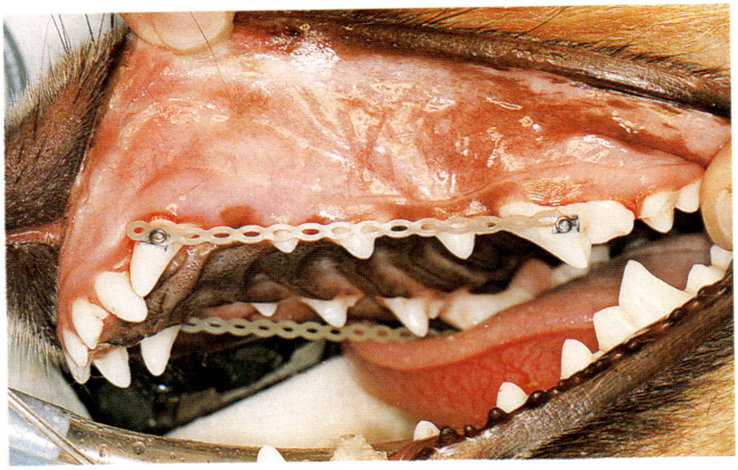

Photo 82.

Elastic power chain attached by buttons cemented on to canine tooth and fourth premolar. Used to correct rostrally deviated canine tooth.

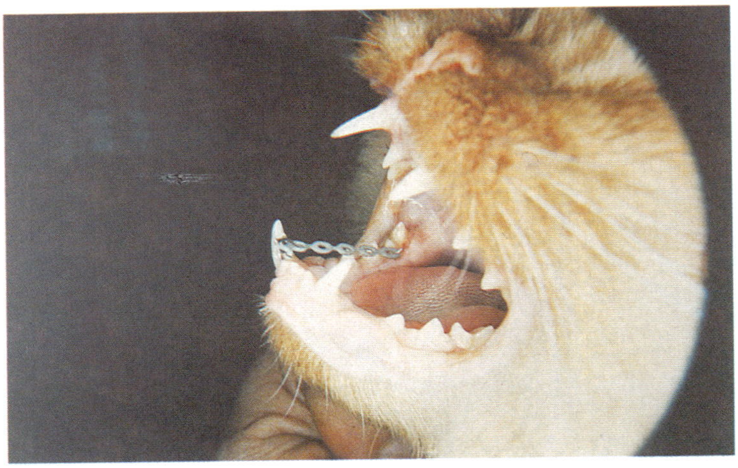

Photo 83.

Rostrally deviated mandibular canine tooth. Elastic power chain attached to canine tooth with a button and to molar with a hook made from ends of wire twisted around tooth.

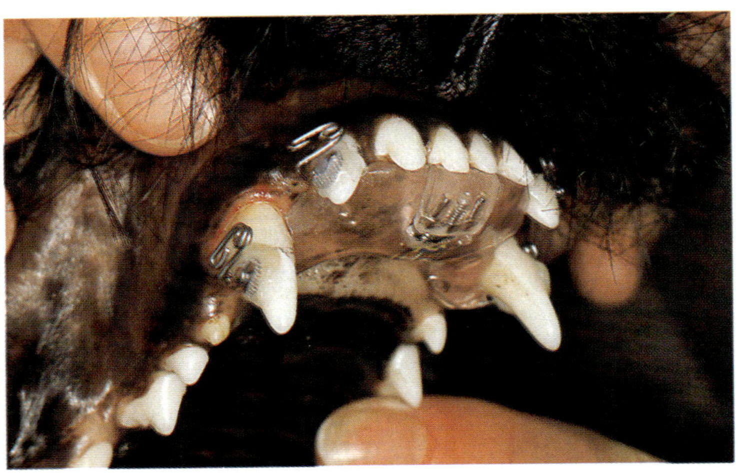

Photo 84.

Expansion screw in removable acrylic plate. Plate is held in place by four spring clamps above bonded buttons.

Photo 85.

Expansion screw bonded with composite to mandibular right canine tooth. Wires on other end are twisted around canine tooth before bonding. Mylar tape protects oral mucosa. Turning screw will expand tips of lingually displaced canine teeth.

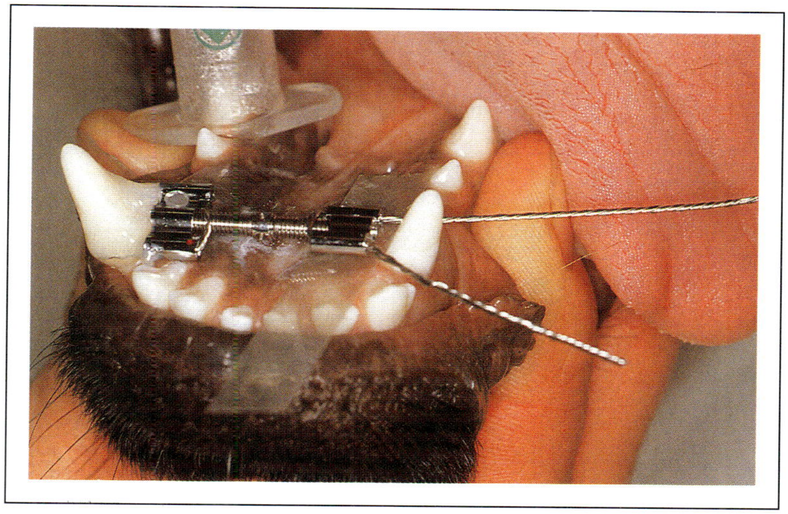

Photo 86.

Braces around maxillary incisors. Slotted brackets are bonded to teeth and square arch wire placed in slots. Tension over caudally displaced central incisors will move them rostrally.

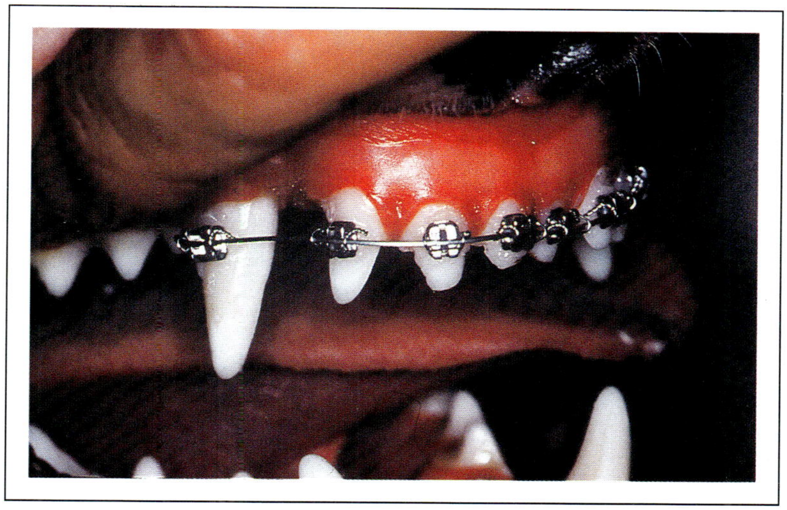

Photo 87.

Bite wing appliance bonded on to maxillary incisors (made of composite and wire). Rostrally deviated mandibular central incisors will be guided caudally.

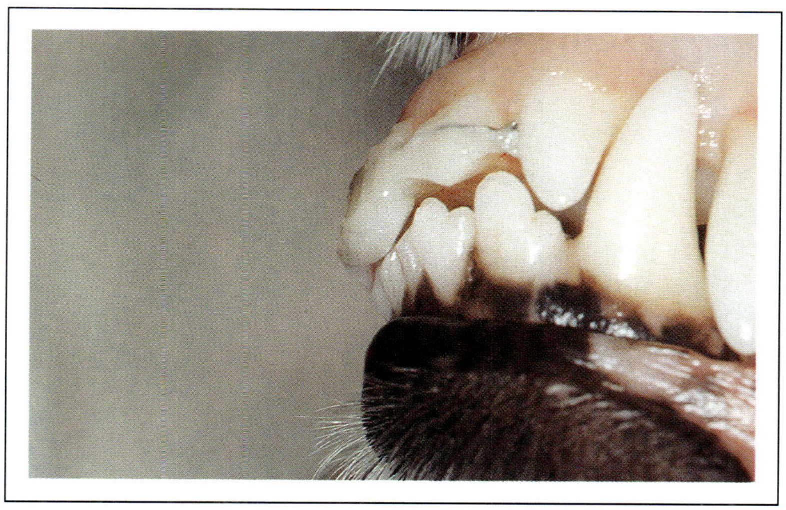

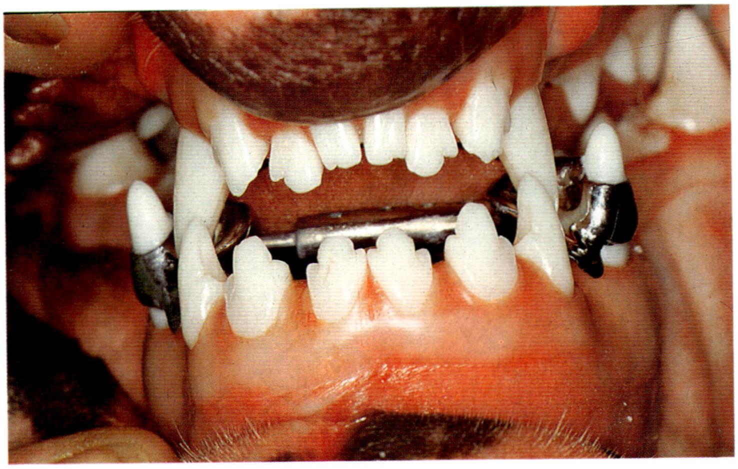

Photo 88.

Lingually displaced mandibular canine teeth. Inclined plane will cause the tips of these teeth to move buccally, when mouth is closed.

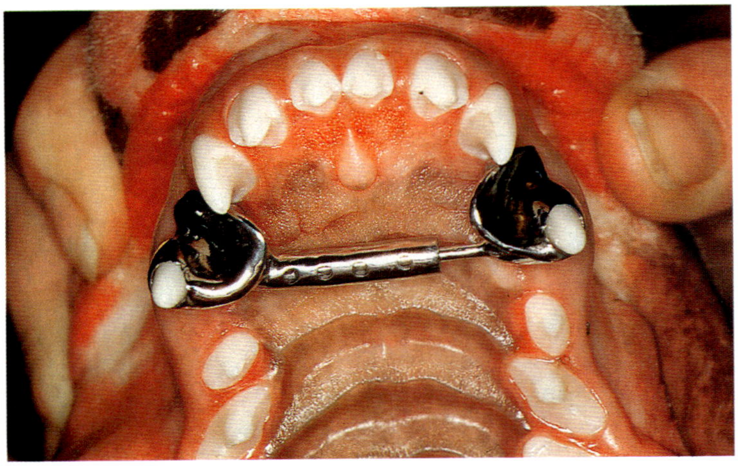

Photo 89.

Cast bilateral telescoping inclined plane appliance, cemented on to maxillary canine teeth.

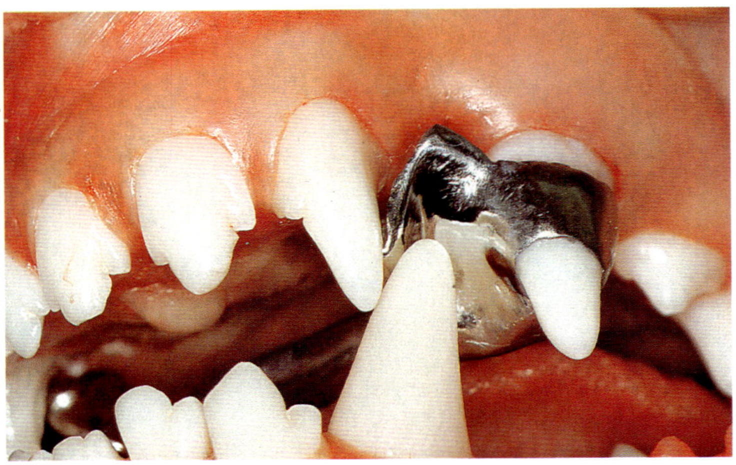

Photo 90.

Inclined plane guiding mandibular canine tooth into normal occlusion.

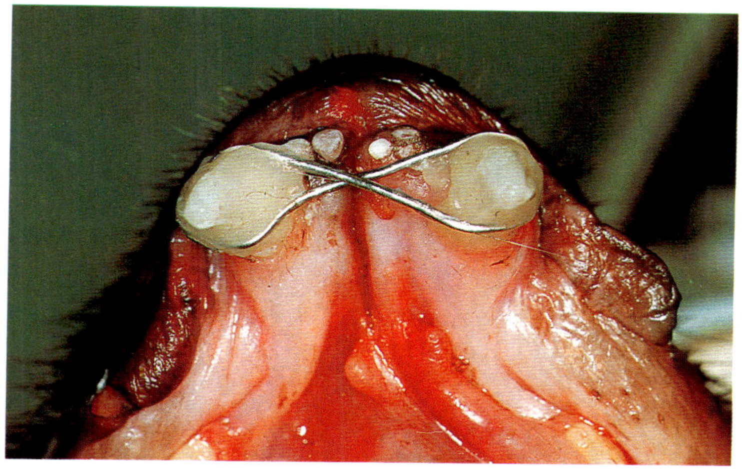

Photo 91

Fractured symphysis of mandible of cat. Figure–of–eight wire is bonded on to canine teeth with composite for stabilization of the fracture.

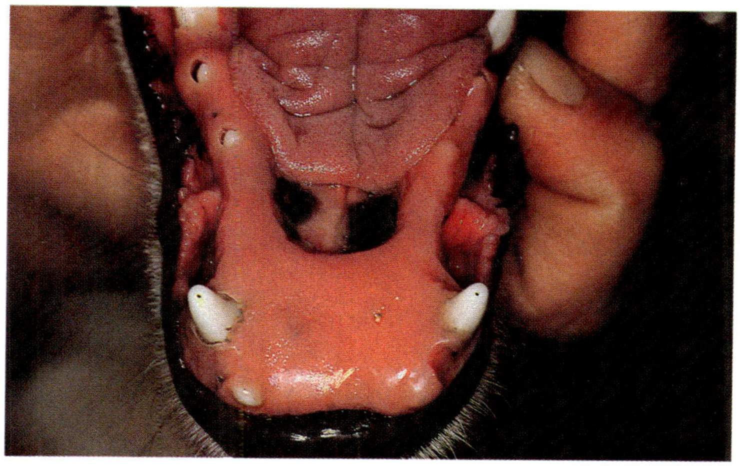

Photo 92.

Acrylic splint over anterior teeth and premolars for stabilization of rostral mandibular fracture.

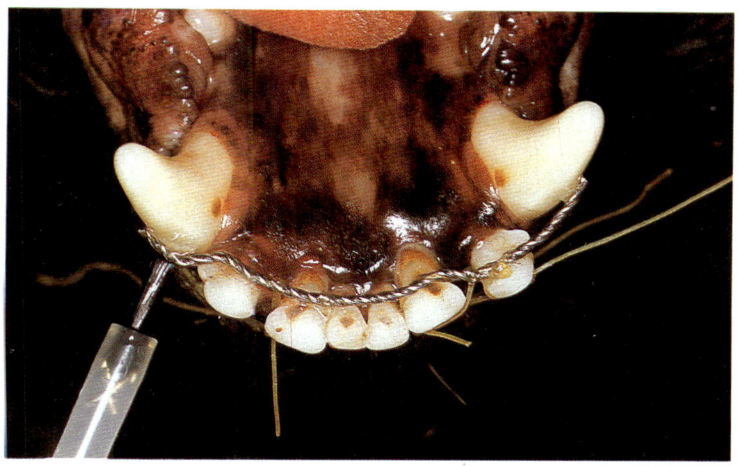

Photo 93.

Stabilization of loose incisors due to periodontal disease. After wire is tightened, it is covered with composite, forming a splint.

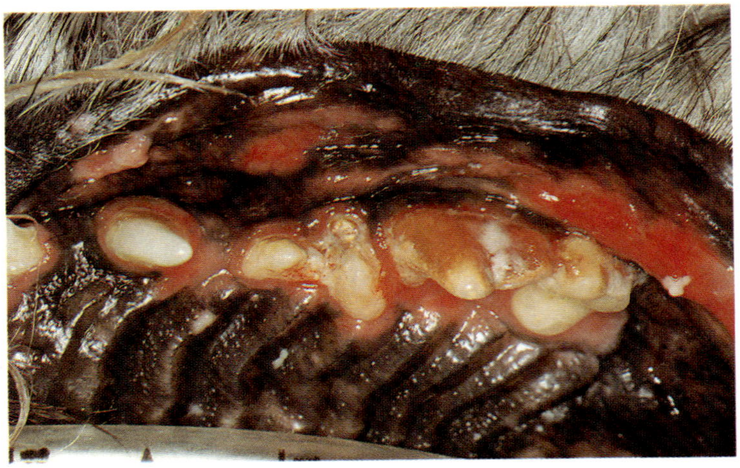

Photo 94.

Ulceration on the buccal mucosa due to long–standing contact with calculus and infected gingival area.

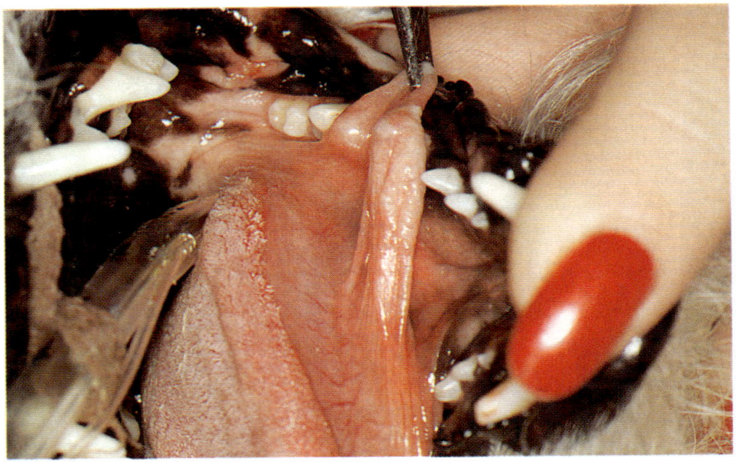

Photo 95.

Abnormal proliferative sublingual mucosa. This loose fold of tissue is constantly caught between the caudal teeth causing "Chewing gum–like" syndrome

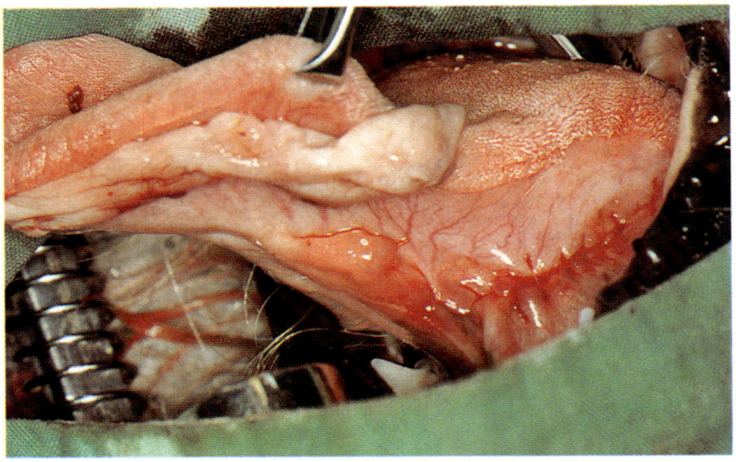

Photo 96.

Abnormal fold of sublingual mucosa resected (upper left). Continuous suture pattern in sublingual mucosa where the fold was removed (lower right).